RISK ASSESSMENT METHODS

Approaches for Assessing
Health and Environmental Risks

RISK ASSESSMENT METHODS

Approaches for Assessing Health and Environmental Risks

Vincent T. Covello
School of Public Health
Columbia University
New York, New York

and

Miley W. Merkhofer
Applied Decision Analysis, Inc.
Menlo Park, California

Plenum Press • New York and London

Library of Congress Cataloging-in-Publication Data

Covello, Vincent T.
　　Risk assessment methods : approaches for assessing health and environmental
risks / Vincent T. Covello, Miley W. Merkhofer.
　　　　p.　cm.
　　Includes bibliographical references.
　　ISBN 0-306-44382-1
　　1. Health risk assessment—Methodology.　2. Health risk assessment—Evaluation.
I. Mekhofer, Miley W., 1947–　II. Title.
　　RA427.3.C68　1993
　　614.4—dc20　　　　　　　　　　　　　　　　　　　　　　　　　　93-23209
　　　　　　　　　　　　　　　　　　　　　　　　　　　　　　　　　　　CIP

10 9 8 7 6 5 4

ISBN 0-306-44382-1

© 1993 Plenum Press, New York
A Division of Plenum Publishing Corporation
233 Spring Street, New York, N. Y. 10013

Printed in the United States of America

PREFACE

Much has already been written about risk assessment. Epidemiologists write books on how risk assessment is used to explore the factors that influence the distribution of disease in populations of people. Toxicologists write books on how risk assessment involves exposing animals to risk agents and concluding from the results what risks people might experience if similarly exposed. Engineers write books on how risk assessment is utilized to estimate the risks of constructing a new facility such as a nuclear power plant. Statisticians write books on how risk assessment may be used to analyze mortality or accident data to determine risks. There are already many books on risk assessment—the trouble is that they all seem to be about different subjects!

This book takes another approach. It brings together all the methods for assessing risk into a common framework, thus demonstrating how the various methods relate to one another. This produces four important benefits:

- First, it provides a comprehensive reference for risk assessment. This one source offers readers concise explanations of the many methods currently available for describing and quantifying diverse types of risks.

- Second, it consistently evaluates and compares available risk assessment methods and identifies their specific strengths and limitations. Understanding the limitations of risk assessment methods is important. The field is still in its infancy, and the problems with available methods are disappointingly numerous. At the same time, risk assessment *is* being used. Correctly interpreting risk assessment results requires understanding the limits of the risk assessment methods that are employed.

- Third, this book provides useful guidance for planning and conducting risk assessments. Organized by the basic steps used in all risk assessments, it shows how methods successfully applied in one area (e.g., assessing the risks of nuclear power plants) might be modified to apply to another area (e.g., assessing the risks of cars lacking air bags).

- Finally, this book provides a generalized way of thinking about risk and risk assessment. The models introduced serve as conceptual aids, helpful in learning to think about risks and how they can be quantified. The terms, definitions, and concepts provided clarify the common aspects of all risks and risk assessment methods.

The key to producing these benefits is the *taxonomy of risk assessment methods* that is utilized throughout this book. The taxonomy supplies the organizational structure for our presentation of risk assessment methods. More important, the taxonomy provides readers with a conceptual framework for thinking about risk and risk assessment, a framework that includes: (1) a convenient language for communication between risk assessors and risk managers, (2) a means for clarifying similarities and differences in the capabilities, applicabilities, input requirements, and analytical perspectives of various methods, (3) a means for identifying methods that may be effective for analyzing problems in situations other than those for which the method was originally developed, and (4) an aid in identifying weak links in the sequence of methods needed to conduct a risk assessment.

The taxonomy is used to organize and explore a broad range of risk assessment methods. For example, this book encompasses all of the major methods covered by important previous reviews addressing specific types of risk, including:

- Risks of chemicals [e.g., National Research Council (NAS–NRC, 1980, 1983a, 1986a); Office of Technology Assessment (OTA, 1981); Conway (1982); International Agency for Research on Cancer (IARC, 1982, 1987); Office of Science and Technology Policy (OSTP, 1984); Rodricks and Tardiff (1984); Ricci (1985); Environmental Protection Agency (EPA, 1986a–e, 1989a); Working Group on Risk Assessment and Risk Management (1992)].

- Risks of nuclear power plants [e.g, Nuclear Regulatory Commission (NRC, 1983, 1984, 1987); Covello and Hadlock (1985); Henley and Kumamoto (1991)].

- Risks of other hazardous facilities [e.g., Center for Chemical Process Safety, American Institute of Chemical Engineers (AIChE/CCPS, 1985, 1989); World Bank (1985)].

- Risks of accidental or deliberate release of genetically engineered organisms [e.g., Fiksel and Covello (1986, 1989); Levin and Strauss (1991)].

As the citations above indicate, the emphasis of the risk assessment literature to date has been on risks linked to chemicals (especially carcinogens) and industrial accidents. This book encompasses a broader scope of risk assessment methods, including methods useful in assessing risks from foods, consumer products, ionizing radiation, and natural disasters, and methods for assessing risks to the natural environment as well as to people. Despite this broad coverage, our emphasis remains focused on technology-related health risks, for several reasons. First, risks linked to chemicals and industrial accidents raise inherently important public health and environmental concerns. Second, the assessment of such risks places extreme demands on risk assessment methodology and sets in high relief most of the principles and issues involved. Finally, risks linked to chemicals and industrial accidents are currently the focus of most of the controversy as to whether risk assessment is sufficiently accurate to serve as a basis for policy making (Conservation Foundation, 1985).

The specific focus of this book is on quantitative methods of risk assessment, that is, methods useful for producing numerical estimates of the probabilities and magnitudes of possible adverse health and/or environmental consequences. The emphasis on quantitative methods reflects the great advantage that quantitative methods provide; they express risk in the language of numbers. Numbers are precise—they leave less room for misinterpretation than words do. Numbers also provide more useful inputs for a decision on what to do about risks.

Despite the focus on quantitative methods, the reader will find few mathematical equations in the main text. The discussion deliberately de-emphasizes mathematics so that readers need not become bogged down in mathematical details to obtain the useful insights and understandings that are available. Where equations have been judged useful to some readers, they are presented in tables so as to minimize interruptions to the flow of the discussion. Finally, the focus on quantitative methods does not mean that qualitative methods are ignored. Indeed, to the extent that qualitative methods are useful for the implementation of a quantitative risk assessment approach, they are addressed.

ACKNOWLEDGMENTS. The idea for and the content of this book evolved over a nearly 10-year period. Its genesis was a study of the state of the art of risk assessment conducted in 1984 by the authors for the National Science Foundation (NSF). The authors wish to acknowledge and thank the many individuals who provided assistance or who reviewed all or portions of earlier drafts, without implying that these individuals necessarily agree with its contents. Counting those who participated in the original NSF study, these include: Lee Abramson, Roy E. Albert, Norman Alvares, Bruce N. Ames, Melvin E. Andersen, Elizabeth Anderson, Gerald Anderson, Kenneth J. Arrow, Michael Baram, Nathaniel F. Barr, Delbert S. Barth, David Bates, Patricia Bauman, Ed Behrens, Marcos Bonazountas, Robert J. Breen, Stephen L. Brown, Robert Budnitz, Daniel M. Byrd, David B. Clayson, Morton Corn, J. Clarence Davies, John Doull, Ward Edwards, Alan Eschenroeder, James W. Falco, Joseph R. Fiksel, Baruch Fischhoff, W. Gary Flamm, Lita Furby, B. John Garrick, Jack D. Hackney, Max Henrion, G. Patrick Johnson, Vojin Joksimovich, Robert Kadlec, Ralph Keeney, Daniel Krewski, Lester B. Lave, H. W. Lewis, Vladimir Lieskovsky, William Linn, Lawrence

McCray, Thomas McCurdy, David McNelis, Gail H. Marcus, Ralph F. Miles, M. Granger Morgan, Jeryl Mumpower, Raymond R. Neutra, Gordon Newell, D. Warner North, Ellen O'Flaherty, David Okrent, Elisabeth Pate-Cornell, Thomas Read, Paolo Ricci, Harvey Richmond, Joseph V. Rodricks, Glenn Schweitzer, Abraham Silvers, Nozer D. Singpurwalla, Miller B. Spangler, Richard D. Stewart, Robert Tardiff, Melvyn Tockman, Curtis Travis, Chris Whipple, Roger Williams, Jim R. Withey, Ron Wyzga, Alvin Young, and Constantine Zerog. In addition, we are indebted to the late Joshua Menkes for his help and contributions, and to Ms. Marcia Szabo for typing the manuscript.

This book was prepared under the partial support of the National Science Foundation under Research Grants PRA-8511329 and SES-8606906. The views and opinions expressed herein are those of the authors and do not necessarily represent a position of the National Science Foundation.

CONTENTS

CHAPTER 1

INTRODUCTION TO RISK ASSESSMENT

1.1. INTRODUCTION

Health and environmental risk assessment is a relatively new field. It is being developed along diverse fronts by experts in distinct disciplines including epidemiology, toxicology, engineering, and statistics. Each of these disciplines has generated at least a few books about risk assessment. However, nearly all such books focus narrowly on specific subsets of available risk assessment methods: namely, those methods that have been developed specifically to address the types of risks with which the author's discipline is most concerned. Thus, risk assessment literature has become specialized and fragmented.

While the specialization and fragmentation of the risk assessment literature may be acceptable to the specialist, it is not useful for the reader with a more general interest in risk assessment. For example, the existing literature makes it difficult to see how the methods described by one author can be extended and generalized to assess the types of risks not addressed by that author. Thus, it is easy to miss opportunities to use efficient or effective methods that have not been developed specifically for a selected area of application.

This book identifies the unifying principles underlying available risk assessment methods and is designed to serve as a useful resource for those interested in risk assessment. This first chapter presents generalized definitions, terminology, and concepts needed for a comprehensive understanding of the field of risk assessment. Subsequent chapters provide detailed descriptions, comparisons, and evaluations of the numerous risk assessment methods that are currently available.

1.2. DEFINITIONS AND TERMINOLOGY

Due to the fragmented way in which the field has developed, there is currently no consensus over the appropriate definitions of *risk* or of *risk assessment*. Rather, competing definitions with relatively narrow applicability have been proposed. Our broad scope and desire for a unifying framework demand that we adopt more general definitions for these terms. We offer, accordingly, what are believed to be useful definitions for the principal topics that will be addressed.

1.2.1. What Is Risk?

Risk is, at minimum, a two-dimensional concept involving (1) the possibility of an adverse outcome, and (2) uncertainty over the occurrence, timing, or magnitude of that adverse outcome. If either attribute is absent, then there is no risk. More formally, we define risk as follows:

> **Risk** A characteristic of a situation or action wherein two or more outcomes are possible, the particular outcome that will occur is unknown, and at least one of the possibilities is undesired.

Although this definition is not standard in risk assessment texts, it is consistent with the way most people think about risk. People talk about risk when there is the chance, but not the certainty, that something they don't want may happen. For example, people talk about the risk of losing their jobs, the risk that a loved one may be in an automobile accident, and the risk of losing money in the stock market. People don't talk about the risk of winning the lottery because, although winning the lottery is uncertain, it is not undesirable. Similarly, people don't talk about the risk of making their monthly auto payment. They may not like to make the payment, but because they know exactly how much and when they will have to pay, there is no uncertainty. In everyday thinking the term *risk* implies something that is both uncertain and undesired.

Most technical writing adopts some more narrow definition of risk. The word *risk* was used originally by economists as a means to distinguish a situation in which the probabilities of possible outcomes are known from a situation in which the probabilities of outcomes are not known. Thus, a gamble whose outcome is determined randomly according to some specified statistical distribution would be, according to these writers, a "risk" rather than an "uncertainty" (Knight, 1921). More common today is the definition of risk as the probability of occurrence for an undesirable outcome—usually death (e.g., Ritter, 1981; Wilson, 1984). Authors adopting this view discuss the risk of death being some number X. Other authors define risk as the total number of deaths (e.g., Zentner, 1979).

The defining of risk as the product of probability and consequence magnitude is slightly more common than the defining of risk as probability or as magnitude of consequence. Accordingly, several authors have defined risk to be the sum of the possible alternative numbers of fatalities weighted by their probabilities (i.e., the expected value of the number of fatalities) (e.g., Hammer, 1972; Lowrance, 1976). More complex definitions of risk have also been proposed. For example, some authors [e.g., the Nuclear Regulatory Commission (NRC), 1975] define risk by envisioning a model that is assumed to behave similarly to the system under study and computing the frequency with which the model predicts various outcomes. The term *risk* is used to describe the model results, and the term *uncertainty* is used to characterize the degree of confidence in the results based on the confidence in the model.

Although better established, none of the previous conflicting definitions of risk are sufficiently broad to support a comprehensive understanding of risk assessment. Therefore, we have adopted the more general definition given above.

1.2.2. What Is Risk Assessment?

The following definition of risk assessment reflects the scope that we have established for this study:

Risk Assessment *A systematic process for describing and quantifying the risks associated with hazardous substances, processes, action, or events.*

Comparing this definition with our definition of risk allows us to infer the appropriate output of a risk assessment. Taking into account the focus of this volume on human health and the natural environment, our definition of risk implies (1) the possibility of adverse health or environmental consequences, and (2) uncertainty over the occurrence, magnitude, or timing of those consequences. Various numerical measures are available for quantifying the occurrence, magnitude, and timing of health and environmental consequences, while uncertainty is best quantified using the well-established methods of probability theory.

Thus, risk may be quantified by identifying the possible adverse health or environmental consequences and estimating their magnitude (e.g., the intensity, amplitude, size), the timing of those consequences, and their probabilities of occurrence. Risk assessment, therefore, can be defined as a systematic process for generating a probability distribution or similar quantification that describes uncertainty about the magnitudes, timing, or nature of possible health or environmental consequences associated with possible exposure to specified substances, processes, actions, or events. In turn, a *risk assessment method* can be defined as any self-contained systematic procedure conducted as part of a risk assessment—that is, any procedure that can be used to help generate a probability distribution for health or environmental consequences.

Debate over the definition of risk assessment relates mostly to establishing its appropriate scope, particularly with reference to related activities, such as *hazard identification or assessment, risk evaluation,* and *risk analysis.* In this book, risk assessment is viewed as one component of risk analysis, as illustrated in Fig. 1. In our view, risk analysis consists of three stages: (1) hazard identification (identifying

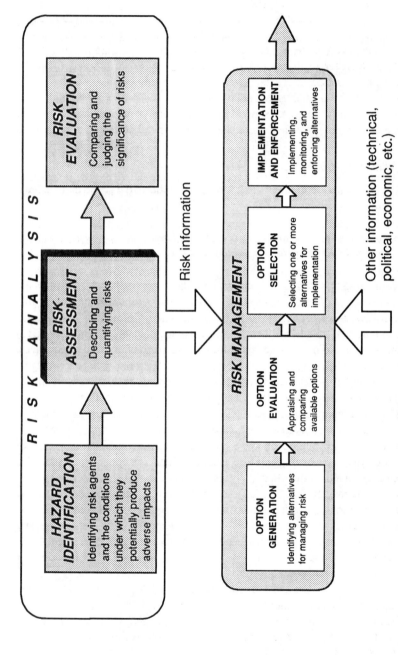

FIGURE 1. The three stages of risk analysis—hazard identification, risk assessment, and risk evaluation—provide key information for risk management.

risk agents and the conditions and events under which they potentially produce adverse consequences to people or the environment), (2) risk assessment (describing and quantifying the risk), and (3) risk evaluation (comparing and judging the significance of the risk). The purpose of these activities is to provide an important part of the information needed to support *risk management* (identifying, selecting, and implementing appropriate actions to control the risk).

1.3. A MODEL OF RISK ASSESSMENT

In general, a risk exists when three conditions are satisfied. First, a source of risk must be present—that is, a system, process, or activity must exist that can release or otherwise introduce a risk agent into the environment. The *risk source* might be, for example, a nuclear power plant, a dam, the spinning blades on a power lawn mower, or a new drug. Second, an *exposure process* must exist by which people or the things they value may be exposed to the released risk agent. Exposure might result from wind dispersing radioactive particles vented from a nuclear power plant, from people building homes below a dam, from a person accidentally touching the spinning blades of a lawn mower, or from the use of a new drug in the medical treatment of patients. Third, a *causal process* must exist by which exposures produce adverse health or environmental consequences. Adverse consequences, for example, may consist of cancers resulting from exposure to radioactivity, property damage and drownings due to water released in a dam failure, amputated fingers resulting from a lawn mower accident, or undesirable side effects from a new drug.

Each of these three conditions—releases from a risk source, exposures, and consequences—may be thought of as links in a *risk chain* (Merkhofer, 1987a). As shown in Fig. 2, quantification of risk requires the quantification of knowledge and uncertainty about each link in the chain.

Because the level of risk depends on the specific nature and characteristics of the *risk source*, the *exposure process*, and the *consequence process*, a comprehensive risk assessment must address each of these components comprehensively. Risk assessment must determine, characterize, and quantify the following factors: (1) the potential of the source to release a risk agent; (2) the intensity, frequency, and duration of exposure, and the nature of the populations (or other valued entities) that might be exposed; and (3) the relationship between exposure and the resulting health or environmental consequences. Finally, the combined influence of these factors on risk must be determined, characterized, and quantified. The final outputs of this process are estimates of the magnitudes of possible adverse health or environmental consequences, including always a characterization of the probabilities, uncertainties, or degree of confidence associated with these estimates.

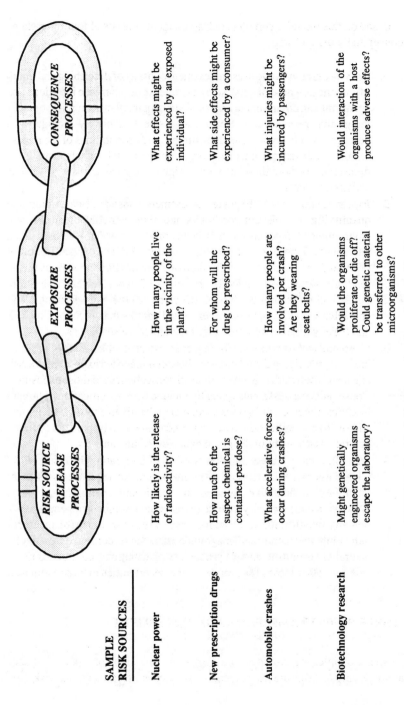

FIGURE 2. The risk chain and examples of questions asked in risk assessment.

SAMPLE RISK SOURCES

	RISK SOURCE RELEASE PROCESSES	EXPOSURE PROCESSES	CONSEQUENCE PROCESSES
Nuclear power	How likely is the release of radioactivity?	How many people live in the vicinity of the plant?	What effects might be experienced by an exposed individual?
New prescription drugs	How much of the suspect chemical is contained per dose?	For whom will the drug be prescribed?	What side effects might be experienced by a consumer?
Automobile crashes	What accelerative forces occur during crashes?	How many people are involved per crash? Are they wearing seat belts?	What injuries might be incurred by passengers?
Biotechnology research	Might genetically engineered organisms escape the laboratory?	Would the organisms proliferate or die off? Could genetic material be transferred to other microorganisms?	Would interaction of the organisms with a host produce adverse effects?

Based on this model, a complete risk assessment consists of four interrelated but conceptually distinct steps:

1. *Release assessment.* Release assessment consists of describing and quantifying the potential of a risk source to release or otherwise introduce risk agents into an environment accessible to people, plants, animals, or other things that people value. Release assessments typically include (a) a description of the types, amounts, timing, and probabilities of the release of toxic substances, kinetic energy, or other risk agents, and (b) a description of how these attributes might change as a result of various actions or events.

2. *Exposure assessment.* Exposure assessment consists of describing and quantifying the relevant conditions and characteristics of human and environmental exposures to risk agents produced or released by a given risk source. Exposure assessments typically include (a) a description of the intensity, frequency, and duration of exposure through various media (e.g., air, water, soil, or food), (b) routes of exposure (e.g., ingestion, inhalation, or absorption through the skin), (c) the number, nature, and characteristics of people and other valued entities that might be exposed, and (d) any other conditions that might affect consequences.

3. *Consequence assessment.* Consequence assessment consists of describing and quantifying the relationship between specified exposures to a risk agent and the health and environmental consequences of those exposures. Consequence assessments typically include (a) a specification of human fatalities, illnesses, or injuries sustained under given exposure scenarios, and/or (b) a specification of ecological damage or adverse effects on the natural environment under given exposure conditions.

4. *Risk estimation.* Risk estimation consists of integrating the results from release assessment, exposure assessment, and consequence assessment to produce quantitative measures of health and environmental risks. These measures typically include (a) estimated numbers of people experiencing health impacts of various severities over time, (b) measures indicating the nature and magnitude of adverse consequences to the natural environment, and (c) probability distributions, confidence intervals, and other means for expressing the uncertainties in these estimates.

1.4. THREE BRIEF EXAMPLES OF RISK ASSESSMENT

Brief examples are provided to illustrate the four steps of risk assessment: release assessment, exposure assessment, consequence assessment, and risk estimation. These abbreviated examples emphasize basic approaches, but not the specific methods underlying each step in the assessment. Section 1.5 provides a more detailed example of risk assessment, including descriptions of some specific methods used for release assessment, exposure assessment, consequence assessment, and risk estimation.

1.4.1. Example 1: Nuclear Power Plant Risk Assessment

Risk assessment has been used frequently to estimate the probabilities of possible consequences of accidents at a nuclear power plant. By conducting the four steps of risk assessment, the analyst constructs a model of the process by which a nuclear power plant creates risk. Figure 3 illustrates the major components of a model constructed for such a risk assessment.

Release assessment, the first of four steps, often constitutes the major portion of a nuclear power plant risk assessment. This is because a nuclear power plant is a complicated facility, and the model needed to estimate the probabilities and nature of possible releases of risk agents, especially radioactive material, is necessarily complex. Furthermore, the release assessment must be tailored to the specific plant in question, whereas the exposure and consequence assessments are more generic (the necessary models and data can sometimes be borrowed from other work). The specific objective of the release assessment is to estimate the probability that different types of accidents or system failures might occur and what radioactive materials would be released in each situation.

Release estimates are derived by constructing a model of the risk source, which in this case is the power plant. The model accounts for events that might initiate an accident or system failure that could damage the plant's reactor. Examples of initiating events are individual component failures (e.g., valve and pump failures) and errors by human operators. Such initiating events may result in thermal and hydraulic stresses on the plant's containment system, including the concrete vessel that encloses the reactor. By estimating the probabilities of initiating events, and the probabilities that such events lead to releases with various characteristics, the probabilities and nature of possible releases are quantified.

Exposure assessment, the second step, is concerned with the transport and fate of radioactive material that might be released into the environment. Data of various kinds including site-specific meteorological data (e.g., prevailing wind patterns), information on the local terrain (e.g., topographical data on land contours), and data on the location of local populations are used to account for the movement and decay of released material and the potential exposures to people and the things that people value. Exposures are often distinguished as acute or chronic. *Acute exposures* are those that occur within a short period of time following a release and may be different for different population groups (for example, people who are evacuated from an area immediately, people who are evacuated somewhat

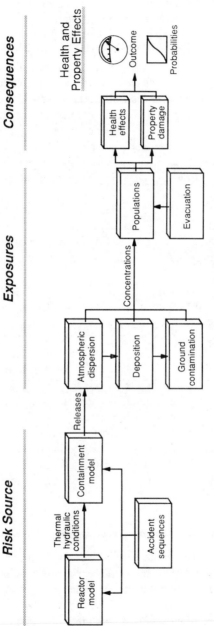

FIGURE 3. Major components of a model for a nuclear power plant risk assessment.

later, and people who are not evacuated). *Chronic exposures* accumulate over a period of years following a release and may result from people living on contaminated land or consuming contaminated agricultural products.

Consequence assessment, the third step, is concerned with estimating human health effects and other adverse consequences associated with exposure. Three categories of human health effects are often included in consequence assessment: (a) immediate fatalities and illnesses that would occur within days or weeks after exposure to large, acute doses of radiation; (b) latent cancer fatalities and nonfatal cancers that would occur 2 to 40 years after exposure to radiation; and (c) genetic damage that could affect succeeding generations. The magnitudes of the various health effects are derived from dose-response relationships based on laboratory and epidemiologic data and from estimates of the amount of radiation actually received by humans (e.g., through inhalation of radioactive material in the atmosphere, as external irradiation from a radioactive cloud or contaminated soil, or from ingestion of contaminated food or water). Economic costs may also be estimated as part of consequence assessment. Such costs may be quite large and include the costs of evacuation, crop damage and lost agricultural production, decontamination, and population relocation.

Risk estimation, the last step in a nuclear power plant risk assessment, consists of integrating the results of the release assessment, exposure assessment, and consequence assessment to produce summary measures of risk. More specifically, this step is concerned with generating probability distributions that describe the uncertainty over the magnitude of possible health and other consequences associated with nuclear power plant accidents or system failures. One approach to accomplish this step is (a) linking the models for the risk source, exposures, and effects, and (b) repeating the estimation of adverse consequences while changing values in the models that represent the critical uncertain variables, such as the accident sequence, wind direction, and evacuation effectiveness. The result of this process is a curve showing a probability distribution of adverse health and other consequences. This curve, together with associated error and confidence measures, provides the principal output of the risk assessment; a quantitative measure of the risk.

1.4.2. Example 2: Poultry Products Risk Assessment

Various inspection programs have been designed to help ensure the safety of poultry products delivered to the marketplace. Nevertheless, human diseases such as salmonellosis have been linked to the consumption of poultry products contaminated with pathogenic microorganisms. Because the effects of these diseases are usually short-lived and often confused with other illnesses, only a fraction of the cases are reported. The pain and discomfort produced, however, can be severe; in some cases the diseases can be fatal. Risk assessment can be used to quantify and

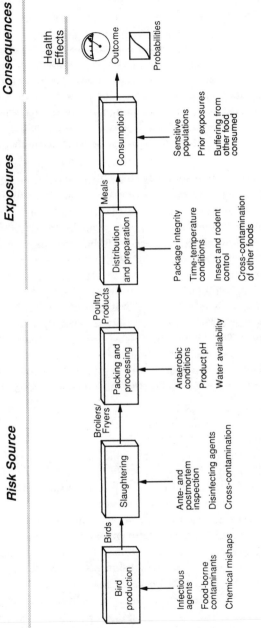

FIGURE 4. Major components of a model for poultry products risk assessment.

describe the risks involved and to explore the extent to which risks might be reduced through the implementation of alternative inspection procedures. Figure 4 shows the components of such a risk assessment model.

As in the previous example, release assessment is a major component of the risk assessment. In this case, release assessment is concerned with estimating (a) the frequency with which various poultry products provided to the marketplace are contaminated with pathogenic microorganisms (or their toxins), and (b) the amount of such contaminants. Although generally thought to be less significant risk agents, toxic chemical residues that accumulate, for example, as a result of the accidental contamination of feed with pesticides, might also be estimated as part of the release assessment.

The model for the risk source contains three submodels: one focused on bird production, one on slaughtering, and one on packing and processing. The poultry production submodel accounts for the various mechanisms by which the production of live poultry may affect the wholesomeness of poultry products. Such mechanisms include (a) pathogenic contamination during breeding and hatching via genetic or egg-borne transmission (from breeder flock), and (b) contamination during growth through exposure to infectious agents in feed and water, pesticides, or vaccines. The slaughtering submodel accounts for activities at the slaughterhouse that affect product wholesomeness. Examples of such activities are (a) the use of disinfecting agents and sanitary dressing techniques, and (b) postmortem inspection procedures. The packing and processing submodel accounts for (a) the rate of cross contamination produced through contaminants on workers' hands, cutting boards, knives, and other sources, (b) the effectiveness and extent of efforts to minimize cross contamination, and (c) the conditions of packaging.

Exposure assessment focuses on estimating poultry consumption and conditions under which people consume contaminated poultry products. This estimation is based on a model of product distribution, food preparation, and consumption practices. The model estimates the extent to which microorganisms in raw poultry products multiply, spread, and possibly cross contaminate other foods during transport, in retail outlets, and after purchase by the consumer. Critical variables for this model include the microbial load at the time of shipment, the internal temperature at the time of loading, and the air temperature and movement in transport vehicles, storage warehouses, refrigerators, and display cases. The major factors contributing to outbreaks of food-borne diseases that originate during the preparation of food in food service establishments and homes are as follows: (1) leaving cooked foods at room temperature for extended periods of time, (2) storing cooked foods in large containers during refrigerated storage, and (3) preparing food a day or more before serving it. Other contributing factors include inadequate cooking or reheating of food, contamination of food by infected persons, and inadequate cleaning of equipment.

Consequence assessment is concerned with quantifying the adverse human health consequences of consuming contaminated poultry products. Current understanding of the relationship between human health and the ingestion of salmonellae, other pathogenic microorganisms, and toxic chemicals is still rudimentary. Nevertheless, it is known that the severity of reaction is affected by a variety of factors including prior exposures of an individual to specific microorganisms, other foods that are consumed at the same time (some of which may provide a buffering effect), variations in individual susceptibility due to age or illness, and the availability and accessibility of effective medical care.

The risk estimation stage of the assessment integrates the results of the release assessment, exposure assessment, and consequence assessment to produce summary measures of risk. For example, data on the frequency of contaminated products, combined with estimates of the likelihood of cross contamination, inadequate food preparation, and medical-care scenarios, can be used to generate estimates of the incidence and severity of poultry-related salmonellosis. These estimates in turn can be used to evaluate the potential effectiveness of different risk-management procedures in reducing risk.

1.4.3. Example 3: Risk Assessment of an Air Bag Passive-Restraint Standard

Risk assessment can be used to estimate the extent to which fatalities and injuries might be reduced by the enactment of a national air bag passive-restraint standard for new cars. Such an assessment must account for the effectiveness and usage of both current and proposed restraint systems. Figure 5 shows the components of such a risk assessment model.

In this case, the risk source can be regarded as both the automobiles and the system of roads and highways on which the automobiles travel. Automobile accidents release accelerative forces and materials possessing kinetic energy (e.g., flying glass) into the passenger compartment. Release assessment in this case is concerned with estimating the frequency and characteristics of the various types of accidents for which the effectiveness of the current seat-belt system and the proposed air bag passive-restraint systems might differ. An air bag will deploy in front-angle crashes (which cause the majority of occupant fatalities) but will not deploy in most side, rear, and rollover crashes. Thus, release assessment must account for the fraction of all accidents that would produce deployment of the air bag. The total number of accidents might be estimated by a simple extrapolation from current data. Alternatively, a more complex analysis might account for the effect of possible changes in the maximum speed limit, changes in the relative size of the 15–25-year age group (which is more accident-prone than other age groups), and for continued improvement in car design and highway construction.

Exposure assessment is concerned with whether occupants in automobile crashes use restraint systems and the extent to which these systems protect them

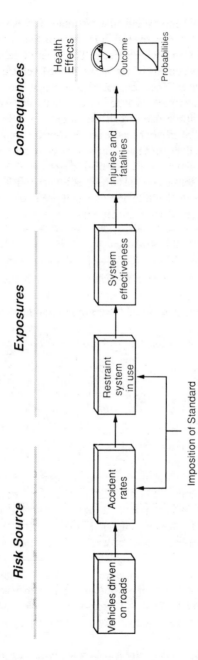

FIGURE 5. Major components of a model for a risk assessment of an air bag passive-restraint system.

from exposure to the kinetic energy and other traumatic forces released in a crash. Air bags redistribute crash forces over a larger area of the occupant's body and provide facial protection from flying objects. The level of safety achieved also depends on whether the occupants of air bag–equipped vehicles are wearing lap belts at the time of a crash. Thus, exposure assessment must account for the likelihood that occupants in various types of accidents are wearing seat belts. Accident data indicate that the rate of belt use in crashes is lower than the rate observed in roadside surveys, in part because accident-prone groups (e.g., teenagers and drunk drivers) are less likely to be wearing seat belts in crashes than the average motorist. Data also indicate that rates of seat belt usage are lower at night, when a disproportionate share of serious crashes occur and when enforcement of mandatory seat belt laws is more difficult. In addition, belt use in cars equipped with air bags may differ from that in cars without air bags.

Consequence assessment is concerned with estimating the fatalities and injuries attributable to various kinds of accidents with and without restraint systems. Automobile accidents produce a diverse set of injuries that may be classified in various ways. One widely used classification system is the National Traffic Safety Administration's Abbreviated Injury Scale (AIS), which provides five categories of injuries ranging in severity from simple cuts and bruises to paraplegia and death. Data from accident reports and tests involving dummies are used to estimate the probability that an accident will produce various levels of injury with and without seat belts and with and without air bags.

Risk estimation integrates the results of the release assessment, exposure assessment, and consequence assessment to quantify the risk. In this case, risk estimation basically consists of multiplying fractions—the fraction of all cars equipped with air bags times the fraction of accidents that cause air bags to deploy times the fraction of injuries that will be averted or made less severe by the presence of an air bag. However, the method also must account for more subtle dependencies and correlations (e.g., between seat belt use and accidents), uncertainties, and changes over time. A comparison of the estimates of the numbers of injuries and lives lost under the current seat belt policy with estimates of the numbers of injuries and lives lost under an air bag policy can provide important information for deciding among alternative automotive safety systems.

1.5. A MORE DETAILED EXAMPLE OF RISK ASSESSMENT: RISKS OF EXPOSURES TO AIR POLLUTION UNDER ALTERNATIVE EMISSIONS STANDARDS

The four essential steps in a risk assessment (release assessment, exposure assessment, consequence assessment, and risk estimation) are illustrated below through a more detailed example: a risk assessment of air pollution under alternative national standards for ambient air quality. Drawn from a study by one of the authors (Merkhofer, 1982), the example is presented for illustrative purposes only. Chapters 2–5 of this volume provide detailed discussions of alternative methods that, depending on the situation, may be more appropriate than those illustrated in this example.

1.5.1. Problems Involved in Setting Air Quality Standards

The Clean Air Act requires the Administrator of the Environmental Protection Agency (EPA) to set national standards for primary ambient air quality. The act states that the standards must be set at a level that will "protect the public health" with an "adequate margin of safety" (Section 109, 42 U.S.C. 7414). The EPA Administrator is responsible both for determining which adverse health effects must be avoided and for defining an adequate margin of safety.

Because health is the only basis for setting standards under the Clean Air Act (Gage, 1979), the EPA Administrator's objective is to identify for each air pollutant a least-stringent standard that protects public health with an adequate margin of safety. To this end, risk assessment is needed for estimating the health consequences of air pollution and the associated uncertainties.

1.5.2. Developing a Model for Estimating Health Consequences

Conducting a risk assessment of air pollution emissions under alternative standards requires the construction of a model for estimating the health consequences to be expected under each standard. The model must account for relevant characteristics of the risk source, exposure processes, and effects processes. Models were constructed for the emissions of air pollutants (the risk source), the atmospheric conversion, dispersion, and transport of air pollutants to sensitive populations (exposure processes), and the health consequences of exposures to elevated concentrations of air pollutants (effects processes).

1.5.2.1. Release Assessment: Modeling the Sources of Air Pollutants. In this example, release assessment involves the construction of a model for the emissions of air pollutants. The model must estimate the nature and geographic distribution of emissions that would occur over time under any given national standard for ambient air quality. An ambient air quality standard usually specifies an averaging time (i.e., the time period over which continuously varying concentrations are to be averaged for the purpose of measurement and enforcement), a maximum level, and an expected number of instances in which concentrations are permitted to exceed the maximum level over a given period of time. For example, the ambient air quality standard for ozone is 0.12 ppm hourly average concentration, with one or less expected days per calendar year when maximum hourly concentrations are permitted to exceed 0.12 ppm.

The primary activities and processes that must be addressed by the emissions model are those that have a direct or indirect influence on air quality. Therefore, the emissions model must account for (1) the production and consumption processes that produce gas by-products to which air pollution can be traced, (2) emissions containment and control technologies that determine the actual quantities of pollutants released to the atmosphere, and (3) actions taken by state or local regulatory bodies that influence emissions either directly (e.g., by influencing industry decisions to use technologies to contain and control pollutants) or indirectly (e.g., by altering the demand for the products that produce pollutants as unwanted by-products). The model must (a) be spatially disaggregated to account for the geographic distribution of emissions, (b) reflect variations in emissions over time, and (c) reflect the dynamics of bringing an area into compliance.

A wide variety of modeling methods can be used to relate a given standard to a spatial pattern of emissions. For example, Fig. 6 shows the geographic distribution of emissions in an analysis of sulfur oxide emissions standards for Florida (Merkhofer and Korsan, 1978). For this analysis projected emissions were

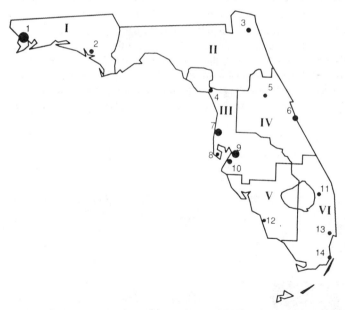

FIGURE 6.   Major point sources of Florida SO$_2$ emissions. Dot size is proportional to emissions of SO$_2$. Roman numerals denote air quality regions designated by the U.S. E.P.A. (Merkhofer and Korsan, 1978).

aggregated into 14 point sources. Each point source was assumed to emit a plume of sulfur dioxide (SO_2) at a rate determined by current and projected electricity sales growth coupled with assumptions regarding the reductions in emissions that would occur under different standards.

1.5.2.2. Exposure Assessment: Modeling Exposures to Air Pollutants.

Exposure assessment is concerned with developing models of exposure processes. In this case, the exposure model must (a) convert emissions to atmospheric concentrations of pollutants expressed as a function of time and space, and (b) account for sensitive individuals who live or work in areas with elevated levels of air pollutants.

Many different types of air quality models are available for converting emissions to ambient concentrations. The appropriate modeling technique for estimating the effect of emissions on atmospheric concentrations depends on the pollutant, its sources, and the meteorology, climate, and geography of the region being modeled. One approach is to use empirical data and statistical methods to construct regression or time-series models that correlate historical emissions to measured pollutant concentrations. Another approach is to use models that simulate physical processes of atmospheric transport, chemical reactions, and deposition of the pollutant. Accounting for atmospheric chemical reactions is important if it is not the emittant that produces adverse health effects, but a product of an atmospheric chemical reaction for which the emittant is a precursor. When causal models are used, they are usually calibrated by adjusting the model's parameters so that the concentrations predicted by the model match actual monitored data.

Figure 7 illustrates the assumptions adopted in the air quality model utilized in the Florida analysis (cf. Fig. 6). The model was based on the assumption that each source emits a plume that disperses pollutants in accordance with local wind

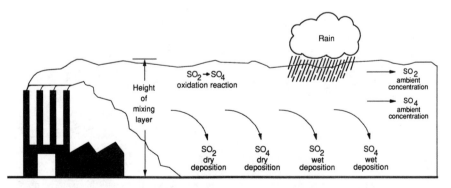

FIGURE 7.   A model for the relationship between sulfur oxides emissions and ambient concentrations.

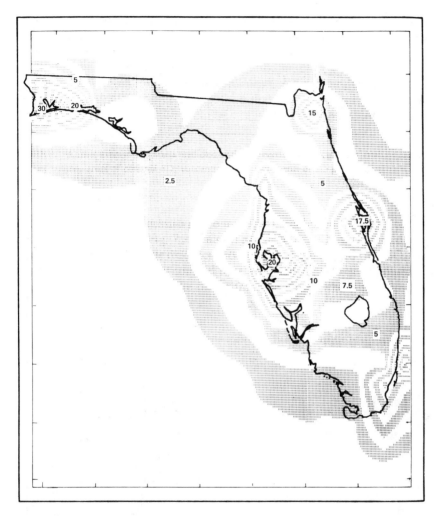

FIGURE 8.   Annual average SO_2 levels predicted by the emissions-to-ambient concentrations model. Contours indicate areas of constant SO_2 concentrations at increments of 2.5 $\mu g/m^3$ (Merkhofer and Korsan, 1978).

directions and speeds (a Gaussian plume model as described in Chapter 3 of this volume). As illustrated in Fig. 7, the model assumed that SO_2 is converted at a constant rate to various sulfate oxidation products (SO_4) and that SO_2 and SO_4 are both removed to the ground at constant rates beginning at the time of emission. Figure 8 provides a sample of the output from the model when the emissions patterns shown in Fig. 6 were assumed. Such contour plots provide a convenient way of summarizing output data and permit comparisons of predicted values with data obtained by monitoring. Short-term (24-hour) average SO$_4$ concentrations were derived in the analysis by scaling historical frequency distributions observed at selected monitoring sites to match the annual averages predicted by the model.

Translating ambient concentrations into exposures requires the identification of potentially sensitive individuals and determining how many of these individuals reside or work in areas with elevated ambient concentrations. Population groups

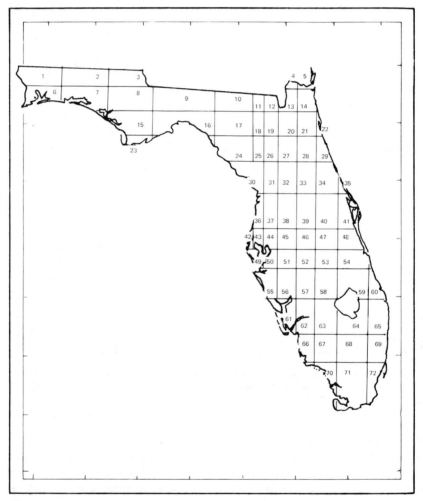

FIGURE 9.   Cells defined for estimating Florida SO$_2$ and SO$_4$ exposures (Merkhofer and Korsan, 1978).

typically sensitive to air pollution include bronchial asthmatics, people suffering from emphysema, young children, and the elderly. A common approach is to divide the geographic region of interest into cells. Cells are selected so that ambient concentrations can be assumed to be approximately uniform within each cell. Demographic data on the location and growth rates of populations of sensitive individuals may then be used to determine the exposures that occur within each cell. Figure 9 shows the cells that were used in the Florida analysis. To account for the distribution of sensitive individuals in this analysis, base-rate estimates for various health effects associated with exposures to elevated levels of SO_2 and SO_4 were obtained for each cell. Table 1 shows the data that were used.

More detailed exposure models may be needed if the objective is to assess variations in exposures to people that occur during a normal day of activities. For example, the exposure model may be constructed of submodels designed to represent the nature, timing, and environments of activities (e.g., exercise activities) engaged in by sensitive individuals. Microenvironment exposure submodels account for pollutant concentrations in localized areas (e.g., those occurring indoors or within vehicles) and other specific environmental factors that influence the health responses of sensitive individuals.

1.5.2.3. Consequence Assessment: Health-Effects Models. Consequence assessment, in this case, involves the development of models of the effects of exposures to air pollutants. Exposures to air pollutants at moderate to high concentrations have been shown to aggravate asthma, emphysema, and chronic bronchitis, reduce resistance to bacterial infection, and cause discomfort such as coughing, chest tightness, and irritation of the mucous membranes of the respiratory tract. The effect of a given concentration or dose is a complex function of (a) synergistic, additive, or antagonistic factors (e.g., synergism between smoking and exposure to atmospheric pollutants), and (b) the distribution of exposure over time (e.g., duration and cumulative exposure).

Considerable flexibility exists for specifying and defining adverse health effects represented in dose-response relationships. For example, health effects might be defined as coughing spells, prolonged chest discomfort, or a specific percentage reduction in pulmonary function. Each such specification may be appropriate—the goal is to use specifications and definitions that are meaningful to risk managers, are consistently interpreted, and offer a reasonably complete description of the health consequences that may be associated with the pollutant.

Lack of knowledge currently precludes defining precise functional relationships among the many factors that determine adverse human health effects of exposures to air pollutants. Consequently, the dose-response relationships used in risk assessments of air pollution are by necessity highly simplified. The simplest approach is to use a simple dose-response curve (e.g., linear, linear with threshold,

TABLE 1. Estimated Total Numbers of Cases of Health Effects (1990) Used in Florida SO$_2$/SO$_4$ Analysis[a]

| | Cell[c] | Population | Number of cases[b] | | | | |
			Mortality	Person-days aggravation of heart and lung disease	Asthma attacks	Child's lower respiratory disease	Chronic respiratory disease
	1	6,420	66	24,185	1,688	138	142
	2	36,934	380	139,137	9,713	794	934
	3	91,086	938	343,138	23,954	1,957	2,305
	4	8,459	87	31,867	2,225	182	214
	5	33,682	347	126,886	8,858	724	852
Pensacola	6	358,056	2,614	621,466	94,162	8,797	10,124
	7	55,139	568	207,719	14,500	1,185	1,395
	8	74,343	766	280,064	19,551	1,598	1,881
Tallahassee	9	225,709	1,535	422,918	59,357	4,945	6,734
	10	47,120	485	177,510	12,392	1,013	1,192
	11	76,550	788	288,378	20,131	1,645	1,937
	12	76,550	788	288,378	20,131	1,645	1,937
	13	7,825	81	29,478	2,058	168	198
Jacksonville	14	771,539	6,867	1,141,309	202,899	18,957	22,320
Small towns	15	157,091	1,618	591,791	41,312	3,376	3,975
	16	35,811	369	134,907	9,418	770	906
	17	17,316	178	65,233	4,554	372	438
	18	48,028	495	180,931	12,630	1,032	1,215
	19	37,689	388	141,982	9,911	810	954
	20	35,408	365	133,389	9,312	761	896
	21	72,428	746	272,850	19,047	1,556	1,832
	22	59,166	609	222,889	15,559	1,271	1,497
	23	8,099	84	30,887	2,156	176	207
	24	23,212	239	87,444	6,104	499	587
	25	1,530	16	5,764	402	33	39
	26	168,233	1,565	325,178	44,242	3,509	5,121
	27	33,791	348	127,297	8,886	726	855
	28	2,413	643	235,122	16,413	1,341	1,579
	29	69,332	714	261,187	18,233	1,490	1,754
	30	21,834	225	82,253	5,742	469	552
	31	3,393	35	12,782	892	73	86
	32	6,072	63	22,874	1,597	130	154
	33	119,702	1,233	450,940	31,479	2,572	3,029
	34	38,275	394	144,189	10,066	823	968
Daytona Beach	35	129,331	1,164	545,884	34,011	2,490	3,331
Small towns	36	14,811	153	55,796	3,895	318	375
	37	228,366	2,352	860,298	60,056	4,908	5,778
	38	129,638	1,335	488,371	34,092	2,786	3,280
	39	92,317	951	347,776	24,278	1,984	2,336

(continued)

TABLE 1. (*Continued*)

	Cell[c]	Population	Mortality	Person-days aggravation of heart and lung disease	Asthma attacks	Child's lower respiratory disease	Chronic respiratory disease
				Number of cases[b]			
Orlando	40	593,213	5,339	1,123,223	156,003	14,658	16,474
Cocoa Beach	41	112,638	721	95,529	29,622	3,170	3,151
Clearwater	42	137,500	2,516	821,430	36,160	2,108	3,313
Tampa	43	493,746	6,172	1,022,532	129,845	11,267	14,459
	44	61,240	631	230,703	16,105	1,316	1,549
Lakeland	45	379,100	4,739	1,353,369	99,696	8,200	9,744
Winter Haven	46	262,989	3,471	944,046	69,161	5,725	6,720
	47	16	0	60	4	0	0
Melbourne	48	122,349	1,260	461,912	32,175	2,629	3,096
St. Petersburg	49	680,844	8,238	4,001,731	179,048	10,866	16,265
	50	1,531	16	5,768	403	33	39
	51	6,346	65	23,917	1,669	136	161
	52	44,231	456	166,627	11,632	951	1,119
	53	1,017	10	3,831	267	22	26
	54	69,799	719	262,946	18,356	1,500	1,766
Sarasota	55	361,844	4,849	1,527,282	95,158	7,295	9,082
	56	35,031	361	131,968	9,212	753	886
	57	74,177	764	279,439	19,507	1,594	1,877
	58	52,263	538	196,885	13,744	1,123	1,322
	59	19,603	202	73,848	5,155	421	496
Fort Pierce	60	190,115	2,262	682,451	49,996	4,219	4,800
Port Charlotte	61	391,308	4,030	1,474,131	102,906	8,409	9,900
	62	16	0	60	4	0	0
	63	9,309	96	35,069	2,448	200	236
	64	66,568	686	250,774	17,506	1,431	1,684
West Palm Beach	65	836,722	9,288	3,135,586	220,041	16,985	21,929
	66	56,990	587	214,692	14,987	1,225	1,442
	67	38,275	394	144,189	10,066	823	968
	68	16	0	60	4	0	0
Fort Lauderdale	69	1,030,119	11,743	3,657,159	270,901	20,262	27,984
	70	69,358	714	261,285	18,240	1,491	1,755
	71	9,032	93	34,025	2,375	194	229
Miami	72	822,398	8,635	2,416,864	216,274	17,040	23,004

[a] Merkhofer and Korsan (1978).

[b] The figures cited are based on population estimates, health effects prevalence rates, and local mortality prevalence rates. Other prevalence rates used are as follows: (1) prevalence of heart and lung disease in elderly persons, 0.27; average number of aggravated days per day person, 0.20; (2) asthma prevalence rate, 0.036; attacks per day per asthmatic, 0.02; (3) annual incidence rate for lower respiratory disease in children, 0.07; (4) chronic respiratory disease prevalence rate, 0.02 for nonsmokers (62%) and 0.10 for smokers (38%).

[c] When a cell contains a major city, the name of the city is given.

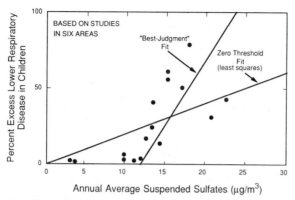

FIGURE 10.   Alternative dose-response functions derived from empirical data.

or sigmoidal). For example, a linear-with-threshold curve assumes that no effects occur if concentrations are below some threshold level, but that the frequency or severity of health effects increases in proportion to concentrations above the threshold. A threshold and slope factor for the relationship could be obtained, for example, by eliciting the judgments of experts. If the experts disagree, sensitivity analyses can be conducted to determine the importance of the uncertainty over alternative thresholds and slopes.

Another possible approach for obtaining dose-response relationships is to infer such relationships from data available from epidemiological, clinical, or toxicological studies. Such studies suggest that short-term exposures to elevated levels of sulfur oxides, especially suspended sulfates, seem to aggravate preexisting heart and lung disorders in the elderly, aggravate asthma, and increase the daily mortality rate. Repeated short-term exposures or elevations of annual average exposures seem to increase the incidence of lower respiratory disease in children and increase the risk for chronic respiratory disease in adults. A simple functional form for each relationship might be assumed (e.g., linear with threshold) and mathematically fit to the available data. Figure 10 shows the results of such a curve-fitting exercise used in the Florida analysis. The example represents a case for which data from several different studies were combined.

In situations where data and/or understanding are sufficient to permit a more complicated exposure model to be developed and where sensitivity analysis indicates that a simple approach is inadequate, dose-response models with multidimensional inputs might be used. For example, if the health impact of exposure to a given concentration of SO_4 is known to depend on the relative humidity, humidity might be included as an input to the model.

TABLE 2.   Base Case Estimates of Florida Annual Health Effects Attributable to SO_4 Concentrations (Assuming Nominal Electricity Sales Growth[a])

	Air quality standard			
	Least stringent	Current	Moderately stringent	Most stringent
Mortality (expected cases)				
1980	4.00	1.33	0.00	0.00
1990	5.66	2.33	0.00	0.00
2000	13.32	8.66	2.33	0.00
Heart and lung (thousands of cases)				
1980	729	447	40	3
1990	987	677	171	11
2000	1553	1273	729	63
Asthma (thousands of cases)				
1980	278	202	39	7
1990	367	287	114	17
2000	516	458	313	60
Lower respiratory (thousands of cases)				
1980	0.00	0.00	0.00	0.00
1990	0.00	0.00	0.00	0.00
2000	0.27	0.00	0.00	0.00
Chronic respiratory (thousands of cases)				
1980	0.20	0.00	0.00	0.00
1990	0.48	0.00	0.00	0.00
2000	5.56	1.60	0.00	0.00

[a]Merkhofer and Korsan (1978).

Dose-response functions are used in risk assessment to convert the exposure profiles generated by an exposure model into health consequences. A simple approach is to use the dose-response functions to estimate the number of health effects for various exposure levels within each geographic cell. Annual average numbers of health effects can then be obtained by weighting and averaging the results according to frequency distributions for exposure levels. Similar health effects can be summed across cells to obtain the total number of adverse health effects of each type occurring as a result of exposure to emissions under each alternative regulatory standard. Table 2 shows the results of the Florida analysis in which estimates of annual health consequences were generated for 10-year intervals. In this example, the first three adverse health effects—premature mortality, aggravation of heart and lung disease, and asthma attacks—were estimated from dose-response functions integrated over frequency distributions for 24-hour concentrations. The remaining two adverse health effects, lower respiratory disease and chronic respiratory disease, were assumed to be direct functions of annual average dosages.

1.5.3. Risk Estimation: Applying the Risk Model to Quantify and Describe Risk

Once the models for representing emissions, exposures, and effects are developed and combined, the resulting risk model can be analyzed to obtain risk estimates. In general, the first step is to conduct a sensitivity analysis to identify those model variables whose uncertainties have the greatest influence on estimated adverse health consequences. In the simplest sensitivity analysis, each input variable in the risk model is varied across a range of values selected to approximate its range of uncertainty while all other variables are held constant at their best-estimate values. The variables whose variations produce the greatest change in the estimated numbers of adverse health effects are identified as variables for which representing uncertainty is most crucial. Because such analyses may not identify crucial uncertainties resulting from interdependencies among variables, selected joint sensitivities may also be measured, a procedure in which two or more of the uncertain input variables are simultaneously varied across their respective ranges of uncertainty. Sensitivity of results to model uncertainty may also be investigated by specifying alternative functional relationships and/or model forms.

The simplest approach to quantifying uncertainty is to estimate minimum and maximum bounds for each uncertain quantity and to use these values along with the risk model to obtain upper and lower estimates for the numbers of each adverse health effect. Such bounds might be generated from the analysis of statistical data or might reflect an expert judgment that the uncertain quantity is "almost certain" to lie within the bounding values. More information is provided if uncertainties are formally quantified using probabilities. Probability distributions for uncertain variables can be generated from statistical data, provided that adequate data are available for a statistical analysis. Often, however, obtaining probability distributions requires eliciting probabilities from experts using probability encoding techniques. Figure 11 illustrates a probability distribution based on expert judgments. The uncertain quantity is the increment to sulfate concentrations resulting from a specified SO_2 emissions level.

Given a risk model and probability distributions that describe uncertainty about each of the crucial input variables of the model, it is relatively easy to design

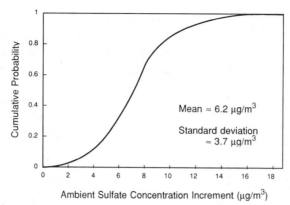

FIGURE 11. Probability distribution illustrating judgmental uncertainty over the increment of ambient sulfate concentration in an urban area 60 km downwind from a power plant emitting 10^4 kg sulfur oxides per hour (North and Merkhofer, 1975).

a computer program that will generate probability distributions for the model's outputs, in this case the adverse health effects associated with the emissions under alternative standards. The results might be expressed as (a) a probability that the total number of adverse health effects under a given standard is less than or equal to a given amount, (b) a probability that the total number of persons experiencing each adverse health effect will equal or exceed a given value for a given time period, or (c) the probability that various sensitive groups will experience different levels of various adverse health effects. These probability distributions provide summary measures of risk and represent the final product of the risk assessment. When these measures are introduced into the standards-setting process, decision makers can balance the estimates of possible health effects, and the uncertainties, against the political, economic, and other considerations that must enter into a final decision.

1.6. OTHER MODELS OF RISK ASSESSMENT

The four-step model of risk assessment proposed in this book—release assessment, exposure assessment, consequence assessment, and risk estimation—is sufficiently general to be applicable to a wide spectrum of risks. Other models, however, have also been proposed. In particular, a model described by the National Research Council (NRC) of the National Academy of Sciences (NAS) (NAS–NRC, 1983a) has been widely used by several government agencies, including the EPA, for assessing the risks of cancer and other health risks that result from exposure to chemicals. According to this model, risk assessment consists of "hazard identifi-

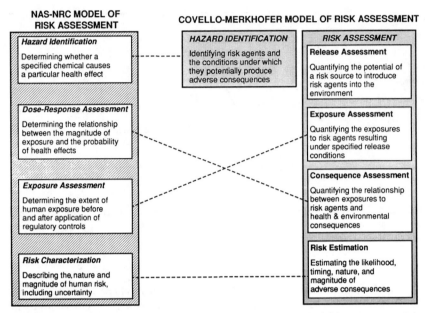

FIGURE 12.   Similarities and differences between the NAS–NRC model of risk assessment and the Covello–Merkhofer model.

cation, dose-response assessment, exposure assessment, and risk characterization." The NAS–NRC report defines these steps as follows:

- *Hazard identification*: The determination of whether a particular chemical is or is not causally linked to particular health effects.

- *Dose-response assessment*: The determination of the relation between the magnitude of exposure and the probability of occurrence of the health effects in question.

- *Exposure assessment*: The determination of the extent of human exposure before or after application of regulatory controls.

- *Risk characterization:* The description of the nature and often the magnitude of human risk, including attendant uncertainty.

The NAS–NRC model of risk assessment and the one proposed in this book are similar, yet have several significant differences. Given the wide acceptance of the NAS–NRC model, it may be useful to clarify these differences; they are summarized below and in Fig. 12.

First, the NAS–NRC risk assessment model includes hazard identification as the first step in risk assessment; our model does not. Instead, our model regards hazard identification as an *altogether separate process that is necessarily conducted prior to risk assessment.* In this view, treating hazard identification as merely one component of risk assessment underplays its importance. The NAS–NRC report describes hazard identification as a major undertaking that produces a qualitative determination of whether exposure to a risk agent can cause adverse health effects. This includes determining cause and effect, weighing the available evidence, and characterizing the nature and strength of the evidence of causation. In fact, approximately half the steps of risk assessment identified in the NAS–NRC report (NAS–NRC, 1983a, pp. 29–33) are hazard identification steps. In our view, hazard identification provides the essential foundation for and must precede risk assessment; it is not simply the first step of risk assessment. Thus, as depicted in Figs. 1 and 12, we have chosen to define the qualitative process of hazard identification as a distinct process; one that is on par with and of equal importance to the quantitative process of risk assessment.

Second, the risk assessment model here proposed identifies release assessment as the first step in risk assessment, while the NAS–NRC model does not include this step. Our model treats release assessment as a separate step since for important types of risk, such as industrial accidents or failures involving large technological systems, quantifying and describing the potential of a risk source to release risk agents into the environment consumes as much or more effort than the other steps of risk assessment. In such cases, obtaining a detailed quantitative understanding of the amount and probability of a release—and how a release might be altered by various actions—is an essential step toward obtaining an accurate understanding of risk.

Third, the NAS–NRC model selects dose-response assessment as the second step in risk assessment. The step we call consequence assessment is similar, yet more general. According to our view, consequence assessment allows for consideration of impacts on the environment as well as on humans.

Fourth, although we have defined exposure assessment similar to the definition adopted for the NAS–NRC model, we have chosen to place exposure assessment prior to consequence assessment in the order of presentation. This makes our model for risk assessment consistent with our concept of the risk chain (see Fig. 2).

Finally, both models view the last step of risk assessment to be one of integration. We have chosen to call this final step risk estimation in order to emphasize the view that risk is a characteristic of the world we live in and that the goal of risk assessment is to communicate that risk estimate in human terms, not to produce some abstract output from a risk assessment model.

TABLE 3. Categorization of Principal Risk Assessment Methods

Release assessment	Exposure assessment	Consequence assessment	Risk estimation
Monitoring	Monitoring	Health surveillance	Relative risk models
• Release monitoring	• Personal exposure monitors (PEMs)	Hazard screening	Model coupling
• Monitoring source status	• Media contamination (site monitoring)	• Molecular structure analysis	Risk indexes
• Monitoring administrative records	Air, surface water, sediment, soil, groundwater	• Short-term tests	• Individual risk
• Laboratory analysis	• Remote geologic monitoring, Aerial photography, multispectral overhead imagery	Animal tests	• Societal risk
Performance testing	• Biologic monitoring Chemical residues, bioaccumulation/degradation, physiology, indicator species	• Acute toxicity studies	Nominal risk outcomes
• Component and system failure tests		• Subchronic toxicity studies	Worst-case analysis
• Accelerated-life tests		• Chronic toxicity studies	Sensitivity analysis
• Accident simulations	Testing	Tests on humans	• Point
• Stress analysis	• Scale models	• Laboratory setting	• Parametric
• Mental movies	• Laboratory tests	• Field setting	• Rank correlations
Accident investigation	• Field experimentation	Epidemiology	• Stochastic
• Field investigation		• Case-control study	• Closed loop
• Laboratory investigation	Calculation of dose	• Cohort study	Statistical methods
• Accident reconstruction	• Based on exposure time	• Retrospective study	Probability encoding
Statistical methods	• Coexisting or decay substances	• Prospective study	• Debiasing
• Actuarial risk assessment	• Material deposition in tissue	• Molecular epidemiology	• Interval method
• Named probability distributions		Animal-to-human extrapolation models	• Probability wheel
• Bayes's theorem		Dose-response models	• Behavioral aggregation
• Statistical sampling		• Threshold	• Mechanical aggregation
• Regression analysis		• Tolerance	
• Extreme value theory			

- Hypothesis testing

Modeling methods
- Engineering failure analysis
- Logic trees, event trees, fault trees, Markov models
- Analytic process models
- Biological models for pests
- Containment models
- Discharge models
- BLEVE models

Pollutant transport-and-fate modeling
- Air
  Analytic models, trajectory models, transformation models
- Surface water
  Dissolved oxygen models, etc.
- Groundwater
  Travel-time models, Absorption models
- Overland
- Food-chain models
- Multimedia models

Exposure-route models

Population-at-risk models
- Census, sensitive groups, trip-generation models, etc.

- Mechanistic
- Time-to-response

Pharmacokinetic models

Ecosystem monitoring

Tests on the natural environment
- Field tests
- Laboratory tests
- Microcosms, macrocosms, mesocosms

Ecological effects models
- Dynamic
- Matrix
- Stochastic
- Markov
- Harvest
- Pollution response

Uncertainty propagation
- Method of moments
- Monte Carlo analysis
- Response surfaces
- Probability trees

Quantitative uncertainty analysis
- Confidence bounds
- Credibility analysis
- Uncertainty partitioning

Qualitative uncertainty analysis

1.7. A TAXONOMIC CLASSIFICATION OF RISK ASSESSMENT METHODS

Risk assessment often requires the application of a large and diverse set of methods. To simplify the task of describing these methods, we have classified risk assessment methods according to the four steps in our model of risk assessment: release assessment, exposure assessment, consequence assessment, and risk estimation. Table 3 lists the principal risk assessment methods described in this book according to their use in the risk assessment process. In summary:

- Methods for release assessment are directed at understanding the potential of a risk source to release or otherwise introduce risk agents into an environment in such a way that exposures to these or other risk agents may occur to people or the things they value. Examples include methods for estimating the probabilities of accidental releases of radioactive materials from a nuclear power plant, the amount of toxic substances introduced into food products, the accelerations produced during automobile crashes, and the pollutants present in the various gaseous and effluent emissions from a coal-fired electric power plant.

- Methods for exposure assessment are directed at understanding the frequency, duration, and nature of human or environmental exposures to risk agents. Examples include methods for monitoring ambient concentrations of air pollutants in urban areas, statistical sampling methods for estimating residual levels of pesticides in food, experiments involving simulated collisions of automobiles using dummies to identify likely points of injury to humans, and modeling methods for predicting the contamination of drinking water by groundwater transport of toxic substances.

- Methods for consequence assessment are directed at clarifying the adverse health or environmental consequences that result from exposures. Examples include animal research to test the toxicity of a new drug, low-dose and interspecies dose-extrapolation methods, biokinetic models of the human body used to simulate injuries produced during automobile collisions, and models to estimate the fish and wildlife losses resulting from the acidification of lakes and streams.

- Methods for risk estimation are directed at integrating the results of a release assessment, exposure assessment, and consequence assessment to produce summary measures of risk. Examples include methods for coupling inputs and outputs of models for releases, exposures, and consequences, and methods for propagating uncertainties through models. Such methods allow risk assessors to quantify possible risk outcomes, including the nature, timing, and magnitude of end consequences such as numbers of deaths, illnesses of various types, and specified impacts to the environment. The estimates should indicate not only the most likely risk outcomes but also the range of possibilities, including worst-case results, and the probabilities of the possibilities.

Within each of these four categories, risk assessment methods differ according to whether they are concerned primarily with constructing and analyzing models or with collecting data that provide the foundation for those models. Thus, some of the methods listed in Table 3 focus on modeling and statistical analysis while others focus on data collection through monitoring and testing. Modeling and statistical methods may be used directly to develop probability distributions for health and environmental consequences. Monitoring and testing methods may not always provide direct measures of risk, but they will provide the essential data and insight necessary for applying the modeling and statistical methods.

Classifying a risk assessment method on the basis of its use in one or another component of the risk assessment process and according to whether the method relates more to models or to data is a matter of judgment. For example, a method's focus on models versus data is a question of degree, since the collection and processing of data is always predicated on some hypothesized underlying model, and models can be neither constructed nor analyzed without data. Furthermore, whether a method is related to release assessment, exposure assessment, or consequence assessment depends on where the boundaries are drawn between releases, exposures, and consequences. For example, pharmacokinetic methods used for studying the distribution of toxic substances in various human organs might be considered part of consequence assessment (if the focus is on consequences for human organs) or as part of exposure assessment (if the focus is on distribution of chemicals within the body). Despite these ambiguities, the four-component classification scheme, coupled with a distinction between methods that rely on monitoring and testing versus those that rely on modeling and statistics, provides a practical if not completely unambiguous way of organizing and distinguishing the vast array of risk assessment methods.

1.8. THE RISK ASSESSMENT PROCESS

We use the categorization scheme discussed in the previous section to organize the descriptions and evaluations of risk assessment methods that appear in the remaining chapters of this book. The scheme allows us to order what would otherwise be a confusing array of sometimes compatible, sometimes competing, sometimes contradictory approaches.

In addition to its usefulness for categorizing methods, our framework has another function. The taxonomy mirrors the basic steps of the risk assessment process. Assuming that a hazard (i.e., a potential source of risk) has been identified, the process begins with the collection of information. Next, models must be constructed to represent the critical links in the risk chain: the risk source, exposure processes, and effects processes. Last, the models must be linked and then analyzed to quantify the uncertainty over possible risk consequences.

The fact that the taxonomy reflects the fundamental steps of risk assessment allows it to serve as a useful framework for understanding and evaluating actual risk assessments. Unfortunately, many risk assessments conducted to date have not attempted to delineate clearly release assessment steps and differentiate them from exposure assessment steps, nor to clearly separate most of the other fundamental steps as we have defined them. Thus, decomposing a risk assessment into release assessment, exposure assessment, consequence assessment, and risk estimation may represent a change in the way many risk assessors approach their work. Our taxonomy is sufficiently natural, however, that the change in thinking is easy to make.

CHAPTER 2

RELEASE ASSESSMENT

Release assessment involves quantifying the extent to which a risk source releases or otherwise introduces risk agents into the human environment. This chapter describes the major types of release processes and risk agents encountered in risk assessment and evaluates the various methods used in release assessment.

Methods for release assessment focus on describing the characteristics of technologies, products, processes, or systems that have the potential for creating risk. Available methods fall into four main categories: *monitoring, performance testing and accident investigation, statistical methods, and modeling.* The methods that are appropriate for release assessment depend on what information about releases is required for the risk assessment, that is, what aspects of the risk source, risk agents, and release processes need to be quantified in order to quantify risk. For example, if a coal-fired electric power plant is regarded as a source of risk, then release assessment might specify the types, amounts, and timing of pollutants that would be emitted to the air and water or disposed of on or in the ground. If the concern is the failure of a dam, release assessment might estimate the probability of various failure modes and the volume of water that would be released under each. In the case of automobile accidents where the overriding concern is the "release" of violent kinetic energy into the passenger compartment, release assessment might address the energy-dissipating characteristics of the automobile's body structure and the integrity and dynamics of the passenger compartment under various crash scenarios. If the concern is a pesticide used in agriculture, release assessment might estimate the quantities of pesticide used and when, where, and how the pesticide would be applied.

2.1. RISK SOURCES AND RISK AGENTS

Risk sources may release risk agents to the air, soil, surface water, or groundwater. The release can be from a point source (e.g., a chimney), a line source (e.g., automobiles along a road), or an area source (e.g., pesticide spray). Releases occur either as by-products of normal operations or because of accidents. Sources that routinely or continuously release risk agents to the air include incinerators, automobiles, and industrial boilers. Risk sources that threaten surface water include mining operations, electric power plants, and municipal sewage treatment facilities. Risk sources for groundwater include underground petroleum storage tanks, hazardous waste disposal sites, and municipal landfills. Accidental releases include catastrophic industrial accidents (e.g., the 1984 release of methyl-isocyanate gas from the Union Carbide plant in Bhopal, India, and the 1986 radioactive release from the nuclear power plant at Chernobyl), oil spills (e.g., the 1989 Exxon Valdez oil spill off the Alaska coast), and in-plant release accidents involving workers.

In many cases, the risk source is a man-made facility or process wherein risk agents are contained by a physical barrier, and releases occur because containment is not completely effective. In other situations, the concept of risk source and release is more abstract. For example, if the risk involves debris from falling satellites and spacecraft, the risk source is the upper atmosphere, and the risk agent is a mass whose potential energy is released as kinetic energy as it falls to Earth. This example illustrates how the boundary that delineates the risk source may be conceptual rather than physical.

The risk agents released may be either chemical, physical, biological, or forms of energy. Chemical risk agents include corrosive acids and alkalis, hazardous vapors and gases, pesticides, pharmaceuticals, and carcinogens. Physical risk agents, such as atmospheric particulates, flood waters, volcanic ash, and cement dust, are similarly dangerous, but pose a threat more because of their physical rather than chemical properties. Biological risk agents include genetically engineered organisms, such as new microbes designed for agricultural or industrial cleanup, as well as natural bacteria and viruses, such as the AIDS virus. Forms of energy include mechanical energy, acoustic energy, electromagnetic energy, extreme heat or cold, and atmospheric pressure.

Table 4 summarizes various categories of risk agents and sources. Table 5 illustrates the diversity of chemical risk agents by listing some of the many chemicals that are currently of concern. Important special categories of risk agents often addressed in risk assessment include toxic metals, chemical solvents, pesticides, genetically engineered microorganisms, electromagnetic radiation, and radioactivity. We use these types of risk agents frequently in our examples.

2.1.1. Toxic Metals

About 80 elements are classified as metals including arsenic, selenium, and thallium, as well as more familiar metals such as iron, copper, and aluminum. Many metals are present in the environment in forms and at levels considered to be harmful to people. Sources include refineries, chemical plants, cement manufacturing, power plants, smelters, trash burning, and tobacco smoke. Automobiles emit

TABLE 4.   Some Important Categories of Risk Agents and Sources

Risk agent category	Example risk agents	Source/description	Example concerns
Criteria Air Pollutants (air pollutants subject to National Ambient Air Quality Standards Under the Clean Air Act)	Carbon monoxide	Automobiles, other fossil fuel combustion	Headaches, dizziness, drowsiness, nausea/ vomiting, coma, death
	Lead	Leaded gasoline and automobile exhaust	Neurologic and behavioral disorders, especially in children
	Ozone	Formed from atmospheric reactions involving volatile organic compounds (VOCs) and nitrogen dioxide	Respiratory effects, materials damage (esp. textiles, paints, and elastomers), reduced forest growth
	Nitrogen dioxide	Fossil fuel combustion	Respiratory effects, photochemical smog, acid deposition with effects on forests and other ecosystems
	Particulate matter (various sizes and chemically composed particles)	Electric utilities, construction activities, mining, windblown dust	Aggravation of chronic respiratory and cardiac disease, increased acute respiratory illness, decreased visibility, material soiling
	Sulfur oxides	Fossil fuel combustion	Effects on lung function, acid deposition with effects on aquatic and other ecosystems, materials damage
Other toxic air pollutants	Volatile organic compounds	Underground petroleum storage tanks, solvents	Cancer
	Metals such as arsenic, cadmium, and chromium	Industrial boilers and furnaces burning recycled oil, municipal waste incinerators	Lung damage, cancer
	Organic compounds such as PCBs and formaldehyde	Industrial boilers and furnaces burning recycled oil, municipal waste incinerators, electrical capacitors and transformers	Cancer, effects on fish and wildlife, bioaccumulation

(continued)

TABLE 4. (*Continued*)

Risk agent category	Example risk agents	Source/description	Example concerns
	Polycyclic aromatic hydrocarbons (PAHs)	Coal-fired electric power plants, forest fires, tobacco smoke	Cancer
Greenhouse gases	Chlorofluorocarbons (CFCs)	Compounds used as aerosol propellants, foam-blowing agents, refrigerants, solvents	Effects on stratospheric ozone with possible increase of ultraviolet radiation and global climate change
	Carbon dioxide	Combustion of fossil fuels, deforestation	Global climate change, rise in sea level
Radioactivity	Radon	Radioactive gas emitted by soil, rock, and building materials	Lung cancer, property values
	Other naturally occurring radioisotopes	Mining, industrial processing of raw materials	Cancer
	Radioactive production products	Nuclear reactors, weapons production, particle accelerators, medical uses	Cancer
Pesticides	Approximately 50,000 pesticide products derived from about 600 basic chemicals	Agriculture, industry, and household use	Various effects on human health, wildlife
Point-source discharges to surface waters	Chlorination products, ammonia, thermal pollution	Industrial operations, municipal waste management facilities, power plants	Damage to aquatic systems, loss of water recreational facilities
Nonpoint discharges to surface waters	Sediment, excess nutrients, pesticides, acids from mining operations	Runoff from precipitation, agricultural runoff, urban runoff	Erosion, silting of reservoirs, clogging of shipping channels, deposition of toxic pollutants attached to sediments

(*continued*)

TABLE 4. (*Continued*)

Risk agent category	Example risk agents	Source/description	Example concerns
Hazardous waste	Toxics, radioactive waste, particulates, excess nutrients, microbes	Municipal waste management facilities, abandoned toxic waste sites, landfills, surface impoundments, incinerators, solvent recovery facilities	Groundwater, surface water, and air contamination
Chemical spills	PCBs, ammonia, chlorine	Chemical releases from truck, barge, rail, and ship transportation; industrial production and storage facilities; electric utilities	Worker safety, public health
	Petroleum products	Spills from pipelines, storage tanks, production facilities	Effects on public health, wildlife
Structural accidents	Collapse of engineering structures	Failure of dams, mines, in-progress concrete and masonry structures, energy installations, underground tunnels, covered excavations	Lost lives, property damage, destruction of fish or wildlife habitat, soil erosion
Viruses	HIV (AIDS), Herpes simplex, Rhinovirus (common cold)	Submicroscopic infective agents capable of attacking and destroying living cells	Infectious diseases, including AIDS, flu, and the common cold
Genetically engineered organisms	Ice minus	Bacterium with excised gene having ability to promote formation of ice crystals below 0°C	Feared side effects, such as impacts on rainfall, toxicity to local crops
	Strain of *Pseudomonas*	Oil-degrading organisms	Gene transfer, toxic metabolites, impacts on ocean organisms
Explosives and combustibles	Propane, gasoline, dynamite, rice flour	Petroleum refineries and distributors, chemical processing plants, marine terminals, distilleries, grain-handling facilities	Fire, injuries, lost lives, property damage, crop loss

TABLE 5.   Some Chemical Risk Agents[a]

Agent	Source/description	Primary concerns
Acetone	Fingernail polish remover, glues, solvents	Accidental poisoning, irritation of eyes and mucous membranes
Acrylonitrile	Plastic resin in pipes, textiles	Cancer, releases hydrogen cyanide when burned
Aflatoxin	Mold toxin on peanuts and corn	Cancer of the liver
Alar (daminozide)	Sprayed on apples, grapes, cherries, and peanuts to make crop ripen, improve appearance, and increase storage life	Cancer
Alcohol	Alcoholic drinks, medications	Birth defects, neurological impairment
Aldicarb	Carbamate pesticide	Poisoning through skin, spontaneous abortions; residues in watermelons, cucumbers
Aldrin/dieldrin	Organochlorine insecticide	Neurological effects, cancer, environmental effects (fish, birds)
Aluminum	Cooking pots, additive in food, nonprescription drugs	Possible role in Alzheimer's disease
Ammonia	Household cleaning solutions, industry and farming accidents	Irritation of skin, eye, and respiratory passages; pulmonary edema; pneumonia
Antibiotics in animal feed	Improving growth rate of food-producing animals	Increase in occurrence of drug-resistant pathogens
Arsenic	Smelting, used oil, pesticides, wood preservative	Skin, liver, and lung cancer; poisoning
Asbestos	Fireproof insulation, ceiling tiles, brake linings	Lung cancer, mesothelioma, asbestosis
Benzene	Petrochemical and refining industries, constituent of gasoline, tobacco smoke	Bone marrow damage, leukemia, blood disorders, upper respiratory tract irritation, cancer
Benzidene	Manufacture of dye, paper, textiles, and leather	Cancer of the bladder
Benzo[a]pyrene (B[a]p)	Forest fires, cigarettes, wood-burning stoves, cooked foods	Cancer
Beryllium	Oil and coal combustion, mining, production of beryllium metal, cement plants, alloys, ceramics, rocket propellants	Dermatitis, ulcers, inflammation of mucous membranes, chronic berylliosis, cancer
Cadmium	Fossil fuel combustion, fertilizers, shellfish, electroplating, batteries	Lung cancer, emphysema, heart disease, kidney and liver disease
Carbaryl	Carbamate pesticide	Environmental effects (bees)

(continued)

TABLE 5. (*Continued*)

Agent	Source/description	Primary concerns
Carbon black	Photocopy toner, paint pigment, manufacturing	Provides transport vehicle for polycyclic aromatic hydrocarbons (PAHs) and other mutagenic contaminants
Carbon tetrachloride	Dry cleaning fluid, pesticide fumigant	Cancer, liver and kidney disease
Chlorine	Drinking water disinfectant, tanker truck spills	Pulmonary edema, carcinogenic by-products of chlorination
Chloroform	Sewage treatment plants, showering with chlorinated water	Cancer, liver and kidney disease
Chloromethane	Manufacture of polymers and resins, antiknock compounds for gasoline	Possible carcinogen, mutagen
Chromium	Chrome plating, paint pigments, leather tanning, wood preservatives	Lung cancer, liver and kidney damage
Cobalt	Foam stabilizer in beer	Heart damage
Cyclamate	Artificial sweetener	Cancer
2,4-D	Herbicide	Forms nitrosamines in intestinal tract, environmental effects (fish)
DDT	Organochlorine insecticide	Cancer, reproductive effects, environmental damage (eggshell thinning)
Diazinon	Organophosphate insecticide	Environmental effects (birds, fish)
Dibromochloropropane (DBCP)	Soil fumigant	Sterility
Diethylsilbesterol (DES)	Drug to prevent miscarriage	Birth defects, cancer of the vagina
Dioxin (Agent Orange)	Herbicide used in Vietnam; contaminant in herbicide, cardboard containers	Chloracne, cancer, birth defects
Ethylenebisdithiocarbamates (EBDCs)	Class of carbamate pesticides	Cancer, birth defects
Ethylene dibromide (EDB)	Fumigant for grain, dye production, scavenger in leaded gasoline	Bromide poisoning, cancer
Formaldehyde	Foam insulation, pressed wood materials	Irritation of eyes and respiratory system, cancer
Heptachlor/Chlordane	Organochlorine insecticide	Cancer, environmental effects (plants, bees, fish)
Hexachlorophene	Disinfectant	Neurological effects in infants

(continued)

TABLE 5. (*Continued*)

Agent	Source/description	Primary concerns
Hydrogen cyanide	Plastic manufacturing, petroleum refining	Acute cyanide poisoning
Kepone (chlordecone)	Organochlorine insecticide	Neurological effects, sterility, environmental effects
Lindane	Organochlorine pesticide fumigant	Neurological effects, possible carcinogen, environmental effects (fish, birds)
Malathion	Organophosphate pesticide	Environmental effects (fish)
Mercury	Thermometers, dental fillings, trace contaminants of ores and fuels	Memory losses, tremors, neurological damage, exposures to fetuses
Methyl ethyl ketone (MEK)	Lacquers, varnishes, industrial solvent	Irritation of eyes, mucous membranes, skin
Methylene chloride (DCM)	Paint strippers and aerosol paints, used in decaffeination of coffee	Cancer
Methylmercury	Organic compound of mercury, industrial and commercial releases accumulated in fish and shellfish	Neurologic damage, reproductive effects, bioaccumulation
Naphthalene	Mothballs	Accidental poisoning of infants
Nickel	Coins, metal products, metal refineries, food	Skin reaction, cancer
Nitrobenzene	Production of aniline	Destruction of blood hemoglobin, coma
Nitrosamines	Formed from precursors, amines, nitrogen oxides, and nitrates in air, water, and food	Cancer
Parathion	Organophosphate pesticide	Respiratory effects, environmental effects (bees, fish)
Phenol	Manufacturing, disinfectant in petroleum and other industries	Skin and eye irritation
Polybrominated biphenyls (PBBs)	Fire retardant, plastic parts	Mislabeled animal feed
Polychlorinated biphenyls (PCBs)	Cooling fluid in transformers and capacitors, plasticizers	Chloracne, cancer, other health effects, environmental effects (mammals, birds, fish)
Saccharin	Artificial sweetener	Cancer
Tetrachlorethylene (PCE)	Dry cleaning fluid, chlorination of acetylene, degreasing metals	Smog, eye irritation, possible carcinogen, liver damage, explosion
Thalidomide	Sedative	Birth defects

(*continued*)

TABLE 5. (*Continued*)

Agent	Source/description	Primary concerns
Toluene	Petrochemical and refining industries, constituent of gasoline, cigarette smoke, model glue	Irritation to skin and eyes, kidney and liver damage
Trichloroethane (TCA)	Drain cleaners, shoe polish, spot removers	Possible mutagen
Trichloroethylene (TCE)	Metal degreasing	Cancer
2,4,5-Trichlorophenoxy acetic acid (2,4,5-T)	Herbicide	Chloracne, birth defects, cancer, environmental effects (fish)
TRIS	Flame retardant in children's sleepwear	Cancer
Vinyl chloride	Production of polyvinyl chloride, PVC pipes, plastic packaging	Angiosarcoma (a rare type of tumor), lung cancer, birth defects

[a]Adapted from OECD (1985), Williams and Burson (1985), Environ Corporation (1986), and Harte *et al.* (1991).

metals, particularly lead emitted by older vehicles using leaded gasoline. Water in pipes can leach out accumulate metals from the plumbing. Metals are also used extensively in the workplace—in welding, grinding, soldering, painting, smelting, and storage battery manufacturing. Trace metals are metals that tend to be present in very low concentrations. Heavy metals are metals whose densities are at least five times greater than water (e.g., cadmium, lead, and mercury).

Once in the human body metals create adverse effects at the cellular level. Some metals disrupt chemical reactions, while others block essential biological processes. Still others bind to nutrients in the stomach, thereby preventing the absorption of nutrients into the body (Pounds, 1985). Brief contact with high concentrations of metals can cause lung damage, skin reactions, and gastrointestinal symptoms. Some metals accumulate in the body over time, reaching toxic concentrations after years of exposure. Many metals including arsenic, beryllium, cadmium, chromium, and nickel are carcinogens. Lead exposure in children has been linked to low IQs. Exposure to methylmercury and lead can cause gross deformities in development (Friberg *et al.*, 1986).

2.1.2. Solvents

Solvents (e.g., chlorine, methyl ethyl ketone, and acetone) are chemicals used to dissolve other substances. Solvents often pose a high health hazard—some are flammable, others explode easily, some are corrosive, and most are toxic. Halogens (chlorine, fluorine, bromine, and iodine) are often added to solvents to reduce their tendency to catch fire or corrode tanks. The most commonly used halogenated solvents are the chlorinated ones (e.g., methylene chloride, trichloroethane, trichloroethylene, and tetrachloroethylene). Major sources of solvents include cleaning operations in the electronics and machining industry, thinners for paints and glues, and dry cleaning. Solvents are also used in many household products, for example, acetone is used as fingernail polish remover.

Exposures to solvents can cause damage to the skin, liver, blood, central nervous system, and sometimes the lungs and kidneys (Andrews and Snyder, 1986). Inhaling solvent vapors can lead to lung and throat irritation, pulmonary edema, dizziness, lightheadedness, blurred vision, nervousness, sleepiness or insomnia, nausea, vomiting, disorientation, confusion, irregular heartbeat, unconsciousness, and death. Repeated exposures to some solvents can lead to chronic bronchitis, permanent liver and kidney damage, and permanent neurological problems. Many commonly encountered chlorinated solvents, including benzene, trichloroethylene, tetrachloroethylene, and methylene chloride, are suspected carcinogens. A few (e.g., glycol ethers) have been found to cause birth defects and reproductive problems.

Many volatile solvents contribute to the formation of urban ozone, while others [including chlorofluorocarbons (CFCs), trichloroethane, and carbon tetrachloride] contribute to stratospheric ozone depletion. Chlorinated solvents are often persistent in soil and water, leading to bioconcentration and groundwater pollution. Trichloroethane degrades in soil to form the more toxic chemical vinyl chloride (Lave and Upton, 1987).

2.1.3. Pesticides

It should not be surprising that pesticides are important risk agents, considering that pesticides are designed to kill. The target pests for pesticides include insects (insecticides), plants (herbicides), molds and mildews (fungicides), rats and mice (rodenticides), mites and ticks (acaricides), slugs and snails (molluscicides), bacteria (bactericides), birds (avicides), and algae (algaecides). Pesticides come in the forms of aerosols, sprays, dust, granules, or as baits. Because of their extensive use and the manner in which they are applied, pesticides are found everywhere—in drinking water, food, air, and soils.

Insecticides include organochlorines [e.g., DDT, polychlorinated biphenyls (PCBs), lindane, aldrin/dieldrin, heptachlor, Kepone, dioxin], organophosphates (e.g., diazinon, malathion, parathion), carbamates (e.g., aldicarb, carbaryl, methomyl), botanicals (e.g., nicotine, rotenone, pyrethrum extracts, camphor, turpentine), and fumigants [e.g., naphthalene, ethylene dibromide (EDB)]. Organochlorines are chlorinated hydrocarbons—synthetic combinations of chlorine, hydrogen, and carbon. They act as neurotoxins, that is, they tend to stimulate the nervous system in insects and mammals, causing tremors and convulsions. As a class, organochlorine pesticides are less acutely toxic to humans than other insecticide classes, but have greater potential for chronic toxicity. Most organochlorine pesticides are now banned or restricted because of their persistence in the environment, tendency to accumulate in the tissues of living organisms, and toxicity to nontarget species.

Organophosphates are chemicals derived from phosphoric acid. They break down rapidly and do not accumulate in tissues, but are often extremely toxic and nonselective. For example, one drop of parathion, if placed in the eye, would be fatal to humans (Koren, 1991). More instances of acute poisoning have occurred with organophosphate insecticides than with any other insecticide class (Stopford, 1985). Organophosphates operate by interfering with the nervous system in a complex way that ultimately affects the respiratory and circulatory systems by binding to and, thereby, blocking the activity of acetylcholinesterase, an enzyme that controls the stimuli to nerve ends.

Carbamates, the most widely used pesticides, are derived from carbonic acid. Carbamates are similar to organophosphates in that they operate by inactivating acetylcholinesterase. However, the bond formed is not as stable, so that the effect is relatively brief. The carbamates are generally fairly safe for use around nontarget organisms with the exception of honeybees and many aquatic invertebrates. Botanicals are compounds produced naturally by plants as defense mechanisms, such as pyrethrum extracted from the flowers of *Chrysanthemum cinerarifolium*. Botanicals tend to be highly specific to pests and have a very low toxicity to humans. The main disadvantage of botanical pesticides is that they are usually expensive. Fumigants are volatile compounds that are applied as gases. They readily penetrate the skin and membranes that line the human respiratory and gastrointestinal tracts, act as narcotics (i.e., induce sleep or unconsciousness), and may be highly toxic to humans.

Herbicides (e.g., 2,4-D and 2,4,5,-T, atrazine, dicamba, paraquat, linuron) vary greatly in their selectivity, persistence in tissues and the environment, and ability to be absorbed by plants. Fungicides include carbamate derivatives [e.g., mancozeb, maneb, metiram, and zineb—known as ethylenebisthiocarbamates (EBDC)] which generally pose low risk to humans from brief exposures, but are often contaminated with ethylene thiourea, which is toxic to the thyroid gland and may cause cancer, mutations, and birth defects.

2.1.4. Genetically Engineered Microorganisms

Genetic engineering is the technology used to alter the genetic material of living cells, thereby enabling changes to be made to the inherited characteristics of plants, animals, and microorganisms. The methods of genetic engineering range from traditional techniques (such as natural mating methods for selective breeding) to the advanced recombinant DNA techniques, wherein genetic material is manipulated directly. The ability to produce organic materials with new characteristics offers diverse application opportunities including the production of pharmaceutical products (e.g., human insulin, growth hormones, antibodies, and vaccines), food processing (e.g., fermentation, development of edible microorganisms), and agriculture (e.g., plant breeding). However, genetic engineering may pose serious risks; for example, a new organism may cause harm, or an introduced gene may be transferred to other organisms, causing harm.

Initial concerns about genetic engineering focused on the safety and security of the laboratories in which it is conducted. More recently, attention has shifted to the special risks associated with genetically engineered microorganisms designed for use in the environment. Potential environmental uses of genetically engineered organisms include biological pesticides, mineral leaching and recovery, enhanced oil recovery, and pollution control. To fully understand the commercial potential of such products, the organisms must be tested in the field. Field tests inevitably result in the use of large volumes of microorganisms and decreased control.

Nonindigenous organisms introduced into an ecosystem may displace or disrupt existing biological communities. They may harm individuals of an indigenous species or whole populations by causing infectious disease. Genetic material may be transferred from the introduced organisms to indigenous organisms, with unanticipated effects. For instance, if drug resistance were to be transferred to clinically important bacteria, the range of antibiotics available for treating infections could be reduced. A transferred characteristic may create a selective advantage for the modified microbe, allowing it to increase its population and substantially alter the microbial ecosystem. Finally, introduced organisms will consume and alter chemicals encountered in the environment. The altered forms, or breakdown products, are called metabolites. The metabolites produced by the organisms may themselves be toxic and persistent in the environment. For example, a potential concern regarding microorganisms intended to biodegrade toxic chemicals is the buildup of intermediary metabolites that are more toxic, more mobile, and/or more resistant than the original chemicals (Strauss, 1991).

2.1.5. Electromagnetic Radiation

Radiation is a form of energy that can be thought of both as a wave and as a stream of particles. Electromagnetic radiation includes radio waves, microwaves, infrared, visible, and ultraviolet light, X rays, gamma rays, and cosmic rays. Such radiation is propagated through space in the form of packets of energy called photons, which travel at the speed of light. The energy of the photon is directly proportional to its frequency. Thus, for example, ultraviolet light has a higher frequency and more energetic photons than visible light, while gamma rays and X rays have still higher frequencies and even more energetic photons.

As it moves through space, electromagnetic radiation interacts with atoms composing matter. Photons in the higher-energy ranges such as X rays and gamma rays can ionize atoms by stripping away the atom's orbital electrons. Radiation of this energy level is termed *ionizing*. Radiation associated with the lower-energy portions of the electromagnetic spectrum is termed *nonionizing*. Nonionizing radiation includes ultraviolet radiation, microwaves, and low-frequency electromagnetic fields.

The major source of ultraviolet (UV) radiation is the sun, although sunlamps, tanning booths, and accidental laboratory and industrial exposures are also sources. Effects of exposure include sunburn, premature aging of the skin, and temporary loss of vision, as in snow blindness. Skin cancer can also result from UV exposure. Since the biological effects of UV radiation do not appear until some time after exposure has occurred, people can receive an excessive amount of UV radiation before becoming aware of the extent of the damage. If exposure is sufficiently high, systemic effects such as fever, nausea, and malaise can occur. UV radiation is of increasing concern due to the apparent ongoing degradation of the stratospheric ozone layer caused by emissions of CFCs and other volatile chemicals. Stratospheric ozone greatly diminishes the amount of UV radiation that reaches us from the sun.

Microwave radiation sources include radar, satellite telecommunication systems, industrial welding, and, of course, microwave ovens. Microwave radiation can cause health damage by heating tissues. Sufficient exposure can produce thermal burns in the skin and eyes. Microwave radiation can also cause nonthermal effects, such as virus activation, interference with enzyme synthesis or cell division, damage to the nervous and immune systems, and changes in cardiac rhythm. The most common symptoms of excessive exposures reported in the workplace include headaches, fatigue, dizziness, confusion, and insomnia (WHO, 1981). Exposures to high-power densities, as in the wave guide of a microwave transmitter, can be lethal.

Low-frequency electromagnetic fields (EMFs) result wherever ordinary alternating current (ac) flows through transmission lines or electric appliances. The major sources of exposures to people are overhead transmission lines, large motors, electric blankets, and computer terminal screens. Exposures may increase the incidence of certain kinds of cancer, although a relationship has not yet been clearly established or explained. EMFs may affect the immune and endocrine systems, the latter of which provides growth-regulatory signals, with the possible result of changes in the flow of calcium through cell membranes (OTA, 1989).

2.1.6. Radioactivity

Unstable radioactive isotopes provide the most significant source of ionizing radiation. *Isotopes* are versions of the same basic element composed of different numbers of neutrons. For example, uranium-238 and uranium-235 are isotopes of uranium (the number following the name of the element denotes the total number of neutrons plus protons; all uranium isotopes contain 92 protons). Radioactive isotopes are unstable, that is, they emit particles and thereby decay to become other isotopes. The three main types of particles emitted are beta rays (electrons), alpha rays (nuclei of helium atoms), and gamma rays (photons). Radioactive isotopes differ from one another in terms of their half lives (i.e., the time it takes for half of the material to be converted to another isotope), the type of radiation emitted (alpha, beta, or gamma), and the energy level of the emitted radiation.

Other differences in radioactive materials important to risk assessment include whether the material is a gas, liquid, or solid, how it interacts chemically with the body, and the isotopes to which the material decays. Internal exposures can result if radioactive materials enter the body through ingestion or inhalation. Outside the body, materials that emit beta particles are more dangerous than those that emit alpha particles, since alpha particles typically cannot penetrate the skin. Inside the body, however, alpha particles present a greater hazard because they produce more highly concentrated damage. Some radioactive materials tend to concentrate in single organs, such as iodine in the thyroid gland.

Various measures have been adopted to describe and quantify radioactivity. The *becquerel* and *curie* are measures of the amount of radioactivity expressed in a way that depends on the rate at which radiation is being emitted. One becquerel of radioactive material is an amount of the material that produces one atom decaying per second. One curie of radioactive material is equal to 37 million becquerels (which is the number of nuclei that decay per second in 1 gram of radium). The *gray* and *rad* are measures of the amount of energy absorbed by an object exposed to radiation. An object is said to receive 1 gray (Gy) of radiation when every gram of that object has absorbed 10,000 ergs of energy from the passing radiation. A rad is 1/100 of a gray. The *sievert* (Sv) and *rem* (one one-hundredth of a sievert) are also measures of exposure. With these measures, radiation exposures associated with the particles are multiplied by an *adjustment factor* to account roughly for the differing degrees of biological damage caused by the different particles. The adjustment factor is 1 for beta and gamma particles, but 20 for alpha particles.

Most human exposure to radiation is associated with natural background radiation resulting primarily from the decay of isotopes in the earth's crust. In many parts of the U.S., for example, the most significant background source is radon gas produced from the decay of radioactive radium. Radon and its decay products can collect in the indoor air of homes and other buildings. The total natural background dose of radiation to people (including radon) is about 3 millisieverts (.003 Sv) per year (Eisenbud, 1984). Major sources of ionizing radiation associated with technology include medical and dental uses, as well as nuclear reactors, which require mining and processing of uranium fuel and storage or treatment of spent fuel. Waste from nuclear weapons production and past atmospheric testing is also a source. Radionuclides released from nuclear facilities include tritium, iodine-131, and plutonium-239. Tritium is a radioactive form of hydrogen used in nuclear weapons. It is a gas, has a half-life of 12.3 years, and decays by emitting beta particles. Iodine-131 is formed when uranium undergoes fission, has a half-life of 8.1 days, and emits beta particles. Plutonium-239 is a decay product of the uranium fuel used in nuclear reactors and is the principal fuel used in nuclear weapons. It decays by alpha particle emission and has a half-life of 24,000 years.

Effects of short-term exposures to very high doses of ionizing radiation (e.g., several sieverts) are immediately observable and include vomiting, hemorrhaging, hair loss, cataracts, sterility, and possible death. Long-term or repeated short-term exposures at much lower levels produce no immediately observable effects, but over time can result in cancers, genetic damage, blood abnormalities, metabolic diseases, and physical abnormalities in offspring (BEIR, 1990).

2.2. MONITORING

Monitoring involves "the assembling of data sets, usually for the purpose of detecting some change in the status of some variable of interest" (Hayne, 1984). When applied to release assessment, monitoring is aimed at collecting data on characteristics of a risk source. Most risk-source monitoring is focused on information related to releases or release potential, including physical and chemical conditions, emission rates, and source geometry and geology. Monitoring assembles data through a process of repetitively observing one or more characteristics or indicators of a risk source according to some prearranged schedule in space and time (Munn, 1973).

Examples of monitoring activities used in release assessment include collecting data on the integrity of hazardous waste at a disposal site, compiling records of the total production and import of toxic chemicals, and analyzing data on the safety status of the federal air traffic control system. Monitoring does not always require collecting new information. Monitoring administrative records, such as the required registration of chemicals, drugs, and pesticides, can sometimes provide important information about sources of risk. The information submitted to obtain a permit or to register a toxic material, for instance, can help identify the nature and amount of specific risk agents likely to enter the environment (Whyte and Burton, 1980).

Monitoring is usually a sampling process. Instead of measuring the status of a variable at all times or locations, selected measurements (samples) are taken. The samples are intended to provide a basis for inferring the characteristics of the system that produced the sample values. (The statistical methods that enable such inferences to be made are described in Section 2.4.) Critical issues in designing a monitoring system include determining where and how to take representative samples, deciding how to handle the samples en route to laboratories, selecting analytical methods to investigate the presence or absence of conditions of interest, choosing a procedure and format for aggregating and presenting the results of the analysis and for conveying the degree of confidence in the data, and determining how to interpret data on the presence, quantity, transformation, and migration of conditions of interest (Schweitzer, 1982).

Selecting appropriate answers to these questions requires considering the needs of the risk assessment that the monitoring is meant to support. An important example is monitoring to support risk assessment at hazardous waste sites (Saltzman, 1987). A major concern for hazardous waste sites is leachate resulting from percolation of hazardous liquids, or water infiltrating through contaminated soil. Key questions may be whether such a release has occurred and, if so, what are its characteristics. A monitoring system designed to identify and distinguish site-related contamination from naturally occurring background levels of chemicals could help answer these questions.

A consideration relevant for a hazardous waste site monitoring system is whether contaminants have reached the water table. Since underground contaminants move very slowly, if the potential contamination source is above the water table any released contaminants may not yet have reached groundwater. Thus, monitoring a hazardous waste site requires collecting both soil and groundwater samples. Additional samples for measuring background concentrations would be collected near the site in areas that could not have received contamination from potential releases at the site, but which have the same basic characteristics as the site. Thus, a prerequisite for identifying appropriate monitoring locations would be a good geographical and geological understanding of the site and its relation to nearby areas.

Surface samples are often obtained by driving a porous ceramic cup into the soil and allowing water to infiltrate the cup. To obtain underground samples, holes and test wells must be drilled. During the drilling, sensing devices are used to identify distinct water-permeable layers, and cement grout is used to prevent mixing between layers. Various sensing and sample acquisition devices are lowered into the holes. Simple bailers are used to obtain grab samples, and pumps are employed to obtain samples of groundwater. Continuous sampling may be conducted using absorbents such as activated carbon.

Samples taken from the site are analyzed in the laboratory to quantify basic characteristics such as acidity, alkalinity, and electrical conductivity and to identify and test for specific compounds of concern such as heavy metals and organic compounds. Methods such as distillation, extraction with solvents, and addition of reagents are first used to separate and concentrate the test compounds. The compound may then be analyzed using spectrophotometry, titrimetry, electrometry, and other standard analytic methods. Spectrophotometric methods involve mixing the test compound with a reagent designed to produce a colored product whose light absorption characteristics indicate the presence of certain chemicals. With titrimetric methods measured amounts of reagent of known strength are added to the sample until slight excess is shown by an appropriate indicator chemical or device. Electrometric methods immerse specially designed electrodes permeable to the test component into the prepared sample solution to measure electrical potentials or currents. Other analysis methods include atomic spectrometry (wherein elements are identified based on the energy levels of their orbiting electrons), gas and liquid chromatography (used to separate out volatile and nonvolatile compounds), and mass spectrometry (wherein a separated pure component is identified by its characteristic mass spectrum).

Quality assurance is an important component of hazardous waste site monitoring systems. The quality assurance program should include (1) testing or qualifying laboratory and field sampling procedures and analytic devices, (2) routine calibrations of all instrumentation, (3) a laboratory cross-check program, (4) regular replicate sampling, (5) procedural audits, and (6) documentation of laboratory and field procedures and quality-assurance records. As a rule of thumb, approximately 10 to 15 percent of the samples processed in a laboratory are resubmitted for analysis as "blind" duplicates (Moeller, 1992). Standard solutions (large bulk samples that have been analyzed so frequently that their chemical content is well established) are routinely used to check the accuracy of new data.

Although monitoring is useful for every component of the risk assessment process, special opportunities may exist for applying monitoring to release assessment. Specifically, when the risk source is a technological facility, a means for monitoring the characteristics of the source can be designed and built into the facility. An example is the monitoring system used in a nuclear power plant. Federal law requires that such systems be designed to permit ongoing determination of compliance with regulations governing the use, production, and emission of radioactivity. Nuclear power plant monitoring includes programs for measuring releases from the plant, as well as radiation fields within the plant. For example, radiation fields within the plant are derived from wall-mounted monitoring units, and portable units may be used in surveys. Fixed release monitors are used to sense and provide a temporal record of radioactivity released via stack effluents or liquid discharges during normal operation, refueling, or accidents. Process monitors are designed to keep track of the flow of materials within the plant.

The sensitivity of nuclear power plant monitoring systems, and the value of monitoring in identifying risks, is illustrated by an incident involving radiation monitors at a nuclear power plant owned by the Philadelphia Electric Company (Krimsky and Plough, 1988). The monitors, which were designed to identify radioactive contamination on the clothes of workers leaving the plant's power block, were installed in December 1984. One employee tripped the radiation monitor every time he left the plant. When the source of the contamination could not be identified, the worker conducted an experiment: one morning he entered the plant, turned around, and immediately walked back out through the monitor, without ever entering the plant's power block. When the radiation alarm went off, it was clear that the radiation was originating outside the plant. Subsequently, it was discovered that the employee's home contained excessively high levels of radioactive radon gas. This incident played a critical role in focusing public and scientific attention on the problems in buildings of radioactive contamination caused by naturally occurring radon.

In addition to monitoring instruments, the monitoring system for a large-scale technological facility generally includes data-handling systems for reading and collecting data from individual instruments, performing necessary conversions, and organizing and summarizing the resulting information. Typically, such integrated systems are also capable of partially checking individual instruments. For example, an electronic test pulse may be sent and used to identify certain types of instrument failures. In addition, such monitoring systems generally incorporate quality-assurance programs that include controls for the acceptance testing of instrumentation, routine calibration and replicate sampling, laboratory cross-checking, procedural audits, and program documentation.

Most risk-source monitoring is, of course, conducted in close proximity to a suspected risk source. In some cases, however, analysis of contaminants obtained at great distances from a source may provide release assessment information. One example involves the analysis of radioactive cesium, which can originate from a fallout from nuclear weapons testing or a release from a nuclear power plant. The type of source can be determined by measuring the ratio of cesium-134 to cesium-137, both of which are products of the nuclear fission process. Cesium-134 tends to be produced in a nuclear reactor but not in the detonation of a nuclear device. Hence, the source is probably not a release from a nuclear power plant if the fraction of cesium-134 is very low.

2.2.1. Strengths

Monitoring provides a useful means for quantifying the current status of a risk source, thereby establishing a baseline for identifying problems and for projecting what might happen in the future. Another important use of monitoring data is to help calibrate release models.

Because monitoring focuses on current and past status, it is most useful for assessing current risks. It can also help in assessing the risks that would remain following regulatory actions that do not affect the risk source, that is, regulatory actions that accomplish risk reduction through altering exposure or consequence processes. For example, if a hazardous waste site is deemed difficult or impossible to clean up, regulatory actions may focus on restricting people from living within a given distance of the contaminated area. In this case, data on site releases (e.g., release rate, concentrations, degree of toxicity, and decay rate) provide important information about the risk source. If the rate of transport for releases can be estimated and the location of populations is known, then the time at which exposures would occur can be estimated and compared with the time it takes for the risk agents to become diluted or to decay to the point at which they no longer pose any danger. Thus, release monitoring provides a basis for assessing the risks resulting under regulatory alternatives that limit exposures.

Monitoring is also useful for release assessments when regulatory actions alter the risk source in a predictable way. For example, if regulation requires installing technology for purifying the emissions produced by some production process, and if the technology is known to have some level of efficiency (e.g., 90 percent), then extrapolation from monitoring data can provide the basis for assessing risk with and without the proposed regulation.

2.2.2. Limitations

The most serious limitation of monitoring is its focus on the past. By definition, nothing can provide "evidence" of the future. For many risks the principal concern is not the continuation of the status quo but a fundamental change that will produce substantially greater danger. Sometimes monitoring can identify trends that foreshadow a significant increase in the risk posed by a hazardous system; however, monitoring is less useful if the cause of increased danger is a discrete event that is not easily detectable from the behavior of the system prior to the occurrence of the event.

Another difficulty concerns the effectiveness of monitoring for ascertaining system status. Although technological facilities such as nuclear power plants contain extensive monitoring systems, the data they provide do not always succeed in providing correct or precise information on the status of the facility during accidents. For example, implementation of appropriate actions during the 1979 accident at Three Mile Island was delayed while engineers sought to correctly interpret conflicting data on the state of the plant's reactor (U.S. President's Commission on the Accident at Three Mile Island, 1979). Even if the implications of monitoring data are readily apparent, monitoring has a significant limitation when applied to rare events. Events such as a nuclear reactor core meltdown or an extreme flood that occurs once in 100 years produce too few observations to provide much opportunity for learning from monitoring.

Another limitation relates to natural or legal barriers to monitoring a risk source. For example, government agencies may be able to monitor water quality downstream from a factory that discharges wastes into a river, but legislation protecting the confidentiality of industrial processes may prohibit analyzing concentrations of risk agents directly in the outflow pipes of the factory. In such situations, where there are barriers to monitoring a quantity of interest, monitoring must focus on related, more readily measurable quantities referred to as indicators. Unless there is a close relationship between the indicator and the quantity of interest, biases may be introduced. For example, monitoring the transport of all hazardous waste may be desirable, but will provide data only on shipments that are properly documented and recorded.

Another limitation is that monitoring is often time-consuming and expensive. If monitoring requires the use of complex measurement devices and depends on the collection of data over a long period of time, the development and implementation of a monitoring program can result in considerable capital and operating expense. Also, if many independent risk sources are present, as is the case for most environmental pollutants, it may be impossible to monitor them all. Accurately monitoring even a single risk source can be expensive; for example, determining the amounts and nature of emissions that come from the stack of a coal-fired electric power plant can cost several hundreds of thousands of dollars per year. Very low release rates can also create a situation in which monitoring does not reveal the presence of a risk agent. For example, even if release rates are too low to measure, they may still pose a risk to human health through the bioaccumulation of risk agents in food. For some risk agents, monitoring is technically difficult. For example, when monitoring electric and magnetic fields, the mere presence of people and their monitoring equipment may alter the environment in such a way as to make accurate measurements difficult.

2.3. PERFORMANCE TESTING AND ACCIDENT INVESTIGATION

Monitoring systems for release assessment are usually designed to collect measurements of the status of a risk source while it is functioning in its normal way. Sometimes it is useful to gather information while deliberately subjecting the risk source or its component systems to stress, that is, to investigate the behavior of a system under conditions that are extreme or otherwise of special concern.

Performance testing entails collecting data about a system under controlled, usually stressful, conditions. Such testing is especially useful in characterizing risk sources that contain common electrical and mechanical components. If performance testing has generated sufficient data about specific types of components, statistical methods can be used to derive the operating and failure characteristics of similar components being used in the technological system under study. In situations where the failure of individual components is of less concern, the complete system might be subjected to performance tests. Even if only limited experiments can be performed, such testing can still be useful. In these cases, however, engineering analysis and judgment necessarily play a larger role than statistics in inferring which characteristics of components are of greatest concern in assessing the system's risks.

Automobile safety is one area in which performance testing has been used for extensive investigation of a risk source. Estimating the change in the number and severity of passenger injuries that will result from a change in an automobile's safety system requires an understanding of the vehicle's response during a high-speed crash. In a typical impact, which lasts less than 100 milliseconds, the automobile's structure undergoes large deformations, accompanied by buckling, fracture, tearing of metal, and complex deformation of joints (Bhushan, 1975). The behavior of the risk source is further complicated by the dependence of the vehicle's response on impact velocity, angle of incidence, and the characteristics of the obstacle with which the vehicle collides. The models developed to account for these considerations are based on the empirical results of experiments. Because full-scale experiments are expensive and time-consuming, much of the research relies on scale models (e.g., see Holmes and Sliter, 1974).

If the reliability of a component or subsystem of a risk source is very high, accelerated-life tests are often used to avoid lengthy tests or the need to test many units to obtain useful failure data. With accelerated-life tests, the unit is subjected to operating conditions designed to produce a large number of failures in a short period of time. Key to the design of accelerated tests is ensuring that the same failure mechanisms occur under the more stressful conditions as under normal conditions. Then, the only change is that time is effectively accelerated. For example, if corrosion failures occur at typical temperatures and humidities, then the same type of corrosion may happen much more quickly in a humid laboratory oven at elevated temperature.

Accelerated testing requires interpreting failure data obtained under extreme conditions. The problem is analogous to one arising in animal testing for health consequence assessment (see Chap.4). Just as data from animal tests conducted at unrealistically high doses must be translated to the low dose range experienced by people, data from accelerated tests must be translated to predict a unit's performance under normal conditions. Acceleration models (Tobias and Trindade, 1986) are used to translate the results of accelerated performance tests to more realistic, lower-stress conditions of use. Section 2.4.1 describes some of the available acceleration models.

Accident investigation is another release assessment method (Cox and Moller, 1980; Kadlec, 1989). The occurrence of a single major accident, such as the 1984 methyl-isocyanate release in Bhopal, India, or the large industrial fire that same year in Mexico City, does not by itself offer much basis for revising statistical estimates of the probability of similar accidents elsewhere. An investigation into such accidents, however, can provide much useful information for risk assessment. An important element of accident investigation is determining exactly what caused a system to fail. For example, although the cause of death in an automobile accident may have been contact with the steering column, the cause of the accident may have been a high blood-alcohol level coupled with the demand for a quick reaction time at a particularly difficult curve in the road.

The approach in accident investigation is to reconstruct the accident based on postaccident information. In the case of accidents involving automobiles, postaccident information includes the damage to the automobiles, skid marks, damage to other obstacles, and the distances traveled by the automobiles after impact. On the basis of the physical characteristics of the automobiles involved, such as the center of gravity and moment of inertia, the investigator is able to estimate the energy lost due to relative sliding, rotation, and deformation and thus can estimate the speeds and directions of motion when the collision occurred.

To help guide an accident investigation, the investigator often employs a method known as *mental movies* (Brenner, 1980). A mental movie is a reenactment of the accident that is played out in the investigator's mind. Mental movies provide a framework for arranging events into temporal and spatial order and serve as a visual reference in which the continuity of event sequences can be tested. Gaps in the movie indicate unknowns that the investigator needs to resolve to understand or explain the accident.

Other methods used by accident investigators include structuring methods (such as flow charts and logic trees), examination methods (such as chemical and thermal analysis, metallurgical testing, and reconstruction of surviving parts), and simulations (crash simulations, explosive tests, and other reenactments of hypothesized accident scenarios).

2.3.1. Strengths

Performance testing and accident investigation can provide important data about risk sources and release processes that are not readily obtainable from standard monitoring methods. In particular, methods based on the investigation of technologies under unusual conditions, such as those causing failures and accidents, can provide better understanding of the root causes of risks. For example, on November 7, 1940, when the first bridge constructed across the Tacoma Narrows at Puget Sound in Washington State collapsed in a mild gale, it dramatically altered awareness of the risks associated with the unstable oscillation of suspension bridges. Subsequent testing involving physical models provided the basis for the development of improved theory and, ultimately, bridge designs with aerodynamic and mechanical properties that resist undamped oscillations (Farquharson, 1950).

2.3.2. Limitations

A principal limitation of performance testing for release assessment is the difficulty of determining and then simulating the conditions that are of greatest concern in risk assessment. Applicability of the results depends on the assumption that the items or systems being tested and the conditions under which the tests are conducted are relevant to the risk being investigated. In accelerated testing, for example, every step in the sequence of chemical or physical events leading to a failure must occur exactly as at lower stresses. Oftentimes this is difficult to ensure. For example, simulation studies have been used to estimate the error rates of operators of technological systems in crisis situations. The test results, however, may be very different from those actually exhibited under the high levels of stress generated by a genuine crisis.

In the case of accident investigation, a principal difficulty is the episodic nature of accidents, which means that investigators must develop a protocol for their investigation on the spot. Identifying the underlying causes of an accident can be difficult because the evidence required for such inferences is often obscured or obliterated during the accident. Because a "control" system (i.e., an identical system that did not produce an accident) may not exist, it may be impossible to systematically compare situations that did and did not lead to a system failure. Furthermore, it is often hard to conduct the investigation in a timely and orderly way because emergency treatment of the injured must take precedence over risk assessment research.

2.4. STATISTICAL METHODS

Statistical inference provides a means for converting repeated measurements of a risk source, such as measurements obtained from monitoring or performance tests, into a form that is useful for predicting future events. Sometimes, statistical methods and monitoring data are all that is needed for risk assessment. This is the case in situations where exposure and consequence processes are simple, for example, when the risk is an event that produces the same health consequences every time it occurs. The most important example is an accident that produces a fatality. If every time an accident occurs one individual is present and the result of the accident is nearly always death, then it is not necessary to decompose the risk into a source, exposure, and consequence—the frequency of the accident provides a measure of the risk of dying.

A similar situation arises in the case of frequent accidents, such as automobile crashes and fires, for which considerable health-consequence data have accumulated. In such cases, basic injury and fatality data may be analyzed directly to quantify the risk. This type of analysis is often termed *actuarial risk assessment* or *historical risk assessment* (Vesely, 1984). The statistics usually estimated are the fatality rates (frequencies) for different cross sections of the population and for different causes. Actuarial data and other statistical records rarely identify the prerequisite causative factors, but they have the advantage of being relatively reliable, easily understood, and widely accepted.

Usually, the relationship between the risk source and consequences is sufficiently complex that simple statistical analysis alone is insufficient for quantifying risk. Nevertheless, statistical methods may provide a useful means for analyzing the risk source. For example, monitoring data on temperature and pressure or data on the frequency of component failures often can be analyzed statistically to help project both the likelihood that the risk source might release risk agents and the magnitude of such releases.

2.4.1. Statistical Models

The underlying assumption in statistical methods is that a statistical model can be used to describe the outcomes of situations that occur repeatedly in the real world. Such models assume that events occur randomly but that something is known about the mathematical character of the processes that produce the events. Typically, this knowledge suggests a functional form or equation for expressing the model.

Tables 6 and 7 list some of the mathematical models frequently used in statistical methods. Table 6 lists statistical models useful for describing the magnitude of uncertain quantities that can take on an infinite number of possible values, for example, temperature. Table 7 lists statistical models useful for describing discrete events, such as the failure of a component. Sometimes continuous models are useful for describing discrete events, such as a model for describing the time between events. Collectively, the tables include both continuous models (such as the exponential, Weibull, normal, and lognormal distributions) and discrete models (such as the Bernoulli, binomial, negative binomial, geometric, and hypergeometric distributions).

The normal and lognormal distributions are often used to express uncertainties in the magnitudes of uncertain quantities. Both are convenient for mathematical calculations and occur frequently in practice; quantities formed by adding uncertain quantities are often normally distributed, and quantities formed by multiplying uncertain quantities are often lognormally distributed. The normal distribution is useful for quantities that can take on either positive or negative values, for example, errors in measured values. The lognormal distribution is useful for nonnegative quantities that generally have low to moderate values but occasionally can have very high values, such as rainfall, spill quantities, explosion intensities, etc.

The exponential, Poisson, and gamma distributions are all useful for describing events that occur in a purely random fashion, including many types of accidents.

TABLE 6. Some Statistical Models Useful for Describing the Magnitude of Continuous Quantities

Name of Model	Equation	Parameters	Description
Normal or Gaussian	$f(x) = \dfrac{1}{\sigma\sqrt{2\pi}} e^{-\frac{(x-\mu)^2}{2\sigma^2}}$	$\sigma > 0$	A symmetric, bell-shaped probability density function. Useful for variables composed of additive uncertainties.
Lognormal	$f(x) = \dfrac{1}{\phi x\sqrt{2\pi}} e^{-\frac{(\log x - \xi)^2}{2\phi^2}}$	$\phi > 0$ $x > 0$	A probability density function of a variable whose log is normally distributed.
Uniform	$f(x) = \dfrac{1}{b-a}$	$a \le x \le b$	A probability density function for an uncertainty whose range can be identified but for which there is no basis for concluding that any values within the range are more likely than any others.
Triangular	$f(x) = \dfrac{b - |x-a|}{b^2}$	$a - b \le x \le a + b$	A probability density function for an uncertainty when values near the middle of the range are more likely than values near the extreme.
Beta	$f(x) = \dfrac{\Gamma(b)}{\Gamma(a)\Gamma(b-a)} x^{a-1}(1-x)^{b-a-1}$	$a > 0$ $b > a$ $0 \le x \le 1$	A probability density function for a variable confined to a fixed range.

The exponential distribution describes the time between the occurrences, the Poisson distribution gives the number of occurrences in a specified period of time, and the gamma distribution gives the time necessary for a specified number of occurrences. The gamma distribution is similar in shape to the lognormal distribution and is also used for expressing uncertainty over the magnitude of nonnegative uncertain quantities. However, the gamma distribution is less "tail-heavy" in the sense that it generally assigns a lower probability to extreme values than does the lognormal distribution. Another similar distribution that is even less tail-heavy is the Weibull distribution, named after W. Weibull (Weibull, 1951). The Weibull distribution is often used in component failure analysis.

TABLE 7.   Some Statistical Models Useful for Describing Events

Name of model	Equation[a]	Parameters	Description
Exponential	$f(t) = \lambda e^{-\lambda t}$	$\lambda > 0$ $t \geq 0$	Probability density function for the time t between failures, assuming a constant failure rate per unit time.
Poisson	$p(k) = \dfrac{(\lambda t)^k}{k!} e^{-\lambda t}$	$\lambda > 0$ $t \geq 0$	Probability mass function for the number of failures k in time t, assuming mean rate of failure is λ.
Gamma	$f(t) = \dfrac{\lambda^n}{\Gamma(n)} t^{n-1} e^{-\lambda t}$	$n > 0$ $\lambda > 0$ $t \geq 0$	Probability density function for the waiting time t until the nth occurrence of an event, assuming a constant occurrence rate of λ per unit time.
Weibull	$f(t) = \dfrac{m}{t} \left(\dfrac{t}{c}\right)^m e^{-(t/c)^m}$	$m > 0$ $c > 0$ $t \geq 0$	Probability density function for the time t between failures, assuming the failure rate is a polynomial function of time.
Bernoulli	$p(x) = \left\{ \begin{array}{l} 1 - p \text{ if } x = 0; \\ p \text{ if } x = 1 \end{array} \right\}$	$x = 0, 1$ $0 \leq p \leq 1$	Probability mass function of an event that either occurs or does not occur and that does not depend on any other event.
Binomial	$p(k) = \dbinom{n}{k} p^k (1 - p)^{n-k}$	$n = 1, 2, \dots$ $0 \leq p \leq 1$ $k = 0, 1, \dots, n$	Probability mass function for the number of failures k in n trials, assuming the probability of failure in each trial is p.
Negative binomial	$p(m) = \dbinom{-k}{m} p^k [-(1 - p)]^m$	$k > 0$ $0 \leq p \leq 1$ $m = 0, 1, \dots$	Probability mass function for the number of failures m encountered before the kth success, assuming the probability of failure on each trial is p.
Geometric	$p(k) = 1(1 - p)^k$	$0 \leq p \leq 1$ $k = 1, 2, \dots$	Probability mass function for the number of trials required to obtain the first failure, assuming the probability of failure on each trial is p.
Hypergeometric	$p(k) = \dfrac{\dbinom{g}{k}\dbinom{p}{n-k}}{\dbinom{g+b}{n}}$	$n = 1, 2, \dots$ $g = 0, 1, \dots, N$ $b = 0, 1, \dots, N - g$ $k = 0, 1, \dots, n$	Probability mass function for the number of failures k in n trials, assuming the total number of components $N = g + b$ contains g good components and b bad components.

[a]Two special symbols are used to simplify notation: $\Gamma(n)$ is known as the gamma function (also used in Table 6) and $\dbinom{n}{k}$ denotes the number of combinations of n objects taken k at a time. Mathematically:

$$\Gamma(n) = \int_0^\infty t^{n-1} e^{-t} \, dt \text{ for } n > 0 = (n-1)! \text{ if } n \text{ is an integer.} \qquad \binom{n}{k} = \frac{n!}{k!(n-k)!}, \; n! = n(n-1)(n-2)\dots(2)(1).$$

Also useful for describing random events are the Bernoulli and binomial distributions. The Bernoulli distribution gives the outcome of an event that either does or does not occur according to some specified probability. The binomial distribution is useful for determining the probability of a given number of event occurrences. The negative binomial, geometric, and hypergeometric distributions describe related quantities defined according to outcomes of Bernoulli events.

The uniform, triangular, and beta distributions are all useful when the possible values for an uncertainty are restricted within a specified range, for example, the location of a leak along a section of pipe. The uniform distribution is appropriate when all possibilities within the range are equally likely. The triangular distribution is convenient if values near the middle of the range are more likely than values near either extreme. The beta distribution is more complicated mathematically, but extremely flexible in its ability to represent variability over a fixed range.

2.4.2. Estimating the Parameters of Statistical Models

As illustrated by the tables, statistical models involve one or more parameters. Before a statistical model can be applied, numeric values for its parameters must be specified. The "correct" values for the parameters are generally considered to be unknown *a priori* but estimable from empirical data. Typically, the first step is to find a *point estimate*, a single value for each unknown parameter that is in some sense "best." Once point estimates for the model's parameters have been found, the model may be used to provide statistical predictions and forecasts.

For many statistical models, the methods for computing parameter estimates from available data have been established by convention, according to statistical criteria such as minimum mean-squared error, unbiasedness, etc. The method of estimation together with the mathematical form of the underlying model determine the data required. Generally, the simplest statistical models are the least demanding in terms of the types of data required for estimating their parameters.

There are two fundamentally different approaches to estimating the parameters for statistical models: a "classical" approach and a Bayesian approach. (A detailed discussion of the philosophical differences underlying these two approaches appears in Chapter 5.) The major practical distinction between these approaches is that the classical approach requires that parameter estimates be derived solely from available data, while the Bayesian approach requires additional information about likely parameter values that is unrelated to the available data.

With the classical approach, data collection is regarded as a process analogous to random sampling, that is, the data collected are interpreted as a sample of the larger universe of possible observations that could have occurred. The data obtained from the sample are regarded as revealing information about the universe of possibilities. For example, if each observation is a number and the average or mean value of the observations in the sample is calculated, then the sample mean is a statistical estimate of the mean of the universe of possibilities. The unknown "true" mean of the universe of possibilities is often one of the parameters necessary for a statistical model. Thus, the sample data provide a way of obtaining a point estimate of a necessary model parameter.

With the Bayesian approach, the unknown "true" value of each model parameter is regarded as a random variable whose uncertainty is described by a "prior" probability distribution. The *prior probability distribution* is based on an initial state of knowledge. Bayes's theorem specifies how the prior probability distribution should be updated to produce a *"posterior" probability distribution* that accounts for the additional data. If $p(H)$ is the prior probability that hypothesis H is true, $p(D)$ is the probability that datum D will be observed, and $p(D|H)$ is the conditional probability that D will be observed given that H is true, then Bayes's theorem states that the posterior probability that H is true given that D has been observed is:

$$p(H \mid D) = \frac{p(D \mid H)}{p(D)} \times p(H)$$

The probability $p(D|H)$ is often called the "likelihood," since it specifies the likelihood of obtaining the data given the hypothesis. The quantity $p(D)$ can be regarded as merely a normalizing factor, because the posterior probabilities of the alternative hypotheses must sum to unity. Thus, Bayes's theorem states that the posterior probability is proportional to the prior probability and the likelihood of the data. With the Bayesian approach, either the mean or the median of the posterior distribution for the parameter is commonly used as the point estimate. An example of the use of Bayes's theorem in parameter estimation is given in the next section.

2.4.3. Component-Failure and Initiating-Event Models

Two important classes of statistical models are used in release assessment: (1) *component-failure models*, which are designed to estimate the probability that some component or aspect of a system will fail, and (2) *initiating-event models*, which are designed to estimate the frequency of some specific event of interest.

Component-failure models may be subdivided into *failure-on-demand models* and *failure-in-time models*. Failure-on-demand models are used to represent components that are in a dormant state until the moment of need, at which time they are activated (e.g., a pressure-release valve). The simplest failure-on-demand model is the *binomial model*, which assumes that a failure occurs with constant probability p per opportunity, independent of whether or not a failure occurred at any other opportunity. To quantify the binomial model, a point estimate must be provided for the parameter p.

With the classical approach, the point estimate for the failure probability p is the number of failures k that have occurred in the total number of opportunities n. Thus, the empirically measured fraction of times that a failure has occurred, k/n, is the usual classical point estimate for the binomial model. With the Bayesian approach, the parameter p must be assigned a prior distribution. Often, the prior distribution is based on "generic data," failure data that is nonspecific to any particular plant or application.

An example of each approach is provided by Apostolakis (1981). Suppose that a diesel generator used in the safety system of a new plant is tested, and it is found that the generator failed to start in 5 of 227 tests. Assuming that there are no trends in the data (for example, an initial 222 successes followed by 5 failures), a binomial failure model might be a reasonable basis for estimating the probability of future failures. A classical point estimate for the failure probability would be 5/227, or about 0.022. Thus, based on the classical approach and assuming that the propensity for a failure in future attempts to start the generator will be identical to historical attempts, 0.022 is the estimated probability that the generator will fail to start the next time an attempt is made to start it.

With the Bayesian approach, the necessary prior probability distribution can be chosen to be the frequency distribution of failure rates reported in the literature for diesel generators from various manufacturers and under various operating and maintenance conditions: a distribution that is well approximated by a lognormal

TABLE 8. An Application of Bayes Theorem: Diesel Generator Failure to Start[a]

Failure Rate (hypothesis)	Prior probability	Likelihood	(Prior probability) × (likelihood)	Posterior probability
0.0087	0.0500	0.0343	0.0017	0.0206
0.0115	0.0587	0.0750	0.0044	0.0529
0.0154	0.0967	0.1320	0.0128	0.1535
0.0205	0.1350	0.1734	0.0234	0.2815
0.0274	0.1596	0.1544	0.0246	0.2963
0.0365	0.1596	0.0820	0.0131	0.1572
0.0487	0.1350	0.0218	0.0029	0.0353
0.0649	0.0967	0.0023	0.0002	0.0027
0.0866	0.0587	0.0001	0.0000	0.0000
0.1155	0.0500	0.0000	0.0000	0.0000
	1.0000		0.0831	1.0000

[a] Apostolakis (1981).

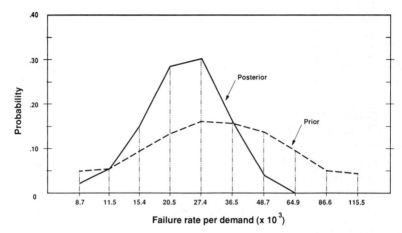

FIGURE 13.   Prior and posterior probability histograms for diesel-generator failure to start (Apostolakis, 1981).

distribution. The mean of this distribution is 0.04. To obtain the posterior distribution, the prior distribution can be discretized and Bayes's theorem applied, as shown in Table 8. The first column shows the discrete failure rates selected, which serve as alternative hypotheses for Bayes's theorem. The second column shows the prior probabilities of each failure rate, as determined by the lognormal distribution. The third column shows the likelihoods (conditional probabilities of obtaining the data), which are derived from a binomial distribution (Table 7) with the number of failures k equal to 5 and the number of trials n equal to 227. The fourth column is just the product of the prior probabilities and the likelihoods, and the last column shows the posterior probabilities obtained by dividing the entries in the fourth column by 0.0831, which normalizes the posterior probabilities so that they sum to unity.

Figure 13 illustrates the results of the Bayesian approach. As shown by the posterior curve, the effect of the plant-specific data is to shift the distribution of the failure rates toward lower values and to reduce its dispersion. The mean of the posterior distribution is 0.025. Thus, based on the Bayesian approach and using the mean of the posterior distribution as a point estimate, 0.025 is the estimated probability that the generator will fail to start the next time an attempt is made to start it.

Even if no generic data are available for deriving a prior distribution, the Bayesian approach may still be used. In the absence of statistical data, a prior distribution can be generated subjectively using engineering judgment and formal probability encoding methods (see Chapter 5). Another approach is to use a "noninformative prior," that is, a prior distribution selected to minimize the effect of the prior on the posterior distribution.

The method of analyzing failure-in-time models is very similar to that of failure-on-demand models. The failure rate is defined as the probability that the component will fail per unit time given that it has not yet failed. In general, the failure rate is a function of time, but the simplest failure-in-time model assumes the failure rate is constant. With this assumption, the exponential model gives the distribution of time between failures, and the gamma model gives the distribution of time required for any specified number of independent failures to occur.

To quantify the exponential or gamma failure models, the failure rate λ must be specified. With the classical approach, a point estimate for λ may be obtained by dividing the total number of failures f by the total time of observation T (i.e., f/T). If failure rates cannot be assumed to be constant, more complicated models may be used. For example, the Weibull model gives the distribution of time between independent events occurring at a rate that varies with time.

Initiating-event models are generally applied to represent events that initiate other events or processes that may ultimately lead to the release of a risk agent. Usually, initiating events are assumed to occur randomly in time at a constant rate. Under such assumptions, the appropriate model is the Poisson model, which gives the probability distribution for the number of initiating events occurring over a specified interval of time. Similar to the exponential and gamma models, the Poisson model requires an estimate of the occurrence rate to quantify its parameter.

2.4.4. Models for Events of Varying Magnitude

To represent events of varying magnitudes (e.g., events producing different magnitudes of releases of risk agents), various named probability distributions such as those summarized in Table 6 often serve as statistical models. In such cases, empirical data are typically used to estimate values for the parameters of the distribution—the parameter values are selected to fit the distribution to empirical data. The distribution describes uncertainty over the magnitude of the event, but not uncertainty over whether or when the event might happen. To describe both uncertainties, one of the event models in Table 7 may be selected and its parameter values estimated as a function of event magnitude, thereby creating an estimate of the frequency of all events producing a given magnitude of release. By choosing successively larger release magnitudes and calculating frequencies of events producing releases greater than these values, a plot of frequency versus release magnitude can be obtained. Often constructed in engineering risk assessments, this type of curve is called a *complementary cumulative distribution* or *risk profile.* (see Chapter 5 for additional discussion of this and other means for displaying risk estimates.)

Various other statistical models are available for representing and evaluating situations in which data are available for the quantity in question and for a number of related variables. In *regression analysis*, for example, models are constructed for forecasting one or more dependent variables based on measurements of one or more independent variables. In the simplest case, the statistical model assumes that the dependent variable y is proportional to one or more independent variables x plus a random error term u that averages to zero. The form of the model is $y = ax + b + u$. Classical and Bayesian methods exist for estimating the coefficients a and b of the linear regression equation from corresponding measurements for the independent and dependent variables. These estimates, $\hat{a}$ and $\hat{b}$, are then used with the equation to provide forecasts y_t given a new set of values, x_t, for x; i.e., $y_t = \hat{a}x_t + \hat{b}$.

Nonlinear regression equations may be used if the dependent variable is not linearly related to the independent variables. The potential for a risk source to release risk agents is often a nonlinear function of some risk-source characteristic. For example, Lindow *et al.* (1988) used nonlinear regression analysis to develop a statistical model for representing the quantity of bacterial pesticide spray released from a nozzle. The form of the equation is $n = ae^{-bd}$, where n is the number of cells deposited per square centimeter, d is the distance in meters, and a and b are the parameters. When the model was fit to data obtained from testing, values of a between 0.3 and 0.45 and values of b between 17.4 and 29.2 were found to provide the best fit.

A common complication for statistical methods occurs when the available data are for events with certain characteristics but the events of concern have other characteristics. Sometimes the data involve conditions that are more extreme than typical, as in failure data obtained from accelerated tests. Other times, the data represent typical conditions but the risk of concern relates to events under extreme conditions. For example, the concern may be the frequencies of extremely high wind velocities, but the bulk of monitoring data may be for winds of lower velocities. *Extrapolation methods* (sometimes called *distribution techniques*) use statistical models to bridge the gap between the conditions of interest and those related to the data. The standard statistical models, including the exponential, Weibull, and lognormal models, are often used for this purpose. Other statistical models have been devised for specialized applications. For example, the *Arrhenius model* is an acceleration model often used to translate thermal stress data obtained from accelerated testing at high temperatures (Tobias and Trindade, 1986). Extrapolation methods assume that events occur under typical and extreme conditions according to the same physical mechanisms and processes.

Extreme value theory (Gumbel, 1957; Vesely, 1984) is sometimes applied if the maximum (or minimum) states of a large number of processes are involved in producing the risk and if dependency among the processes is not strong. Extreme value theory has been used to predict frequencies of catastrophic floods, and similar methods have been used to predict maximum fire, tornado, and hurricane characteristics that might occur in given time periods. The basic estimation process involves a model obtained by fitting a frequency-versus-magnitude curve to past data. As with other statistical methods, the model is specified except for one or more unknown parameters. Based on past events with measured characteristics, the parameters are estimated and the resulting specified function is used to predict the frequencies of events with more extreme characteristics. As an example of the method, empirical data suggest that the quantity of hazardous material R released in an industrial accident is related to the frequency f of the accident according to an equation of the form $\log R = a \log f + b$ (Withers, 1988). The parameters a and b may be obtained from data emphasizing high-frequency, low-release accidents. Withers used the approach and data from three chemical plants to obtain values for a and b for the hazardous chemicals propylene, chlorine, and ammonia.

2.4.5. Hypothesis Testing

As noted earlier, statistical methods play an important role in the design of sampling and testing strategies for monitoring and performance testing. *Hypothesis testing* is one such method used for this purpose (e.g., see EPA, 1988a; EPA, 1989b). A typical hypothesis test compares two competing claims, a *null hypothesis* and an *alternative hypothesis*. For example, in the context of monitoring for release assessment at hazardous waste sites, the null hypothesis might be that on-site concentrations are not statistically different from background levels, suggesting that no release has occurred. The alternative hypothesis might be that on-site concentrations are statistically higher than background levels, suggesting that a release has occurred.

There are two types of errors that can result from hypothesis tests. A *Type I error* occurs if the null hypothesis is rejected when it is true (e.g., concluding that contaminant concentrations on-site are higher than background levels when in fact they are not). A *Type II error* occurs if the null hypothesis is not rejected when it is false (e.g., concluding that contaminant concentrations are not higher than background levels when in fact they are). A good sampling strategy is one that will produce an acceptably low probability of Type I error, denoted α, and an acceptably low probability of Type II error, denoted β. The impact of sampling strategy on both α and β must be considered jointly because the consequences of the two types of errors may be very different. In the example, a Type I error could lead to unnecessary and costly remediation efforts, while a Type II error could result in failure to identify and address a real problem.

To facilitate the design of sampling strategies, the concepts of *significance level* and *power* are used. A sampling strategy is said to have a level of significance α (e.g., $\alpha = .05$) if the probability of Type I error is, at most, α. The power of a sampling strategy is defined as the probability of rejecting the null hypothesis, which equals α if the null hypothesis is true and $1 - \beta$ otherwise. Thus, a sampling strategy for the example with a statistical significance of .05 and a power of .90 would have a 5 percent chance of concluding that on-site concentrations are above background levels when they are not, and a 90 percent chance of concluding that concentrations are above background levels when they in fact are. Power curves, published in textbooks on applied probability, give the probability of rejecting the null hypothesis as a function of the number of samples, α, and the parameters of the underlying statistical model.

Any of the simple statistical models for component failure, initiating events, and events of varying magnitude can be used as the basis for developing a sampling design for hypothesis testing. Once a model is selected, the test hypotheses must be defined in terms of the parameters of the statistical model. For example, a sampling strategy for comparing on-site measurements with background levels might assume that on-site measurements follow one of the named probability distributions (e.g., lognormal model). The null hypothesis might then be that the mean of the sampled distribution equals average background. The alternative hypothesis would be that the mean of the distribution sampled is greater than average background levels. This is termed a *one-sided test* because the alternative hypothesis is defined as all values that lie on one side of a specified value. In the case of failure testing, the binomial model is often used. For example, the null hypothesis might be that the probability of failure is equal to some value, and the alternative hypothesis might be that the probability of failure is less than or greater than that value—this is an example of a *two-sided test*. Common one- and two-sided hypothesis tests are defined both for the case of sampling from one population (e.g., on-site measurements only) and from two populations (e.g., sampling both on-site and off-site).

Specifying the sampling strategy involves specifying acceptable probabilities of Type I and Type II errors, the number of tests N in the sample, and the rule or criteria for deciding between the two hypotheses. For example, if the alternative hypothesis is that the mean of the population is greater than some specified amount, μ_0, the rule would be to accept the hypothesis if the sample mean is at least an amount δ above μ_0 (i.e., $\mu_0 + \delta$). For a fixed sample size N, larger values of δ lead to smaller probabilities of Type I error (α) and larger probabilities of Type II error (β), as might be expected. Formulas, tables, nomographs, and computer programs are available for computing the appropriate δ, or other decision rule, that leads to a given level of significance for a specified sample size N. Power curves then provide a useful visual aid that fully summarizes the characteristics of the sampling strategy.

2.4.6. Selection and Interpretation of Statistical Models

Selection of the underlying statistical model is crucial to the application of any statistical method. In some cases, such as component-failure and time-to-failure models, the models have become quite standardized. Even in these circumstances, however, it is essential to verify the appropriateness of the model that underlies a selected statistical method. For example, if components are wearing out or otherwise degrading with time, then the various failure models that assume a constant failure rate may be inappropriate, including the exponential, Poisson, and gamma models. Important considerations for choosing a model include physical and engineering justifications and the nature of the available data. Statistical methods of significance testing can be used to investigate the reasonableness of the statistical models. Hypothesis testing methods may be used to support the selection of a statistical model. Despite the many methods available for aiding the model selection process, the choice ultimately reduces to making a judgment.

The role of judgment in selecting a statistical model is illustrated by the methods that have been proposed to account for plant-to-plant variations in observed failure data. As monitoring activities have collected data on the operating characteristics of similar systems and components installed at different plants, it has become apparent that component and system failure probabilities vary from plant to plant (e.g., due to the use of different designs or maintenance practices). For this reason, it would be incorrect to simply pool the data to compute some presumed underlying "true" parameter value for use in estimating the probability of failures at a new plant. Instead, one must develop a statistical model that takes into account the similarities and differences between the plants for which data are available and the plant that is of interest. Shultis *et al.* (1981), for example, assume that the failure rates for similar components at various plants represent a random sample from a beta distribution. Easterling *et al.*(1985) similarly model the failure probabilities from plants as outcomes from some probability distribution, but make no *a priori* assumption for the form of that distribution. Instead, they use estimates of the distribution's mean and variance to construct intervals within which failure rates are predicted to fall. The creative, if somewhat ad hoc, nature of the approaches used in these examples illustrates that use of statistical techniques seldom eliminates the need for the analyst to make judgments that potentially affect conclusions.

Once an appropriate statistical model has been developed, care must be taken in interpreting the estimates provided by that model. Statistical estimates are, in general, subject to four sources of potential error. First, the random nature of statistical models almost guarantees that the best forecast from the model will not exactly match actual future outcomes. This randomness is represented in a regression analysis, for example, by the u term in the regression equation. Second, the process of estimating the parameters of the statistical model (e.g., the p in the binomial model; a and b in the simple regression model) introduces errors because the estimated values will not exactly equal "true" values. Third, additional errors are introduced to the extent that the data contain measurement errors. For example, if values for the independent variable x in a simple regression analysis contain measurement errors, additional error is introduced into the regression forecasts. Fourth, errors are introduced to the extent that the statistical model is an oversimplified or incorrect representation of reality. Straightforward formulas exist for quantifying all but the last of these four sources of errors.

Of the sources of error mentioned above, error in the estimation of model parameters is affected most significantly by the quantity of data available. Thus, for example, the observation that exactly 100 failures occurred in 1 million hours of operating experience would provide a more reliable basis for estimating the failure-rate parameter for an exponential model (and, in turn, a more reliable statistical estimate for the probability distribution for the time between failures) than would the observation of 1 failure in 10,000 hours.

The most common method by which the accuracy of statistical estimates may be conveyed is through *confidence intervals*. The exact meaning of and methods for computing confidence intervals depend on whether the classical or Bayesian approach to parameter estimation is used (and whether the analyst adopts a classical or judgmental interpretation of probability) (see Chapter 5). Interpretation of a confidence interval is relatively easy with the Bayesian approach. A confidence interval is established by specifying upper and lower limits for the unknown parameter. The confidence level corresponding to these limits is just the fraction of the probability distribution that lies between these two limits. Thus, a 90 percent confidence limit for a failure rate consists of an upper limit, p_U, and a lower limit, p_L, such that the probability is .9 that the true value lies within these bounds.

With the classical approach to parameter estimation confidence intervals are closely related to the concept of *standard errors*. The key to understanding standard errors and classical confidence intervals is the recognition that if the process of collecting the data for a statistical analysis were repeated over and over, random variations in the data would cause the computed parameter estimates to vary. The amount of this variability could be quantified by calculating a statistical variance, that is, by computing the sum of the squares of the deviations of the estimates from their mean value. The larger the variance, the less reliable the point estimate. Although the variance associated with a statistical estimate cannot be known without repeating the data collection process, this variance can be estimated from the form of the statistical model and the original data. The square root of this estimated variance is termed the *standard error of estimate*, and straightforward formulas and tables exist for standard errors for all of the models mentioned above and for many other statistical models.

Standard errors may be used to construct confidence limits of any specified confidence level. For example, the point estimate for the failure rate plus or minus two standard errors provides an approximate 95 percent confidence interval for the true failure rate. In the classical interpretation, the confidence interval and level imply a statement about the different confidence intervals that would be generated if data gathering and analysis were repeated, that is, the confidence level (e.g., 95 percent) approximates the percent of times that the computed confidence interval would include the true value of the quantity. In other words, a classical confidence interval cannot be interpreted as the probability that the true parameter value lies within the indicated interval, but only as the probability that repeated data collection efforts would yield confidence intervals that bracket the true values.

Another way of interpreting a classical confidence interval is as a range of parameter values that are consonant with the data to some specified degree. For example, for a failure probability p, an upper 95 percent confidence limit (denoted p_{U95}) specifies that for values greater than p_{U95}, the observed data are in the extreme upper 5 percent of possible outcomes. Thus, for values greater than p_{U95}, the chance of observing data this "good" (the observed number of failures or less) is 5 percent or less. Similarly, the lower statistical confidence limit on p (denoted p_{L95}) is such that for values less than p_{L95}, the observed data are in the extreme lower 5 percent of possible outcomes. The interval between the lower and upper 95 percent statistical confidence limits is a 90 percent confidence interval.

The same statistical methods used for release assessment are often applicable for exposure and consequence assessment as well. Many issues surrounding the use of statistical methods are independent of whether the methods are being applied to release assessment or to some other component of the risk assessment process. Additional discussion of statistical methods appears in Chapter 5.

2.4.7. Strengths

In situations for which a great amount of data has been collected, such as automobile accidents and fires, statistical methods can be an extremely effective way of quantifying uncertainty about a risk source. Applications of statistical methods do not require models based on engineering or cause–effect knowledge; instead, parameter estimates are based on relatively simple statistical models and the historical patterns of repeated measurements. Measurements, such as those obtained through monitoring or performance testing, can provide the relative frequencies with which a system or its components were in various states; for example, the percentage of time that a valve was open when it should have been closed and closed when it should have been open. Estimates of probabilities of future behavior can be inferred from this data, together with error measures that account for potential inaccuracies attributable to limits in the quantity of data. Although release assessment results generally depend strongly on the underlying statistical model that is assumed, sensitivity analysis can be used to compare the results of different models, which can indicate the robustness of the results to changes in model assumptions.

2.4.8. Limitations

The principal limitation on the use of statistical methods for release assessment is the lack of an adequate data base. For many risk sources, the available data are insufficient to permit estimating reliably the frequencies of releases of risk agents or of other characteristics of concern. For example, the data base supporting the transportation of hazardous wastes is particularly poor. Records of hazardous material shipments are often not kept or are not accessible. Thus, estimates are often based on samples of shipment data that are of uncertain accuracy and validity and subject to considerable judgmental interpretation.

For rare accidents, adequate data for meaningful statistical inference simply may not exist. For example, rupture of the container on a liquified natural gas (LNG) tanker is a serious concern for which there are very few statistical data. In such cases, surrogate data bases must be used, for example, oil tanker container ruptures as a surrogate for LNG tanker container ruptures (Philipson and Gasca, 1982). The problem with using surrogate data is that the data may not reflect important differences between the surrogate and the actual risk sources. For example, suppose the concern is the frequency of collisions of LNG tankers serious enough to rupture cargo tanks. If surrogate data on the frequency of oil tanker accidents were used, an important difference in the hull construction of LNG ships would be ignored (Rasmussen, 1981). Unlike an oil tanker, an LNG tanker has a special triple-hull construction with insulation between two of the hulls to provide thermal isolation. Thus, use of surrogate data would introduce serious errors into the risk assessment.

Even in the case of "insurable risks," where the data are copious and highly accurate, application of statistical methods can be problematic. Estimating the probability that a particular driver will be in an accident or that a particular homeowner will experience a fire requires that the entity be catalogued as belonging to some representative group. This group defines the "universe" for the statistical model. The specification of this group represents a judgment that may be highly subjective. Also, events usually triggered by independent mechanisms may occasionally result from underlying causes that contaminate the data with unwanted dependencies. Examples would include an increase in accidents associated with the distractions caused by the increasing use of audiotape players in automobiles or a spate of fires due to arson.

When statistical methods are applied to reliability analysis, cost restrictions may prevent performance testing from generating sufficient data to use the more general failure models that are most demanding in their data needs. For example, components such as pipes and boilers may have an uncertain life that depends on stress, but cost and time constraints may prevent testing components of all possible ages and at all levels of stress. Thus, a simpler failure model that is less demanding of data may be postulated, and the results of more limited performance testing may be used to make inferences about the numerical values of the model's parameters.

Assuming that the model is accepted and assuming that repetitive items being tested are independent (i.e., that there are no common-mode, causal, failure mechanisms) and identically distributed, then classical probability statements can be made about failure rates at different stress levels. However, if the components under consideration will be used at extreme stress levels where the model has not been calibrated, then probabilistic assessments based on the model may be misleading (Raiffa and Zeckhauser, 1981).

The use of aggregated data can often introduce errors and bias into statistical estimates. For example, a regression analysis might relate the average values of variables (i.e., averaged over time or category) rather than individual measurements. Such aggregations lead to an underestimation of forecasting error because they produce an artificial reduction in the random component of forecasts. Furthermore, as shown by Theil (1971), aggregations generally lead to a bias in forecast values. Theil has shown that the only condition under which the coefficients produced using aggregate data will not be biased by aggregation is when the underlying coefficients for the unaggregated data are all equal.

Another limitation of statistical methods is that the assumptions implicit in the underlying models or their methods of application may involve approximations that introduce subtle errors into the computed results. For example, component-failure models that assume constant failure rates ignore gradual deterioration of the component or possible improvement due to plant modifications, improved maintenance practice, and greater operating experience. Another example is the linear approximation to the exponential distribution. With the exponential model, the probability that a failure will occur by time t is given by $e^{-\lambda t}$, where λ is the failure rate. Since λ is usually very small, this is typically approximated by λt. Unfortunately, the requirement that λ be small (less than $\sim .1$) is sometimes forgotten.

Another example is the lognormal distribution customarily used to represent uncertainty in failure rates in the Bayesian approach to reliability estimation. The example in Section 2.4.3 provided an illustration. The lognormal distribution is convenient mathematically; but, regardless of how its parameters are set, it has a "tail" that indicates finite probability of an actual failure rate that is greater than unity. In most applications, this aberration does not significantly distort the results of statistical analyses. As noted by Apostolakis and Kaplan (1981), however, in some situations serious errors can be introduced. These authors cite a case wherein a component has a failure rate that is assumed to be lognormally distributed and calculate the probability that the system containing the component will fail within a 24-hour period, assuming various levels of redundancy in the component. They find that the computed result is overestimated when the linear approximation is used with the error increasing as the degree of redundancy increases. At triple redundancy, the probability of system failure in their example is about 1.5 in

10,000. However, the result computed using the linear approximation with the lognormal distribution is more than a factor of 4 higher; 7 in 10,000.

2.5. MODELING METHODS FOR RELEASE ASSESSMENT

Although even the simplest statistical methods for characterizing a source of risk are technically "models," many risk-source models are considerably more sophisticated. This is especially the case in risk assessments where the risk is derived from a complex but reasonably well-understood man-made or natural system. In particular, complex models are often required for performing release assessment of continuous risks and for representing the continuous elements of a discrete risk. Such models estimate the characteristics, amounts, and locations at which some risk agent is emitted into the environment and how these might change over time and location or with various controls.

Release assessment models separate the risk source from the rest of the environment by establishing various spatial, temporal, and other conceptual boundaries. The risk source, as defined by these boundaries, is then broken down into a set of individual elements, each of which is then analyzed separately. These elements are often associated with the various subsystems or processes within the risk source that exchange energy, materials, or activities. Submodels are then constructed for each element, with the inputs and outputs of these submodels representing the energies, materials, or activities that are exchanged. If more than one element contributes the risk agent, then like quantities are summed to obtain aggregate estimates of the total releases.

A key decision for the design of a release model is the logic or theory assumed to govern the behavior of the various elements that make up the model. The choice often depends on the alternatives that are being considered for reducing releases. For example, suppose a release model is needed to support a regional risk assessment of alternative strategies for reducing sulfur oxides emissions from coal-fired electric power plants. If the control strategy involves regulations requiring plants to install emissions control technologies, then the release model must account for the effectiveness of the available technologies. Engineering and process models might be developed to estimate the releases that would occur from various representative types of plants equipped with the available emission-control technologies. If, on the other hand, the control strategy involves increased taxation of high-sulfur coal, the approach might be to construct an *econometric model* (a model based on economic and empirical data) that would predict the effect of increased prices of high-sulfur coal on sulfur emissions by estimating the extent to which the energy industry would shift to using oil and other low-sulfur energy fuels (e.g., by comparing supply, demand, and price with interfuel competition).

Empirical data often play an important role in the specification of a release model. As an example, data from performance-testing the crashworthiness of automobiles have been used to construct simulation models involving lumped mass and nonlinear resistance assumptions. These models have then been used to predict the response of a vehicle body structure and the motion of occupants in various specified crash situations (King and Mertz, 1973; Kurimoto, Nakaya *et al.*, 1981).

In many applications where time and effort are limited, or where there are insufficient data and understanding to justify detailed models, only the grossest details of the risk source are represented. A general feature of such simplified models is the use of proxy variables. In the absence of mechanistic detail, relationships may be based on plausible associations rather than formal theory and detailed cause–effect logic. For example, to estimate the probability of failure of a crucial aircraft part, the failure probability might be related to the flying time of the aircraft. In effect, the submodel uses flying time as a proxy variable for the complicated stress, temperature, corrosion, and maintenance history of that part. Justification for the use of simple models based on proxy variables is found in the degree of agreement often obtained between the predictions derived from such models and reality. Practical reasons are also important, such as the impossibility of using any alternative mechanistic model if there are only limited data available either for testing the validity of the model or for extrapolating to new circumstances.

2.5.1. Failure-Mode and Effects Analysis (FMEA) and Related Methods

For discrete risks such as accidents, models of the risk source provide a means for estimating the probability and characteristics of failures of systems even if there have been no actual experiences of failure. Such methods are generally based on a specification of the circumstances and sequence of events that must occur for the accident to take place. Many of the methods used for this purpose are largely qualitative in nature but contain some quantitative components. Examples are failure mode and effects analysis (FMEA), preliminary hazards analysis (PHA), fault hazard analysis (FHA), hazards and operability analysis (HAZOP), and criticality analysis (CA). (For detailed descriptions, see Green and Bourne, 1972; McCormick, 1981; AIChE/CCPS, 1985; and Henley and Kumamoto, 1991). These and similar methods used to develop a model of a risk source typically consist of reliability and functional diagrams that show how the system functions and coding schemes that reference the various system components and elements of the analysis to the accompanying diagrams. For example, Fig. 14 shows a diagram of a facility for loading a rail tank car with liquid chlorine. Table 9 shows a partial listing of possible incidents that could potentially produce a release, such as might be produced by a hazards and operability analysis.

To provide an example of how such methods may be used in conjunction with one another to produce a quantitative characterization of a risk source, consider

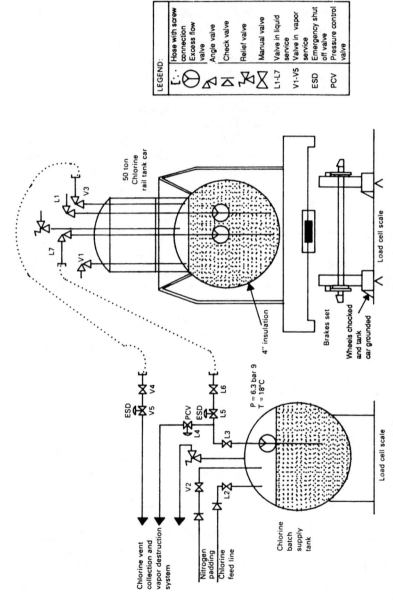

FIGURE 14. Diagram of a liquid chlorine rail tank car loading installation (AIChE/CCPS, 1989).

TABLE 9. Outputs from a HAZOP Review of a Chlorine Rail Car Loading Facility[a]

Deviation	Possible causes	Consequences	Action required
No flow	Manual valves shut ESD valve shut Hose blocked Pipe blocked	Operational delay	Confirm operating instructions suitable for safe corrections of all no-flow cases
High flow	Flange leak	Toxic hazard	1. Minimize flange connections 2. Check suitability of gasket specification 3. Ensure ESD activation point is at convenient location; consider two actuation points 4. Check location of breathing apparatus
	Valve leak	Toxic hazard	Similar to flange leak
	Pipe leak due to impact	Toxic hazard	Minimize activities near chlorine line
	Relief valve malfunction on rail car	Toxic hazard	Inspect relief valve before loading Hazard analysis required
	Hose leak	Toxic hazard	Develop preventive maintenance program for hoses
High level	Weigh scale error	Chlorine passes through relief valve—toxic hazard	Unlikely, existing design and weigh scale system considered adequate
High temperature	External fire from neighboring: 1. Rail line handling flammable material 2. Elevated pipeline with flammable material	1. Relief valve lifts—passes large vapor flow 2. Shell failure cata-strophic rupture—toxic hazard	Hazard analysis required. Fire protection facilities adequate, approximately 60 minutes to control pool fire. Catastrophic rupture unlikely before fire brought under control.
High pressure	Nitrogen supply overpressure	Relief valve lifts and emergency vent—toxic hazard	No action required; pressure control system on nitrogen supply and PCV to emergency vent adequate
Other: Corrosion	Internal corrosion of tanks or pipe fittings	Liquid or vapor leak; toxic hazard	Periodic internal inspections (1–5 year intervals) should detect any incipient corrosion

[a]Derived from AIChE/CCPS (1989).

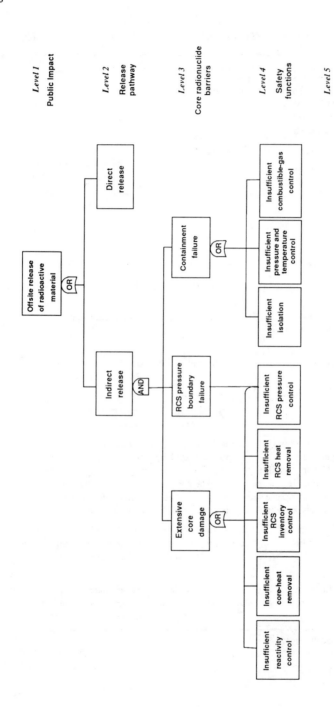

FIGURE 15. Master logic for a fault-tree diagram of a nuclear reactor (derived from NRC, 1983).

the combined use FMEA, FHA, and CA (Hollenback, 1977). FMEA studies a system or subsystem to determine what failures of which components will result in what effect. An FHA studies a system or a subsystem to determine the impact of its failure on other portions of the system or subsystem and to classify quantitatively hazards. A CA studies a system or subsystem to determine the relative magnitude of each potential failure, based on its failure rate and effect on the system or subsystem.

These three methods might be used as follows to characterize chemical releases originating from a planned chlorine rail tank car loading facility (Fig. 14). The FMEA would be applied to determine what would happen during and after the failure of various facility components, such as flow and pressure deviations, temperature changes, pinhole leaks, and spontaneous catastrophic tank rupture. The FHA would be applied concurrently with the FMEA to quantify the damage to other parts and equipment including, perhaps, injuries to personnel. On completion of the FMEA and FHA, critical failure modes would be defined in the CA by assigning criticality numbers representing the relative probability that the failure mode being considered will cause the end consequence of concern (e.g., a toxic cloud blowing downwind). The criticality number is computed from the conditional probability of the end consequence, the probability of the initiating event, and the portion of the system operating cycle during which the equipment associated with the initiating failure event operates. The resulting criticality numbers would be ranked to clarify which components' parts or assemblies are likely to cause the most problems and where additional design work may be needed most.

2.5.2. Fault-Tree Analysis, Event-Tree Analysis, and Related Methods

Fault-tree analysis and *event-tree analysis* are the methods most frequently used for creating models of sources of discrete risks. Fault-tree analysis is based on a specialized model that may be represented as a diagram of binary (yes-no) logic that traces backward in time the different ways that a particular event could occur. Figure 15 illustrates the structure of a fault-tree diagram. Fault-tree analysis (Gottfried, 1974; Fussel, 1980, 1981; Fussell and Burdick, 1977; Vesely *et al.*, 1981) is applicable when the risk source is made up of many parts and the failure rates for the parts may be estimated. For example, fault-tree analysis is well-suited for estimating the probability that the electromechanical safety system in a nuclear power plant might fail, but poorly suited for estimating the failure rate for a steel pressure vessel.

The first step in constructing a fault tree is to define the final failure event whose probability must be quantified, for example, off-site release of radioactive material from a nuclear reactor. Using a functional description of the reactor system, one identifies the events that could logically cause the failure. For example, off-site releases can be caused either directly, by the deliberate venting of radioactive

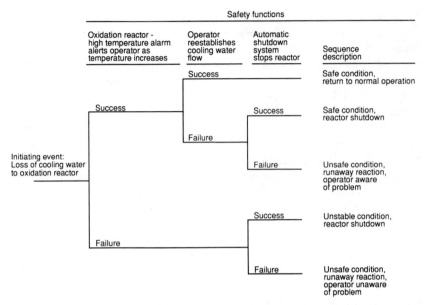

FIGURE 16.   A simplified event tree for assessing the consequences of loss of coolant to a nuclear reactor (adapted from AIChE/CCPS, 1985).

contaminated material, or indirectly, through system failures. This relationship is shown in Fig. 15 by connecting these two release pathways to the final or top-level event through an *OR gate*. The OR gate indicates that either one or the other of these events will produce the top event. If the probabilities of direct and indirect releases are small and independent of one another, then the total probability of release will be the sum of the probability of direct release and the probability of indirect release. Similarly, the Level 2 events are related to lower-level events, and the diagram may be expanded until a level of basic or "primary" events is reached, for example, the failure of individual components such as pressure relief systems, pumps, and electrical components. Failure rates for the basic events are either assumed to be known with certainty or are assumed to be described by probability distributions derived from statistical analysis of component failure data. The probability distribution for the failure rate for the top-level event is then derived from a calculation based on the equivalence between the fault-tree diagram and a corresponding set of Boolean algebraic expressions for the manipulation of probabilities.

Event trees (e.g., see Rasmussen, 1975; McCormick, 1981) are also graphic tree structures. An event tree starts with a particular undesired initiating event, such as the failure of a coolant pump in a nuclear reactor, and projects all possible plant

TABLE 10. Questions Posed by an Event Tree for a Nuclear Power Plant[a]

1. Is AC power available after the initiating event?

2. Does emergency core cooling fail prior to overpressurization of containment?

3. Where is the initial reactor coolant system break?

4. What is the size of the initial reactor coolant system break?

5. Are the steam generators wet or dry?

6. Do the fan coolers fail to actuate before core degradation?

7. Do the containment sprays fail to actuate in the injection mode before core degradation?

8. Do the containment sprays fail to actuate in the recirculation mode before core degradation?

9. Where, if at all, is there a temperature-induced failure of the reactor coolant system during the period of core degradation?

10. What is the size of the temperature-induced reactor coolant system failure?

11. What is the primary system pressure during core degradation? Also, what would be the containment pressure increment from a primary system blowdown?

12. At what level, if any, is containment bypassed during core degradation?

13. What is the rate of blowdown to containment during core degradation?

14. Do the containment sprays fail to actuate during the period of core degradation?

15. Is there containment heat removal during core degradation?

16. At what level, if any, does containment fail due to steam pressurization before vessel breach?

17. What is the containment pressure before vessel breach?

18. Is there a hydrogen burn before vessel breach? Also, what is the pressure increment from such a burn?

19. Does containment fail because of a hydrogen burn before vessel breach?

20. Do the fan coolers fail after the early hydrogen burn?

21. Do the containment sprays fail after the early hydrogen burn?

22. Is there containment heat removal after the early hydrogen burn?

23. What is the mode of vessel breach?

24. Does direct heating of the containment atmosphere occur just after vessel breach? Also, what is the pressure increment from a steam spike alone and from a steam spike plus direct heating?

25. Is there a hydrogen burn just after vessel breach? Also, what is the pressure increment from such a burn?

(continued)

TABLE 10. (*Continued*)

26. Does containment fail due to a steam spike, direct heating, and/or hydrogen burn just after vessel breach?

27. Do the fan coolers fail after vessel breach?

28. Do the containment sprays fail after vessel breach?

29. Is there an oxidation release?

30. Is ac power restored after vessel breach?

31. Do the fan coolers fail late in the accident?

32. Do the containment sprays fail late in the accident?

33. Is there containment heat removal late in the accident?

34. Has the inventory of the refueling water storage tank been injected into containment?

35. What is the amount of water injected into containment?

36. Do significant core-concrete interactions occur after vessel breach?

37. Is ac power recovered late in the accident?

38. What is the containment pressure late in the accident?

39. Does a later hydrogen burn occur?

40. What pressure rise would occur if combustible gases were to burn late in the accident?

41. Would containment fail due to a late hydrogen burn or steam production?

42. In what way, if at all, does containment fail due to gradual pressurization from boil-off of water or noncondensible gases or hydrogen burning?

43. Do the fan coolers fail after the late hydrogen burn?

44. Do the containment sprays fail after the late hydrogen burn?

45. Is there containment heat removal very late in the accident?

46. Does basemat melt-through occur, given no prior containment failure?

47. Does containment depressurize after basemat melt-through?

48. What is the ultimate containment failure mode, if any, resulting from core-concrete interactions?

---

[a]Adapted from NRC, 1987a.

responses to that event. Each branch in an event tree represents a possible state (often simply success or failure) for the plant's subsystems that would be called upon as the accident progresses. Such states might include the conditions in the reactor vessel, the type and degree of core melt, and the status of containment safety and mitigation systems. Figure 16 illustrates a simplified event tree. Tracing a particular path through an event tree provides the answers to questions needed to specify a unique accident sequence or scenario describing the states of the subsystems. Table 10 illustrates some of the questions that would be answered by tracing a specified path through an event tree for estimating the consequences of an initiating event at a nuclear power plant.

The probabilities of the various accident sequences represented in an event tree may be obtained by associating probabilities with the various states represented by the branches in the tree. The probabilities associated with the individual branches may be obtained through statistical methods or fault trees. A series of probability calculations then provides the probabilities of occurrence of the final plant accident states at the plant. Each accident state is then analyzed in terms of the releases that would result. In a release assessment of nuclear reactor accidents, for example, the *accident analysis* involves using models to calculate the pressure, temperature, fluid flow, and neutron flux profiles that are generated in the accident sequence. *Containment analysis* (NRC, 1984) is concerned with identifying and assessing containment-failure modes and predicting the amount of hazardous materials released to the environment under alternative accident sequences; it combines the results of engineering analyses with models composed of fault trees and event trees.

The use of fault trees and event trees in modeling discrete risk sources tends to be complementary; applications range from large event trees and simple fault trees to the exact opposite. The extent to which each is used varies, depending on the system being analyzed and the preferences of and computational resources available to the analyst. Although nuclear reactor safety is the most prominent area of application, fault trees and event trees have been applied to many other areas as well.

In addition to fault trees and event trees, related modeling methods useful for characterizing risk sources include reliability block diagrams (Shooman, 1968), GO methodology (Gately and Williams, 1978a,b), and Markov models (Howard, 1971). Depending on the application, some of these modeling methods are more useful than event trees and fault trees. For example, *Markov models* (discussed in Chapter 4) are very effective at representing systems that involve time-dependent failure rates. Patwardhan *et al.* (1980) have used this type of model to forecast the occurrences of large earthquakes.

2.5.3. Discharge Models

To characterize the materials released in the event of a containment failure, *discharge models* are used. A review of such models, briefly summarized here, is

TABLE 11.   Three Discharge Models[a]

Application	Equation	Parameters
Liquid discharge from sharp-edged orifice	$G_L = C_d A \rho \left(\dfrac{2(p - p_a)}{\rho} + 2gh \right)^{1/2}$	G_L = Liquid mass emission rate (kg/s) C_d = Discharge coefficient (dimensionless = .61) A = Discharge hole area (m^2) ρ = Liquid density (kg/m^3) p = Liquid storage pressure (N/m^2 absolute) p_a = Downstream (ambient) pressure (N/m^2 absolute) g = Acceleration of gravity (9.81 m/s^2) h = Height of liquid above hole (m)
Gas discharge through hole	$G_v = C_d \dfrac{Ap}{a_o} \Psi$	G_v = Gas discharge rate (kg/s) C_d = Discharge coefficient (dimensionless ≤ 1.0) A = Hole area (m^2) p = Absolute upstream pressure (N/m^2) a_o = Sonic velocity of gas at $T = (\gamma RT/M)^{1/2}$ R = Gas constant (8314 J/kg-mol/°K) T = Upstream temperature (°K) M = Gas molecular weight (kg-mol) γ = Gas specific heat ratio (dimensionless = 1.1 to 1.67) Ψ = Flow factor, dimensionless[b]
Gas discharge through pressure relief valve due to fire	$G_{rv} = \dfrac{Q_f}{h_{fg}}$	G_{rv} = Gas discharge rate from relief valve (kg/s) h_{fg} = Latent heat of vaporization at relief pressure (kJ/kg) Q_f = Heat flux input through vessel wall from fire (Btu/hr) = 34,500 $FA^{0.82}$ F = Environment factor, dimensionless A = Total surface area (ft^2)

[a]Derived from AIChE/CCPS (1989).

[b]For subsonic flows: $\Psi = \left\{ \dfrac{2\gamma^2}{\gamma - 1} \left(\dfrac{p_a}{p} \right)^{2/\gamma} \left[1 - \left(\dfrac{p_a}{p} \right)^{(\gamma-1)/\gamma} \right] \right\}^{1/2}$ for $\dfrac{p}{p_a} \leq r_{crit}$,

for subsonic (choked) flows: $\Psi = \gamma \left(\dfrac{2}{\gamma + 1} \right)^{(\gamma+1)/2(\gamma-1)}$ for $\dfrac{p}{p_a} > r_{crit}$,

where r_{crit} = critical pressure ratio = $\left(\dfrac{p}{p_a} \right)_{crit} = \left(\dfrac{\gamma + 1}{2} \right)^{\gamma/(\gamma-1)}$

and p_a = absolute downstream pressure (N/m^2).

provided in a book by the American Institute of Chemical Engineers Center for Chemical Process Safety (AIChE/CCPS, 1989). Discharge models are applicable for modeling both controlled releases, such as an emergency release from a pressurized tank through an emergency relief valve, and catastrophic releases, such as a tank rupture. The models tend to be based on well-developed theories of chemical engineering and thermal dynamics, although empirical relationships are also used to account for considerations for which formal theory is lacking or overly complex.

Key considerations for a discharge model are the size of the hole through which releases occur and the phase of the released material, that is, whether discharge will be in the form of a liquid, a gas, or as a two-phase liquid–gas release. The phase of the release is important because it affects the release rate from a given hole size. A two-phase release can occur if the contained substance is a liquid at the pressure and temperature at which it is contained, but a gas at normal atmospheric pressure and temperature. It can also occur if the release mechanism causes the phase of the substance to change, for example, discharge of a refrigerated liquid through a pathway that brings it into contact with a heated surface. Models for two-phase discharge under various release conditions tend to rely on empirical relationships. Some models, for example, the SAFIRE computer program developed by the American Institute of Chemical Engineers Design Institute (Fauske et al., 1986), are quite complex; however, simplified models are also available (e.g., Leung, 1986).

Table 11 summarizes three common discharge models. The classic model for liquid discharges from a hole is an equation that expresses the emission rate as a function of the hole area, liquid density and storage pressure, and the height of the liquid above the hole (Perry and Green, 1984). Modifications to the basic equation have been suggested to account for obstructions to the discharge, such as pipe fittings (Crane Company, 1981). Pilz and Van Herck (1976) provide a generalized chart showing discharge rates through holes as a function of pressure gradient for a range of common fluids.

Gas discharge models differ depending on whether the source is a containment vessel or a long pipe and whether the discharge is through a hole or a relief valve. Other conditions distinguishing gas discharge models include whether the release is assumed to occur adiabatically (without loss or gain of heat) or isothermally (at constant temperature), and whether the pressure drop is sufficient to cause sonic (rather than subsonic) flow. Table 11 provides a rate equation for gas discharges through a hole. The case of a long pipe is more complicated since frictional resistance within the pipe must be considered, which causes the discharge rate to vary with time even if the containment pressure does not. Discharges through relief valves are typically based on empirical relationships. An important special case is discharge through a pressure relief valve due to fire. Table 11 summarizes the relevant equations, which account for the heat flux through the vessel wall caused by the fire. The National Fire Protection Association Codes (NFPA, 1987) recommend heat flux values to be used under various conditions.

Discharge models are also used to estimate the vapor releases from pools of volatile liquids, such as from a waste holding pond or a waste spill. Wu and Schroy (1979) provide an evaporation model based on heat and mass balance equations, taking into account the thermodynamic properties of the liquid and the thermal properties of the surface on which the liquid rests. The output of the model is the mass rate of vaporization from the pool surface. If the release involves a pressurized liquid to the atmosphere at a temperature above its normal boiling point, the liquid will start to flash, or rapidly vaporize. If the amount of liquid is relatively small and its temperature is well below the ambient temperature, a relatively simple flash model may be used that assumes all of the liquid is rapidly converted to a vapor cloud. More complicated flash models account for two-phase release because the vapor produced may entrain a significant quantity of liquid as droplets, which remain suspended as an aerosol or rain out onto the ground. This affects the subsequent dispersion of the cloud, since the droplets cause the cloud to have a higher mass and, possibly, a lower temperature.

Flash models typically provide the vapor/liquid split from a discharge of superheated liquid. Models for aerosol and rainout must then be used to provide estimates of the characteristics of the resulting cloud, which typically would be input to atmospheric dispersion models (discussed in Chapter 3). Flash models rely on empirical relationships to estimate the fraction of aerosol entrained in the resultant cloud.

Another common application for discharge models is estimating the characteristics of atmospheric releases in situations where released gases may have a significant momentum or a positive buoyancy, such as from the exhaust stacks of power plant stations powered by burning fossil fuels. Plume models are useful for continuous releases, while puff models are used when the release occurs over a very short period of time. Like other discharge models, plume and puff models are designed to provide the initial conditions of a release cloud for atmospheric dispersion models, including temperature, aerosol content, density, size, velocity, and mass.

Discharge models are also available for representing explosions and fires. Explosion models are concerned with estimating the characteristics of the shock wave overpressure effects and projectile effects. Fire models are concerned with thermal radiation effects. Several different types of models for explosion and fire have been developed. For example, flash fire models describe the ignition of cloud formed from the release of a volatile flammable material (Eisenberg et al., 1975). Such models estimate thermal radiation zones, which would provide input for a thermal effects model, or peak overpressure as a function of distance, which would be input to an explosion consequence model. Baker *et al.* (1983) describe a model for the explosive rupture of a gas-filled container. The output is overpressure versus distance for shock wave effects and the velocity and expected maximum range of projectiles generated by the burst vessel. A special case of vessel rupture models is a pressure vessel containing a superheated liquid or liquified gas, such as LPG. A boiling liquid expanding vapor explosion (BLEVE) model may be used in such situations (Moorhouse and Pritchard, 1982; Mudan, 1984; Pitblado, 1986; Prugh, 1988). BLEVE models estimate radiant flux levels, overpressure effects, and fragment numbers, velocities, and ranges.

2.5.4. Strengths

Through the use of modeling methods, important characteristics of a risk source can be deduced from more fundamental factors and their relationships. This is an important advantage, since many risks originate from highly complex systems or processes that cannot be systematically evaluated through performance testing or for which insufficient monitoring data exist to permit important characteristics to be estimated directly. Using models, the rate at which risk agents would be released by a system or the probability that an accident will occur can be estimated, even if the system has not yet been built or if no accidents have yet occurred.

The most important insights gained from models of the risk source are often qualitative rather than quantitative in nature. For example, modeling methods for discrete risks often help identify the failure modes of equipment, errors by operators, maintenance problems, and system dependencies that are most likely to lead to large accidents. Applications to nuclear reactors, for example, have been claimed to be "successful at identifying many, if not all, of the ways a reactor may be vulnerable to severe accidents" (NRC, 1985).

Another strength of using modeling for release assessment is the explicitness of models. Because the assumptions underlying models must be specified (e.g., in computer code) the model's logic may be reviewed and then accepted or rejected by concerned parties. Although the logic of the model may be complex and highly technical, models are usually composed of submodels that lie within the domain of particular professional specialties. Thus, specialists may be relied upon to develop and critique those aspects of the model that fall most directly within their areas of expertise.

2.5.5. Limitations

A release model is by its nature an abstraction—a compromised representation of physical reality. Errors may be introduced through lack of understanding of the cause-effect processes governing the behavior of the risk source and through limitations and constraints associated with the modeling exercise. If understanding of the processes involved in the risk source is extremely limited, then the model for the risk source will be based on plausible rather than proven relationships (derived, for example, from analogies with better understood systems) and may involve proxy variables. Even if such models are validated against past data, failure to account for underlying mechanisms leaves these models open to the danger of being completely incorrect when extrapolated to different circumstances where the previously demonstrated correlations between mechanisms and the proxy variables no longer hold.

Incompleteness and inaccuracies are of special concern when modeling a source of discrete risks, such as accidents. In the case of event trees, for example, the relatively small number of accident sequences that are modeled in detail must be considered representative of a range of related sequences that could occur. The model outputs may be significantly wrong if any of the following occur: (1) important failure modes have been overlooked; (2) multiple failures that might be induced by a single obscure initiating event are missed; (3) partial failure and reduced performance modes that induce risk have been omitted; or (4) catastrophic accidents with a very small probability of occurrence have been excluded.

Accounting for the influence of human actions on the release or production of risks presents special difficulties for modeling. Human behavior is a complex subject that does not lend itself to simple models such as those for component reliability. Nevertheless, human error can be an extremely important cause of accidents. A study of hazardous material transport found that 60 percent of all transport vehicle accidents were attributable to operator mistakes rather than equipment failure (OTA, 1986). Attempts have often been made to incorporate human behavior into failure models. For example, fault trees have been used that classify a human response as either a success or a failure; however, quantifying the likelihood of these outcomes and accounting for the possibility of other operator conditions that might affect the system in more complicated ways are difficult tasks. For example, applications to nuclear power plants have had difficulty quantifying the likelihood that operators might misdiagnose the cause of an incident and thus employ the wrong procedures in attempting to remedy it.

Similar limitations exist in accounting for human behavior as it affects risk sources that continuously or regularly release risk agents to the environment. For example, analyses of the impact of proposed regulations often assume that there will be 100 percent compliance. Immediate and complete compliance, however, is rare, and the actual extent to which those responsible for a source of risk will take actions to comply with government requirements depends on many factors including the costs of compliance, the threat of legal actions, and the penalties for failing to comply.

The need to account for human behavior is not limited merely to operator performance and compliance. Failure to account for unregulated human reactions can also be critical. This is illustrated by Staley's (1987) description of an assessment of the environmental risks associated with alternative regulations regarding sport fishing off the west coast of Canada (Argue *et al.*, 1983). The assessment considered alternative limits on the minimum size of Chinook and coho salmon that could be caught, limits on the number of fish allowed per fisherman, and limits on the seasons in which fishing could take place. In its first version, the model for the risk source assumed that there would be a constant number of fishermen who would fish according to historical patterns, subject only to the restrictions posed by regulations. For example, the model assumed that the requirement to throw small fish back would not increase the effort spent catching larger fish. Under these assumptions the risk assessment predicted that even minor regulations would significantly reduce the annual harvest and quickly restore the stock of game fish. When the model was extended to account for increased effort by fishermen to catch larger fish, however, the conclusion changed dramatically. By ignoring the unregulated response of fishermen, the conclusion of the risk assessment would have been grossly in error and misleading to policymakers responsible for the fishery resource.

Not surprisingly, models of complex technological systems are themselves complex. Fault trees and event trees, for example, can easily become so large that they cannot be displayed in reports. Although logically precise, many models are difficult to understand and are not mathematically unique. Fault trees, for example, bear no resemblance to system flow charts, a more intuitive graphical representation, and many different fault trees can often be developed to represent the same system.

Many other issues regarding the limitations of modeling methods are independent of whether the methods are applied to release assessment or to some other component of the risk assessment process. These issues are discussed in greater detail in Chapter 5.

CHAPTER 3

EXPOSURE ASSESSMENT

Exposure assessment is the process of measuring or estimating the intensity, frequency, and duration of human or other population exposures to risk agents. Exposures may occur in a variety of ways, such as through ingestion (e.g., eating fish contaminated with mercury), dermal contact (e.g., handling toxic substances), or inhalation (e.g., breathing air contaminated by industrial emissions). The appropriate methods and units to be used for exposure assessment depend on the risk agent and pathways for exposure, the level of aggregation adopted for the assessment, and many other factors. For instance, the amount of material ingested is often used as a measure of exposure to toxic contaminants in food, the speed and level of flood water have been used as measures of exposure to dam failure, and the ratio of mosquitoes to human population has been used as a measure of exposure to malaria.

For many risk assessments, exposure assessment is the most difficult task. The reason for this is that exposure assessment often depends on factors that are hard to estimate and for which there are few data. Critical information on the conditions of exposure is often lacking; for example, although industrial manufacturers are generally required to keep records on workers' exposures to toxic chemicals, the levels of exposure and the particular chemicals involved are often not known or not recorded. Exposures to the general population are even less well-documented due to the limited availability of systems capable of measuring the exposures to specific risk agents actually experienced by people.

A major source of the complexity of exposure assessment is the strong influence that individual personal habits can have on human exposure. In the case of food contaminated with risk agents, food storage practices, food preparation, and dietary habits have a major influence on the amount of the risk agent actually consumed. For example, if raw meats have been contaminated with pathogenic microorganisms, a critical factor in predicting health consequences is whether and to what extent the meat is cooked. As another example, to estimate consumer exposure to a pesticide requires data on pesticide residues, data on how many pesticide-treated food products are consumed by an average person, and data on how many people consume large amounts of the pesticide-treated food products.

If the risk agent is absorbed when a consumer product is used, the patterns of use will affect exposure levels. A solvent whose vapor is potentially toxic, for example, may be used outdoors or in a small, poorly ventilated garage. Thus, for risk assessments associated with consumer products, exposure assessment focuses on understanding how the products may be used and how different use patterns affect exposure levels.

If exposure occurs through the air or water, then exposure assessment must consider how the risk agent moves from its source through the environment and how it is altered over time. Chemical risk agents generally become diluted and may degrade after release. The aim of exposure assessment in this case is to determine the concentration of toxic materials in space and time where they interface with target populations (Travis *et al.*, 1983). With some risk agents, understanding the changes that occur following release is all-important. For example, genetically engineered organisms released to the environment will seek to reproduce, spread, and evolve in ways that are beneficial to their own survival. Exposure assessment for genetic engineering is therefore much concerned with the persistence, establishment, and growth of released organisms (Levin and Strauss, 1991).

Physical risk agents such as mechanical force or heat can also be the subject of an exposure assessment. For example, in automotive safety, exposure assessment is concerned with estimating accident involvement rates for various types of vehicles and with the dynamics and biomechanics of occupant motion during a collision.

Another important aspect of exposure assessment is determining which groups in the population may be exposed to a risk agent; some subgroups may be especially susceptible to adverse health effects. Pregnant women, very young and very old people, and persons with impaired health all may be particularly sensitive to toxic chemicals. Some regulatory laws (such as parts of the Clean Air Act) require explicit consideration of the effect of pollutants on "sensitive or susceptible individuals or groups."

Exposure to multiple risk agents often results in portions of the population becoming more sensitive to single agents. Exposure to risk agents that act synergistically greatly complicates risk assessment because most assessments are conducted on individual risk agents. For example, exposure to both cigarette smoke and asbestos results in a rate of cancer incidence much greater than that indicated by carcinogenicity data for each substance individually (NAS–NRC, 1983a). Synergisms also often necessitate that exposure assessment consider the activities in which the exposed individuals engage. For instance, strenuous activity often increases the magnitude or likelihood of adverse reactions to exposures to many air pollutants. Multiple sources also complicate exposure assessments. An individual can be exposed to a single risk agent from several distinct sources. Exposure to lead, for example, can come from breathing air, eating food, and drinking water.

The same concepts of exposure apply to assessing risks that impact the natural environment. Exposure assessment for environmental risks, however, poses additional difficulties. Unlike humans, who may be regarded as point receptors, a sensitive ecosystem may cover a broad geographical area. Differences in the geographical distribution of risk agents are often crucial given that the environment is inhabited by diverse organisms that have differing sensitivities to impacts.

To be comprehensive, an exposure assessment must describe the levels of exposure and all conditions that might be needed to assess the effects of those exposures, including (1) the magnitude, duration, schedule, and route of exposure; and (2) the size, nature, and sensitive subpopulations of the populations exposed. If environmental effects are of concern, then the exposure assessment might also have to describe the spatial distribution of exposures relative to the distribution and differential sensitivities of exposed elements of the natural environment. In addition, a comprehensive exposure assessment must describe the uncertainties in all of these estimates. Finally, given the variety of pathways by which risk agents can be transmitted, a comprehensive exposure assessment may also have to account for the cumulative effects of simultaneous exposures via distinct environmental media.

This chapter presents and evaluates the various methods used in exposure assessment including monitoring, testing, and modeling methods.

3.1. MONITORING METHODS FOR EXPOSURE ASSESSMENT

Monitoring plays a central role in nearly all exposure assessments. Consider, for example, an assessment of the risks posed by a site at which hazardous wastes have been disposed. Soil, surface water, and groundwater contamination levels at various distances from the site may be monitored using conventional field measurement techniques. Remote techniques, such as aerial photography and multispectral overhead imagery, might be used to delineate waste site releases, and ground-penetrating remote sensing technologies may be used to estimate the subsurface distribution of waste materials (Schweitzer, 1982). Air sampling units may be used to sense airborne releases of respirable particulates or gases from volatile organic compounds. In addition, biological monitoring (Gompertz, 1980) may be used to identify possible food-chain problems, e.g., by measuring chemical residues in the tissues of food crops, livestock, or local fish. Finally, wild animals and indigenous vegetation might be sampled to find indications of local contamination.

Monitoring methods used in exposure assessment can be categorized into direct and indirect approaches. *Direct methods* are usually practical only for monitoring human exposures. In the direct approach, individual exposures are measured directly by instruments that accompany the individual, such as personal exposure monitors

(PEMs) (Wallace and Ott, 1982). Depending on the nature of the risk agent and the route by which the individual is exposed, PEMs are designed to measure the concentrations of risk agents in the air, in water, or in food. In the case of water or food, individuals actively test water or food before they consume it. Since it is generally infeasible to provide the entire population of potentially exposed individuals with PEMs, population exposures are usually estimated by obtaining 24-hour exposure profiles from a statistical sample of the population.

An example of the direct approach is provided by an EPA study of carbon monoxide (CO) (Åkland *et al.*, 1985). Several thousand randomly selected individuals were interviewed by telephone and screened to obtain a smaller target sample stratified according to smoking habits, commute times, and other factors likely to influence CO exposures. An interviewer then visited and instructed each individual on the use of a miniaturized personal CO exposure monitor. The monitor was capable of measuring and recording CO concentrations with a time resolution of less than 1 minute. During the next several days, the individuals carried their CO PEMs as they went about their normal daily activities. From the recorded data, it was possible to construct exposure profiles for each person in the sample and to extrapolate the results to the larger populations of the cities in which the people lived. Similar studies have also been conducted to measure exposures to volatile organic compounds (Wallace *et al.*, 1984) and to electric and magnetic fields (EPRI, 1987). The method is also commonly used to measure exposures of radiation workers, who carry dosimeters, film badges, or other radiation-sensitive devices.

In the *indirect approach* to exposure monitoring, factors that affect exposure are measured rather than exposure itself. For example, fixed-site monitors are widely used to measure the concentrations of pollutants in media, especially air and water. Site monitoring is often used in situations where risk agents are routinely released or the release occurs over a sufficient period of time to allow a fixed-site monitoring system to be established. Unlike PEMs, fixed-site monitors can be large, heavy, and sophisticated. Commercially available air-sampling devices include sequential samplers that draw air in at multiple sampling points according to a programmed sequence and time interval. Samples may be collected in parallel and subjected to different analyses. The most powerful versions continuously complete analyses and record final results (Lioy and Lioy, 1983).

A frequent problem in site monitoring is the spatial and temporal variation of concentrations of a risk agent found in media (especially air and water). Thus, the selection of a particular dose-measurement interval, or more generally, the selection of particular sites or measurements, can have a strong effect on the numerical results. Furthermore, if only site-monitoring data are available, exposures for individuals must be derived indirectly, using additional monitoring data on human activity patterns and models to estimate concentrations of risk agents in unmonitored locations.

Great quantities of data have been generated from studies that monitor pollutants in the air and water. Examples include analyses of the plumes from a power plant to determine the nature of transport and transformation processes occurring from a single-point source of emissions (Schiermeier, 1979); studies of air pollution in the city of St. Louis (Strothmann and Schiermeier, 1979); monitoring of PCBs and DDT in western Lake Superior (Vieth *et al.*, 1977); and studies of the dispersion of sewage sludge discharged from vessels off the coast of New York (Callaway *et al.*, 1982). Major air quality databases include the National Emissions Data System (NEDS), which contains data on total suspended particulates (TSP), sulfur oxides, nitrogen oxides (NOx), hydrocarbons, and CO; the Sulfate Regional Experiment, which contains data on TSP, sulfur dioxide, sulfates, and NOx; and the Hazardous and Trace Emissions System (HATRAEMS), which contains data on pollutants not regulated by primary ambient air standards (Roth *et al.*, 1984).

The problem of spatial variation may be addressed in site monitoring through the use of either a random or systematic strategy for locating site monitors. With *random sampling*, monitoring locations are selected in a random manner such that it is not possible to predict the location of any sampling point based on the location of others. For example, sampling points might be established by choosing a series of pairs of random numbers that can be mapped onto a coordinate system established for the area of concern. Randomly locating sampling locations allows the use of simple statistical methods; average concentrations for the area of concern can be estimated by averaging sample data. *Systematic sampling* involves laying out a grid of sampling locations that follow a regular pattern, with the initial reference for the grid located randomly. Systematic sampling ensures that the sampling effort across the area of concern is uniform, and it is efficient if the objective is to search for small areas with elevated concentrations. Systematic sampling, however, calls for the use of more complex statistical methods, including the use of special variance calculations to estimate confidence limits on the computed average concentrations (EPA, 1988b).

To address the issue of temporal variations, consideration must be given to the timing of measurements. Repeated samples from a specified location generally produce time-series data whose temporal correlations must be accounted for through the use of statistical methods for analyzing time series. For example, the concentration of a contaminant in an aquifer measured at a given well on a given day will depend in part on what the concentration in the aquifer was on the previous day. If such correlations are ignored and time-series data are treated as a random sample, confidence limits (e.g., for the estimated mean concentration) will be underestimated. Seasonal variations must also be addressed because weather conditions often affect sample composition; heavy rains may result in sediment loading to water bodies, which could increase contamination or affect the concentrations of other contaminants through adsorption and settling in the water column. Ideally, monitoring should provide a full annual sampling cycle. If this cannot be accommodated, sampling of water bodies should at least encompass seasonal extremes such as conditions of high water/low water, high recharge/low recharge, windiness/calmness, and high suspended-solids/clear water.

Groundwater contamination has been monitored through the EPA's National Pesticides in Groundwater Survey, a multiyear monitoring study of 90 organic chemicals and 70 active pesticides and inert ingredients commonly used in agriculture (Poje, 1987). Chemical contaminants in the U.S. food supply are monitored annually through the FDA's Total Diet Studies, which examine and analyze the purchase of roughly 200 foods sold in grocery stores across the United States. Various data on the kinds and quantities of foods consumed by different population groups have also been collected as part of the U.S. Department of Agriculture's National Food Consumption Survey and the National Health and Nutrition Examination Survey.

Another means for indirectly determining exposures is biological monitoring focused on biomarkers. *Biomarkers* are selected biochemical or physiological responses measured in individual organisms that can be used to quantify exposures and levels of sublethal stress. The most direct biomarkers of exposure are chemical residues in tissue, useful for risk agents that bioaccumulate in specific plants or animals and in specific organs. Metals, for example, often accumulate in the liver and kidneys of animals. Methylmercury accumulates in brain tissue and iodine builds up in the thyroid. Human hair obtained from barber shops has been analyzed to monitor for possible exposures to radioactive strontium (Moeller, 1992). Levels of risk agents in tissue can be used to estimate exposures provided there is some understanding of preferential biological absorption and retention process of the risk agent in organs or organisms and some understanding of the physical decay processes of the hazardous substance or material (such as radioactive decay or biodegradation).

Indirect biomarkers of exposure include delta-aminolevulinic acid dehydrase (delta-ALAD) and various cholinesterases. Delta-ALAD is an enzyme that catalyzes a reaction involved in blood synthesis. Because of its sensitivity to inhibition by inorganic lead, Delta-ALAD activity in blood has been used as an index for exposure to inorganic lead in humans and in rats, ducks, pigeons, and fish (EPA, 1989c). Cholinesterases are enzymes that are sensitive to inhibition by organophosphorous and carbamate compounds. Measures of these enzymes, e.g., in the brain tissue of birds, provide an indirect indicator of exposures for the insecticides that contain these compounds (Hayne, 1984).

Sometimes the main advantage of biological monitoring is that the species monitored does the work of collecting samples. For example, since bees cover large areas and collect pollen from a wide range of plants, honey is sometimes monitored as an indicator of arsenic, cadmium, and fluoride contamination. Population effects on sensitive species may give information about exposure levels. For example, certain species of salamanders have proven to be very sensitive to acid rain, leading some researchers to suspect that their decline is a warning of impending widespread damage to forests. Some species may prove to be useful indicators, not because they are harmed by pollutants, but because they thrive in polluted conditions; elevated levels of the coliform bacteria *Escherichia coli* (*E. coli*) are often found in waters contaminated with sewage. Other population effects that may be measured for indicator species include altered population distribution, altered population processes (such as survival or productivity) and altered parameters (such as age or sex ratio). On an even broader scale are biological community effects, which include changes in such parameters as species diversity and the ratio of food to consumer organisms.

Accident monitoring also provides a means for indirectly determining exposures. In the area of automobile safety, accident monitoring provides accident exposure rates for different population groups, geographic areas, and vehicles. Two basic accident rates are often monitored. The first is the *accident-population rate*, which is the number of accidents per unit of population, where the population may be the total number of persons in some driver group (e.g., drivers aged 18 to 21) or the total number of vehicles being studied; the second is the *accident-travel rate* measured in accidents or collisions per unit of travel (e.g., collisions per 100 million vehicle miles). These two rates are derived from three sets of statistics: the number of vehicles (or persons) in the population being studied, the number of accidents incurred by those vehicles (or persons), and the total amount of travel of the vehicles (or passengers) during the time interval being considered.* Other factors that might be monitored to provide additional information useful for accident exposure assessment include the ages of the driver and occupant(s) (because the young can withstand more trauma than older persons) and whether the collision takes place at night or during the day (since post-crash care is typically less efficient and more scarce at night).

3.1.1. Strengths

Exposure monitoring provides estimates of individual and population exposures and helps define the causal connections between the sources of a risk agent and the resulting levels of exposures to human and other populations. Monitoring

---

*
When these same concepts are applied to health effects assessment, they are known as epidemiological methods (see Section 4.5). Peranio and Katz (1970) note that with the epidemiological perspective, the accident-population rate can be looked upon as an index of the incidence of the "disease" of accidents brought about by motor vehicle use, and the accident-travel rate is an index of the "virulence" of the disease of motor vehicle use.

is a versatile means for exploring exposure processes. It can encompass surveys of (a) the uses and misuses of consumer products, (b) exposures of individuals to accidents involving various activities or technologies, (c) characteristics of the ambient environment, the human environment, the home, and the workplace, (d) characteristics of food and water consumed, and (e) doses absorbed and retained by humans and other populations. In some circumstances, monitoring for exposure assessment provides direct measures of current exposures, especially in situations where exposure involves direct contact with the monitored medium (e.g., contact with chemicals in soil) or where monitoring has occurred directly at an exposure point (e.g., PEMs or site monitoring of a public water supply). More generally, monitoring provides data for setting the parameters of exposure models.

3.1.2. Limitations

The most important limitation in monitoring for exposure assessment relates to the constraints on its ability to provide the basic data needed to apply statistical methods. The logic of most statistical methods (see Chapter 2) is based on an assumption of random samples; data are assumed to provide an unbiased representation of the larger universe of possible observations from which the measurements were taken. In many monitoring systems, however, costs and practicality demand that sampling be performed at convenient sites and times. Thus, monitoring often produces an "index," not an unbiased estimate.

The difficulty of collecting statistically meaningful samples of exposure measurements is aggravated by the great diversity of environmental media and exposure pathways. Selecting the right tradeoffs about where, when, and what to monitor means answering difficult questions. For example, should limited resources for exposure monitoring focus on a "typical" site or should a location be selected where environmental stresses are highest, even though the latter would not provide a representative sample? Should only infrequent, convenient samples be taken (e.g., sampling during daylight hours, excluding holidays and weekends) or should more expensive continuous sampling be used to obtain data on the time correlation among measurements? If the effects of an environmental pollutant depend on a variety of associated factors (e.g., temperature, humidity, and other pollutants present), which additional factors must be monitored to ensure that the collected data prove useful?

Another problem is that the natural variability of the environment over time and space makes it very difficult to translate measurements obtained from fixed monitoring stations into actual exposures experienced by people or animals that move from place to place. To address this issue, field experiments have attempted to correlate exposures estimated from site monitors with those obtained from PEMs. The results show that the concentrations experienced by people engaged in common activities (i.e., driving, walking on sidewalks, shopping in stores, and working in buildings) do not correlate well with simultaneous readings obtained from monitoring networks (Cortese and Spengler, 1976; Wallace, 1979; and Ott and Flachsbart, 1982).

This problem is due in part to the fact that individual behavior has a large influence on exposure. The problem becomes especially acute when monitoring exposures to animals, which generally cannot be equipped with PEMs. For example, the concentration of a chemical in food may not be the concentration actually taken up by wildlife. The ability to detect and avoid contaminated food is well-documented for many species. Chemical residue measurements may provide a means for estimating the exposures of animals that can be subjected to laboratory analysis. The approach may not be so effective, however, for animals in the wild; if an animal becomes sick it may seek a secluded location. Thus, biological monitoring may not provide an accurate assessment of wildlife exposures, due to the impact of the exposure on the animals' availability for monitoring.

Random variability also creates problems by making it difficult to distinguish a risk-signaling trend from random variations. For example, although even a small reduction in the earth's stratospheric ozone would cause a discernable increase in ultraviolet radiation reaching the earth's surface, day-to-day, month-to-month, and year-to-year variabilities in stratospheric ozone make it difficult to detect long-term trends. Pittock (1974), has estimated that a sudden 2 percent depletion of ozone would require an additional 10 years of observation before the event could be identified through statistical methods with 95 percent confidence.

As is the case with monitoring for release assessment, monitoring for exposure assessment may be limited by legal, natural, or technological barriers; for instance, agencies may not have the authority to monitor indoor air pollutants at a factory. Concentrations of toxic chemicals in a food source might be monitored, but not how much is eaten, and how often. The deposition of an airborne pollutant can be measured directly using filter instruments, but monitoring the transmission of the deposited pollutant through soil and groundwater systems is much more difficult.

For some media pollutants, concentrations measured in parts per million or parts per billion may be sufficient to cause significant effects. Such minute levels may be extremely difficult or impossible to measure given the current sensitivity of monitoring technology. With antimony, the lowest level that can be accurately and reproducibly measured is well above reference concentrations suspected of producing cancer risk (EPA, 1989a). Even when low levels of a risk agent can be measured, they may be masked by background levels. With radioactivity, regulations limit exposures near nuclear power plants to about 0.05 mSv per year; however, the average external dose rate from naturally occurring cosmic and terrestrial radiation is 0.6 to 0.7 mSv per year (Moeller, 1992).

3.2. TESTING METHODS FOR EXPOSURE ASSESSMENT

Since it is generally difficult to conduct controlled tests in large environmental systems under artificial conditions, most of the data relevant to exposure assessment are collected under natural conditions. Thus, monitoring plays a larger role in exposure assessment than the closely related methods of testing and controlled experimentation. Nevertheless, laboratory tests and controlled experiments do play a limited but important role in exposure assessment.

One productive application of testing to exposure assessment is in the study of microcosms. *Microcosms* attempt to recreate portions of the environment, e.g., a marine ecosystem, in a laboratory setting. Ideally, a microcosm faithfully mimics the processes occurring in nature. Experiments that could not be conducted in the real environment, such as the introduction of specific chemicals, can be performed in the microcosm in a controlled way. Using a microcosm, the partitioning of a chemical among the various components of the environment, together with the associated chemical and biological conversions, can be studied in a single integrated experiment. Performance testing of microcosms has been applied to marine, freshwater, terrestrial, subsurface, and atmospheric microcosms (OSTP, 1984). The method has also been applied to help predict indoor exposures to air pollutants (Duan, 1981).

Microcosms need not be full-scale re-creations to be useful. Scale models sometimes provide an adequate means of simulating exposure processes. For example, a detailed scale model of an urban area has been constructed for the purpose of accounting for the effect of terrain on pollution concentrations caused by emissions from truck and automobile traffic (Murphy and Davies, 1988). Mobile source emissions were represented by a continuous line source simulator, which was built into the model. The entire model was placed in a wind tunnel, with the dispersion of vehicle exhaust simulated by imposing properly scaled meteorological conditions (wind speed and direction) on the model. The impact of the source was then assessed by measuring concentrations at strategically placed receptors.

In general, laboratory tests are useful whenever conditions relevant to exposure can be replicated and more easily studied in the laboratory setting than in the real world. Depending on what exposure processes are being studied, a vast array of such methods may be available. Fiksel and Covello (1986), classify methods for quantifying the potential of pathogenic organisms to survive, grow, and become dispersed in an environment. These include (1) methods that involve the growth of microorganisms on or in a cultivation medium or host, (2) methods that measure biochemical activity in dilution-to-extinction media (most-probable-number methods), and (3) methods that measure directly by microscopic observation.

Not all test methods are laboratory-based. Performance testing conducted in the field can often help clarify exposure processes. For example, a nontoxic tracer dye might be introduced into a water system to improve understanding of the transport of pollutants. An example of how large-scale field tests can be used for exposure assessment is a planned Department of Energy facility in Nevada designed to explore how winds and gravity affect large-scale releases of cryogenic or pressurized flammable fluids, toxic substances, and heavy gas. A system of sensors and data collection equipment would monitor release characteristics, including rate, volume, temperature, and pressure. An additional system of sensors would acquire data on meteorological parameters, downwind gas concentrations and aerosol characteristics, and blast and fire effects (DOE, undated).

In the case of exposures to accidents, performance testing has been used to study the dynamics and biomechanics of various types of accidents, including automobile-pedestrian collisions (Schneider and Beier, 1974). One technique utilizes anthropometric dummies in full-scale collision experiments. The experiments are designed to collect data on the relative frequency with which various parts of the body are impacted and the resulting accelerations and forces that collisions produce.

3.2.1. Strengths

Testing provides a means for experimentally studying processes that influence exposures to risk agents. By creating special conditions that occur infrequently or that are difficult to study in nature, the researcher can isolate key factors and improve understanding. Data that are collected can be used to provide the necessary inputs for exposure models and to help calibrate these models to faithfully replicate real conditions relevant to the risk assessment.

3.2.2. Limitations

As in other applications of testing and laboratory methods, the principal question regarding their use for exposure assessment is how well such tests are able to replicate the real world. In the case of microcosms, for example, portions of the environment that are omitted from the laboratory re-creation may mask or alter processes critical to determining real-world response. Similarly, anthropometric dummies used to study the impacts and violent forces to which people are subjected in accidents cannot fully account for the infinite variability of both individual characteristics and accident conditions. Validating laboratory test conditions is often extremely difficult and yet is of critical importance to judging the significance of tests.

The complexity of processes relevant to exposure assessment also creates problems of data collection and test design. In the case of microcosms, comparing results of different tests is difficult due to the wide diversity of testing methods currently in use, each with a narrow sphere of applicability. Distinguishing significant effects from normal fluctuations in ecosystem structure is also burdensome and generally requires arduous and long-term data collection, processing, and interpretation.

3.3. MODELS FOR EXPOSURE ASSESSMENT

As applied to exposure assessment, a "model" is a mathematical expression representing a simplified version of the essential elements of exposure processes. Its purpose is to provide a means by which diverse data on relevant factors can be combined to predict levels of human or other exposures in the absence of complete or adequate monitoring or testing data.

In general, an exposure model must account for the intensity, routes, and conditions of exposure, the frequency and duration of exposure, and the segments of the population exposed. The models are often developed by generalizing a physical relationship or phenomenon observed in the laboratory or derived empirically from field measurements. For example, the air monitoring data from St. Louis and the power plant plume studies cited previously have been used to construct models for predicting population exposures to air pollution (OSTP, 1984).

Hundreds of exposure models have been developed for a diversity of risk sources, risk agents, and routes of exposure. These models range from "back of the envelope" calculations to large, user-friendly models implemented on mainframe computers. In recent years, there has been a rapid increase in the number of microcomputer-based exposure models.

Some exposure models address physical risk agents, such as acoustic energy and vibration. For example, models have been developed to represent the transmission of ground motion from the source of an earthquake to a given site, taking into account the magnitude of the earthquake, local soil conditions, and the distance from the epicenter to urban areas or a facility at risk, such as a dam (Patwardhan *et al.*, 1980). Models have also been developed to approximate the dynamics and biomechanics of exposures to mechanical energies that occur during accidents involving consumer products or specific technologies. For instance, based on the collision tests with dummies, models have been developed to study the factors that are most important in determining the accelerations and points of impact that occur during automobile–pedestrian collisions (Schneider and Beier, 1974).

Within the general class of exposure models, the largest category of well-developed models consists of specialized models for describing the transport and transformation of specific pollutants released into the environment. Often referred to as *pollutant transport and fate models*, their objective is to determine the average concentrations of a pollutant for a particular time frame and population group for one or more exposure pathways. The pollutant might be a chemical or biological risk agent, such as a toxic chemical or genetically engineered microorganisms, or it might be a form of energy, such as heated water released by an electric power plant or the ionizing energy of radionuclides released by a nuclear power plant.

The temporal resolution of these models varies from seconds to years, and the exposure pathways considered may include ingestion, inhalation, and dermal absorption. Pollutant transport and fate models are among the most computationally complex of existing exposure models because the processes by which pollutants are dispersed, transformed, and removed from air, water, and other environmental media are extremely complex.

Most pollutant transport and fate models have been developed for specific applications such as estimating radionuclide exposures at locations surrounding a nuclear power plant or estimating exposures from pesticides used in agriculture. The models vary in their data requirements, costs, difficulty of use, types of output, accuracy, and ability to interface with other models. Although a model designed for one application (e.g., radionuclide transport) can seldom be directly applied to another (e.g., genetically engineered microorganisms), it can often be adapted without great difficulty.

Fiksel and Skow (1983) list seven factors that differentiate various pollutant transport and fate models: (1) environmental transport media (e.g., air, surface water, soil groundwater, or biota), (2) geographic scale (e.g., global, national, regional, or local), (3) pollutant source characteristics (e.g., continuous or instantaneous releases from industrial, residential, and commercial point or area sources), (4) risk agents (e.g., a specific compound or a class of related substances), (5) receptor populations (e.g., humans, animals, plants, microorganisms, and habitats, as well as specific subpopulations exposed to high pollutant levels or particularly sensitive to exposure), (6) exposure routes (e.g., ingestion, dermal contact), and (7) time frame (e.g., retrospective, current, or prospective assessment). Several other general reviews of pollutant fate and transport models have been published, including those by Hoffman *et al.* (1977), Miller (1978), and Bolton *et al.* (1985). The subsections below provide brief summaries of the various types of exposure models, organized by transport medium.

3.3.1. Atmospheric Models

Air pollutant transport-and-fate modeling has reached a relatively high degree of sophistication. In general, atmospheric models address the processes of pollutant transport, diffusion, and deposition. *Transport* refers to the movement of a suspended pollutant through air currents. Air currents typically cause emissions from a point source to follow a zigzag course initially, and then to veer off to one side in an arc. *Diffusion* refers to the motion of individual particles and molecules that tends to spread and dilute the pollutant. Diffusion is the same process that causes smoke particles from a cigarette in a still room to spread out slowly to all parts of the room. *Deposition* is the transfer of particulate matter to the ground, water bodies, and vegetation. Deposition is caused by gravity, as individual particles fall to the ground (dry deposition) or as pollutants contained in falling raindrops or snowflakes reach the ground (wet deposition). Models distinguish between wet and dry deposition because the rate of deposition is generally much higher during rain or snow than it is otherwise.

Transport, diffusion, and deposition occur through complex processes. One important consideration is atmospheric stability, that is, conditions that tend to resist or enhance the vertical motion of air. At most times and in most places, the atmosphere gets steadily colder with greater altitude. Since warm air rises, this produces a general upwelling of warm air; however, if for some reason the temperature at the surface becomes cooler than the temperature above, then the dense, cooler air near the surface cannot get enough lift to rise. In this case, an atmospheric inversion occurs, and upwelling stops. Without upwelling, any pollutant injected into the atmosphere at the surface from chimneys and tailpipes builds up in the air near the surface. For emissions into the air from industrial exhaust stacks, momentum and buoyancy usually cause emissions to rise a considerable distance. The height to which emissions will rise depends on the conditions of the release (e.g., velocity, temperature, and stack height) and on atmospheric stability. Atmospheric stability is particularly important for estimating atmospheric concentrations near the ground, because it determines where the plume will first reach ground level.

The primary outputs of atmospheric models are (1) atmospheric concentrations of the pollutant, and (2) deposition rates, both wet and dry. Atmospheric concentrations determine human exposure through direct inhalation. Deposition rates determine how much of the pollutant emitted to the atmosphere reaches the soil, surface water, and groundwater.

Most models simplify the process of computing atmospheric concentrations and deposition by dividing the dispersion process into two phases: initial plume rise and subsequent dispersion and deposition. Plume rise is generally assumed to occur without significant dispersion. For industrial exhaust stacks, the amount of rise is added to the actual stack height to determine the effective stack height. Briggs (1975) has developed equations to describe plume rise under different atmospheric stability conditions, using atmospheric stability and Pasquill stability classes described by Martin (1979) and Hanna *et al.* (1982).

Since so many variables affect the diffusion process, no rigorous mathematical solution has been found. Instead, the most common modeling approach, called the *Gaussian plume model*, is statistical in nature. The model assumes that the plume from an emission source spreads laterally and vertically in accordance with a Gaussian distribution. Gaussian models often assume that wind is distributed uniformly whenever it is within a specific angular sector. Consequently, the estimated pollutant concentration varies according to the downwind distance from the source but is constant in the crosswind direction within each angular sector. To apply the Gaussian approximation, one must assume a distribution of mean wind speeds and directions as a function of atmospheric stability class. The long-term concentration for a particular angular sector is then computed as the sum of the concentrations over all stability classes.

Gaussian models have limited applicability when the terrain is complex or uneven and when release rates are highly variable. They are fairly accurate, however, for predicting ground-level concentrations where reasonably flat terrain exists and where an average, fairly stable release rate can be assumed (Travis *et al.*, 1983). Validation studies have concluded that Gaussian plume models can predict within a factor of two the annual average atmospheric concentrations at distances of 10 kilometers or less over relatively flat terrain (Hoffman *et al.*, 1978). Predictions over time scales of a few hours or days, however, tend to be less accurate.

The Gaussian plume model is widely used for representing the aerial dispersal of particulates. It has also been used to represent the aerial dispersal of microorganisms. For example, Lighthart and Frisch (1976) developed a modified Gaussian plume model to estimate ground-level concentrations of airborne microorganisms dispersed from a cooling tower, sewage treatment plant, or other point source. The model actually superimposes many Gaussian plumes, one for each droplet size category. Lighthart and Mohr (1987) further refined the model by taking into account the survival rate of microorganisms as a function of weather, including temperature, relative humidity, solar radiation, and time in the aerosol.

Another, more computationally demanding class of atmospheric models attempts to compute the trajectory that a pollutant might follow. Trajectories are typically composed of a connected sequence of trajectory segments estimated for fixed intervals of time and based on historical wind data. Running the models requires solving complex systems of equations that represent continuity of motion and conservation of mass. *Trajectory models* are most often used for long-range predictions of atmospheric concentrations. Short-term concentrations are assumed to follow some specified frequency distribution. Distributions often used include lognormal, gamma, and Weibull distributions. The approach typically consists of (1) selecting a frequency distribution to represent short-term concentrations, (2) using a Gaussian or trajectory model to estimate how releases might alter the parameters of the distribution (e.g., mean and variance) from historically observed values, and (3) inferring values for short-term concentrations and probabilities from the revised frequency distribution produced by the estimated parameter values.

To handle cases where the terrain is not flat and clearly has an effect on transport and dispersion, complex terrain models have been developed. In addition to accounting for plume rise, atmospheric stability, dispersion, and deposition, such models account for plume interaction with terrain, including plume deflection around obstacles, plume lifting over terrain, plume impingement on terrain, and terrain contours (Strimaitis *et al.*, 1987).

To represent rapid, short-duration emissions, such as might result from explosions, "puff" transport models have been developed. *Puff transport models* frequently adopt the simplifying assumption that transport and dispersion of a pollutant in the crosswind and vertical directions are uncoupled from the downwind direction. Typically, dispersion in the crosswind and vertical directions is assumed to have a Gaussian distribution. Pollution distribution in the downwind direction is most simply represented as "plug flow," wherein it is assumed that the pollutant is carried by the wind with no dispersion in the downwind direction and no change in the size of the puff. More complicated models account for downwind dispersion and growth of the puff (Overcamp, 1988).

Models for short-term or transient releases that are neither puffs nor continuous plumes have also been developed. One approach is to assume that the short-term release behaves like a succession of puffs. In this case, the results of repeated runs of a puff model are numerically integrated to obtain the desired concentrations. Another approach is to assume a mathematically convenient form for the short-term release that leads to a mathematically convenient form for the concentration as a function of space and time. For example, models have been developed that assume that the release rate of the pollutant from the source decreases exponentially, often a reasonable assumption for a gas leaking from a tank (Wilson, 1979).

Atmospheric models have also been developed for the indoor air environment (OSTP, 1984). Indoor emissions may occur in various ways, including transport of outdoor-generated dust or vapors indoors, or as a result of volatilization of chemicals indoors during use of contaminated water (e.g., during showering, cooking, washing). Accounting for differences in indoor and outdoor concentrations can be crucial. Levels of some pollutants are typically much lower indoors than outdoors (e.g., ozone), while the reverse is true for other pollutants (e.g., styrene). Few models are available for estimating indoor air concentrations originating from outside sources. As a result, most applications make simple assumptions; for instance, indoor concentrations of dust are usually assumed to be some fraction of those outdoors. For vapor transport originating outdoors, concentrations indoors and outdoors are often assumed to be equivalent.

For representing vapor concentrations from indoor emissions, such as where subsurface soil gas or groundwater seepage are entering indoors, *compartmental models* have been developed. Compartmental models account for the multiple sources and sinks of pollutants and the ventilation rates among discrete volumes of air within a building (NAS-NRC, 1982). Such models can be either steady-state or time-segmented to account for dynamics. Indoor models can be as complex as or more complex than outdoor models. For example, even a model of a single room can become quite complex if it incorporates the effects of air filter efficiencies, particulate agglomeration/planting out, nonspecific heterogeneous decay of reactive pollutants, multiple sources and sinks, and varying source strengths (OSTP, 1984).

In addition to transport and dispersion, many atmospheric models account for transformations of airborne risk agents (e.g., photochemical transformations of chemicals or the survival of microorganisms). Such models are necessary in situations where transformation products may pose greater or less hazard than the parent pollutant. The formation of acid rain is one example. Sulfuric acid and nitric acid, the two acids that make up acid rain, are formed in the atmosphere from the gaseous pollutants sulfur dioxide and nitrogen oxides, which are emitted when coal or oil is burned. The formation of these acids in the atmosphere occurs during the chemical reaction of oxidation. Chemical transformation processes and changes in the populations of microorganisms are often approximated by first-order rate reactions. A simple fate model that does not assume constant rate is the Monod equation, often used to represent the growth of microorganisms (Levin and Strauss, 1991). The Monod equation assumes that population growth continues until the available nutrient source is depleted.

To account for more complicated transformation processes, researchers have used more sophisticated models. For example, Stordal and Isakson (1986) have used a two-dimensional atmospheric chemistry model to estimate changes in stratospheric ozone concentrations as a function of atmospheric concentrations of chlorofluorocarbons (CFCs) and other gases. Their model accounts for the following processes: (1) migration of CFCs to the stratosphere, (2) breakdown of CFCs and release of chlorine as a result of ultraviolet radiation, (3) chemical reactions in which chlorine acts as a catalyst to convert two molecules of ozone to three molecules of oxygen, and (4) the return of the chlorine atom to the troposphere, where it is rained out as hydrochloric acid.

3.3.2. Surface-Water Models

Surface-water transport and fate models are similar in several respects to atmospheric transport and fate models. Pollutants in surface water can originate from point sources (e.g., toxic industrial wastes or heated discharges from cooling technologies) or from nonpoint sources (e.g., seepage from groundwater, direct deposition from air, or normal or storm rainfall runoff of pollutants deposited on land). As with atmospheric models, the concentrations produced by surface water depend on the flow and mixing characteristics of the water body and any physical, chemical, radiological, or biological transformations that may occur.

There are, however, certain key differences between surface water and atmospheric models. Pollutants released to water may dissolve (as acids do) or float on the surface (as petroleum products usually do). Volatile pollutants (i.e., benzene and toluene) will tend to escape from water by turning to vapor. Pollutants in dissolved form may be adsorbed from solution onto sediments, or removed by aquatic organisms. Pollutants in the form of particulate matter may settle, or precipitate, to the bottom (as metals often do). Adsorption and precipitation tend to reduce the concentrations in surface water, but create deposits that become long-term pollutant sources through desorption or resuspension processes.

The characteristics of the water body that determine mixing also differ from those important in the atmosphere. Pollutants entering surface water are initially dispersed by currents and local turbulence; subsequent concentrations depend on flushing characteristics. In a lake, for example, the rate at which new water enters from incoming streams and leaves by an outlet stream are important. A shallow lake will tend to be well stirred because wind keeps the waters mixed. In contrast, a deep lake may have a well-stirred surface layer and an unmixed deeper layer. Such lakes are called stratified (i.e., layered). Lake stratification is particularly common in summer when the top 10 feet or so of a lake warms in the sun and floats above the colder, deeper water. Thermal stratification can trap and partition pollutants in the various water layers, causing large concentration gradients and temporarily high concentrations.

Chemical processes can be very important in water. Ionization occurs when water molecules, in effect, pull apart the molecules of the contaminant. The resulting ions are reactive, and readily combine with other ions to create different chemicals that may be more or less toxic, dissolvable, volatile, or likely to bioconcentrate. The rates at which such chemical processes occur often depend on water temperature, oxygen levels, and the acidity of the water. With metals, the less oxygen combined with the metal and the more acidic the water, the more dissolvable the metal. Dissolved metals are more likely to be taken up by plants and ingested by animals. Warmer water typically causes reactions to speed up.

Surface-water models must account for such effects. The objective of most surface-water models is to predict the movement, dilution, partitioning, and degradation of contaminants in surface water. Typical applications include (a) estimating the position and size of plumes and/or mixing zones for point-source discharges; (b) estimating the downstream movement rate, dispersion, and fate of contaminants following spills or other pulse discharge events; and (c) estimating average concentrations as a function of distance for continuous point-source or nonpoint-source discharges. The models are generally designed for specific types of water bodies such as streams, rivers, estuaries, coastal waters, impoundments, reservoirs, or lakes.

Descriptions of the basic principles and uses of dynamic surface-water models can be found in engineering textbooks (e.g., Thomann, 1972); however, implementing these principles can be complicated. Representation of the physical processes responsible for transporting pollutants in water bodies presents many challenges. Models for stratified or partially mixed reservoirs and estuaries can be especially complex. Even calculating the time variation of flow in simple streams can be computationally demanding. Silts and clays are often important pollutant-carrying media, but modeling their deposition and sedimentation processes is difficult. Estuaries also present a particularly difficult case, combining conditions of unsteady flow, uncertain residual circulation, and variable salinity (SETAC, 1987).

Underlying most surface-water models is a set of partial differential equations that describe the movement of water, sediments, and contaminants as defined by the physical laws of conservation of mass and momentum. For example, the concentration of a chemical in a water body might be represented by the *mass-balance equation*. The mass-balance equation states that the rate of change in the concentration c of a chemical in a volume of water V must equal the total inputs of the chemical to the volume minus the total outputs of the chemical from the volume:

$$V\frac{dc}{dt} = \text{Inputs} - \text{Outputs}$$

The various terms that appear in such equations represent specific aspects of relevant phenomena. For example, inputs and outputs would include chemical inflows to and outflows from the water volume from external sources, as well as formations and decays within the volume that are associated with chemical reactions and other processes.

Simpler surface-water models often assume steady-state conditions, complete vertical and lateral mixing, and constant decay rates. The *steady-state* assumption implies that conditions do not change over time but only over distance along the waterway. The assumption of *complete mixing* implies that pollutant concentrations are constant across the entire waterway at all depths and locations. If an assumption of complete mixing is unrealistic, surface-water models often represent the water body as a series of completely mixed, interconnected compartments. Each compartment is then described by a mass-balance equation, with the inputs and outputs for each equation including transfers from other compartments.

For example, a complicated waterway may be divided into reaches, each of which is assumed to be uniform in character (i.e., velocity, depth, etc.). The mass-balance equations are then solved to calculate pollutant concentrations within each reach as a function of distance downstream from the beginning of the reach. The concentrations and flow information at the end of each reach provide the boundary conditions for the next reach and are combined with the appropriate source and flow information for that reach.

Dynamic models have been developed for use in situations where the goal is to simulate contaminant distributions in space and time. The physical and chemical processes represented in these models are the same as in steady-state models; however, dynamic models can simulate the effects of time-varying contaminant inputs and hydrological parameters on contaminant concentrations. Examples include effluent plume models for calculating contaminant concentration or temperature distributions in the vicinity of time-varying point sources (Koh and Fan, 1970), and the various water quality simulation models described by Basta and Bower (1982) and Boutwell and Roberts (1983).

Reviews and evaluations of available surface-water models are presented in the following: Grimsrud *et al.* (1976), Hoffman *et al.* (1977), EPA (1979), Smith *et al.* (1977), Mills *et al.* (1982), Onishi *et al.* (1980; 1981), and Boutwell *et al.* (1986). The models differ according to (a) whether they are steady-state or time-dependent, (b) the types of water bodies to which they apply (c) the number and kinds of pollutants addressed, (d) how transformation and decay processes are treated, and (e) whether they emphasize sediment processes, water quality, or other processes. The review by Onishi *et al.* (1981) groups available models into three categories: (1) *water quality models*, which primarily address the interaction of waste substances and life forms present in water systems, (2) *radionuclide models*, which are designed to track releases of radioactive elements from nuclear power plants, and (3) *sediment models*, which address the movement of sediment through water systems.

3.3.3. Groundwater Models

Groundwater models are used to estimate the fate of contaminants that enter groundwater. Most groundwater models have been developed to analyze the transport of chemicals leached from hazardous waste disposal sites.

Once a contaminant enters the groundwater flow system, its motion is determined largely by underground water-flow patterns. These patterns depend on local geohydrological features such as the location of aquifers (i.e., saturated layers in the soil and rock that are generally more permeable than the geological units directly below them), natural water recharge, infiltration and withdrawal rates, and factors that influence the density of the fluid (such as temperature and brine concentration). Whether or not groundwater flow is present, contaminants can be transported by dispersion through molecular diffusion. In many cases, however, a large proportion of contaminants in groundwater are absorbed into the soil, thus greatly retarding their movement relative to that of the groundwater. In addition, as in other media, contaminants in groundwater can be transformed through chemical reactions or biological breakdown.

The objective of most groundwater models is to calculate the distribution of contaminants in the unsaturated soil around the sources of leached pollutants (such as disposal sites) and in the saturated soil of aquifers. One output of primary concern in risk assessment is the concentration of pollutants in groundwater used for irrigation and drinking. Groundwater models are often complex, due to the many physical and chemical processes that may affect transport and transformation in groundwater. The important mechanisms that may have to be addressed include contaminants leaching from the surface, advection (including infiltration, flow through the unsaturated zone, and flow with groundwater), dispersion, sorption (including adsorption, desorption, and ion exchange), and transformation (including biological degradation, hydrolysis, oxidation, reduction, complexation, dissolution, and precipitation). The fact that not all chemicals may be dissolved in water means that groundwater models may have to represent chemicals that float on top of groundwater or sink to the bottom of the aquifer.

Groundwater transport and fate models typically include two components: a model for groundwater flow and a model for contaminant transport. *Groundwater flow models* define the convective flow field and provide estimates of water velocities or flow paths and travel times. The basic equations underlying flow models are based on theories of groundwater hydrology. For example, the equation used to describe an aquifer system is either one defining a fluid flow continuum in porous media, or one defining a porous media equivalent flow for a fracture flow dominated system (Bolton *et al.*, 1983). Based on the results of the groundwater flow model, the contaminant transport model estimates the migration of contaminants, taking into account dispersion and retention. The *contaminant transport model* may also account for degradation and transformation of the pollutants.

Since groundwater systems are interconnected over vast geographic distances, appropriate limits must be placed on the geographical scale of the groundwater model. This is typically accomplished through the specification of *boundary conditions*, which describe flow and transport conditions along the perimeter of the modeled area. Boundary conditions can include the specification of fluid and concentration fluxes across the boundary and water-table elevation and contaminant concentrations at the boundary. For example, boundary conditions would include the locations of streams, lakes, and pumping wells and their contribution to discharge and recharge of groundwater, the locations of impermeable geological features across which no-flow conditions occur, the quantity of rainfall infiltrating the subsurface, and the concentrations of source contaminants.

Distinct types of models using different assumptions are usually required to describe groundwater flow and contaminant transport in the unsaturated and saturated zones. The *unsaturated zone* normally extends down from the surface to the groundwater table; the *saturated zone* includes the volume below the water table. Flow and transport in the unsaturated zone are typically dominated by vertical movement. Water in an aquifer, however, tends to flow in horizontal directions along the bedding plane of the more permeable geological formation because the resistance to flow is less. The less-permeable (*aquitard*) or impermeable (*aquiclude*) layers below, and sometimes above, the aquifer tend to retard or completely block the vertical flow. As a result, one-dimensional models are often adequate for describing groundwater flow in saturated zones.

Due to their independence, some physical transport mechanisms (i.e., filtration and diffusion) can be treated separately for each contaminant. Other processes, generally chemical in nature (e.g., ion exchange reactions and precipitation), must be modeled simultaneously for all contaminants present in the water, as these mechanisms can interact or compete with each other. Basic retentive phenomena, however, are usually not specifically distinguished in groundwater models. Their total effects are typically represented by a constant ratio between the amount of contaminant retained on rocks or soil and the amount in solution. These linear distribution coefficients are defined either per unit mass of the soil or rock or by unit area of fractures. The *linear assumption* implies that each element migrates independently in a unique chemical form and that retention is instantaneous and reversible.

Hundreds of different groundwater models have been described in the literature, and many have been reviewed, summarized, and tabulated by different authors including: Bachmat *et al.* (1978), Knox and Canter (1980), Lappala (1980), Moiser *et al.* (1980), Science Applications, Inc. (1981); Koines (1982); Nelson (1982); Onishi *et al.* (1982), Oster (1982), Kincaid *etal.* (1983), Boutwell *et al.* (1986), and the EPA (1988c). Each model has its own specific assumptions and limitations. The proper selection and application of groundwater models requires a thorough understanding of the physical, chemical, and hydrogeologic characteristics of the site. The EPA has published various guidance documents for the selection of groundwater models (e.g., EPA, 1988d).

3.3.4. Watershed Runoff Models

Many of the pollutants deposited on plants, rocks, and soil end up largely in lakes and streams. Pesticides and other soluble pollutants, for example, are typically flushed out by rain into water bodies. Even pollutants that adhere tightly to soil particles eventually find their way to water bodies; for instance, heavy metals adhering to soil particles can be transported through soil erosion. *Watershed runoff models* focus on surface transport of contaminants—transport driven by rainfall, overland water flow (runoff), and erosion. These models are generally designed to estimate nonpoint-source pollutant delivery to streams and other surface-water bodies and pollutant infiltration through the soil into the groundwater. Substance-specific factors such as sorption characteristics, solubility (which may depend on soil pH), degradation (such as biodegradation by soil micoorganisms), and volatility (which depends on meteorological conditions) affect rates of removal and delivery to surface water. Thus, watershed models must account for the chemical characteristics of the watershed as well as the basic hydrologic characteristics. The number of soil chemical phenomena included and the sophistication of simulated chemical processes vary widely among available models.

Despite this diversity of components, most available watershed models incorporate the same or very similar mathematics. A simple approach is to base the model on mass-balance equations that consider all important sources and sinks for the pollutant, including atmospheric deposition, deposition in irrigation water, uptake by plants, leaching into subsurface soil, runoff into surface water, and accumulation in surface soil. The model may represent the drainage basin as a whole, without accounting for the spatial distribution of contaminants within the basin, or it may represent the region under study on a grid or map that accounts for variations in hydrologic processes and contamination distributions from point to point throughout the basin. These *grid-type models* generally divide the area under study into subregions within which the mass-balancing equations are applied. For example, the quantity of pollutant in a volume of surface soil at the end of a particular time period might be determined by the background pollutant concentration in the soil at the beginning of the period, the deposition rate, and the rate at which the pollutant leaves the soil volume. Pollutants can leave through runoff, plant uptake, or infiltration into deeper soil layers and groundwater (Bolton *et al.*, 1985).

Processes controlling runoff, soil erosion, and overland contaminant transport are essentially continuous. Thus, watershed runoff models are often continuous simulation models that describe runoff flow and runoff quality within a drainage basin over an extended period (e.g., 1 year). The bulk of contaminant migration over an extended period, however, is often concentrated in a few storm events that produce runoff. Thus, discrete *storm event models* that describe response to a single storm (perhaps in storm-averaged form) tend to be more widely used than continuous simulation models.

Many models of overland contaminant transport are basically modified versions of *erosion models*. Erosion involves two steps: detachment of soil particles from the land surface, and transport of these particles by overland flow. Soil detachment is dependent upon a number of factors, such as particle cohesiveness, organic-matter content of the soil profile, rainfall intensity, vegetative cover, slope gradient, slope length, and soil cultural practices (Wischmeier and Smith, 1978). Thus, erosion models calculate erosion as a function of rainfall, soil characteristics, slope, and vegetative cover. Modifying the models to reflect overland transport of contaminants entails accounting for the properties of the contaminants themselves (e.g., solubility and degradability); simple partition coefficients and first-order rate constants are generally used. For example, Mills *et al.* (1982) describe a model for the overland transport of pesticides based on the universal soil loss equation (Wischmeier and Smith, 1965) but modified to account for pesticide degradation and volatilization. More complex models of runoff and erosion are also available (see Donigian, 1981; Basta and Bower, 1982; Crawford, 1982). In these models the universal soil loss equation is replaced by mechanistic descriptions of hydrological processes such as interception, evapotranspiration, infiltration, percolation, and interflow. Several summaries of overland models have been prepared, including ones developed by EPA (1976), Bolton *et al.* (1983), and Bolton *et al.* (1985).

3.3.5. Food-Chain Models

Small amounts of persistent substances (i.e., substances not metabolized or biodegraded) can reach large environmental concentrations if they are captured by plants and animals and then transferred to other animals and microorganisms in a stepwise fashion through the food chain. This process is known as *bioconcentration* or *bioaccumulation*. Persistent substances include organochlorine insecticides (e.g., dieldrin, and PCBs), heavy metals (e.g., mercury and lead), and radioactive materials (e.g., strontium-90, cesium-137, and iodine-131). Risk assessments often employ food-chain models to account for exposure to such substances.

Bioaccumulation of persistent substances occurs in aquatic organisms as well as in other animals and in certain plants. In the case of aquatic organisms, the accumulation and concentration of toxic materials can occur through processes of absorption and adsorption as well as through metabolic mechanisms. These processes and mechanisms vary according to species characteristics, feeding habits, and environmental variables such as water temperature and salinity (Moghissi *et al.*, 1980). In the case of nonaquatic animals, pollutants may be concentrated within animal organs or products as a result of the animal's consuming contaminated vegetation, drinking contaminated water, or inhaling pollutants. In the case of plants, pollutants may reach the plant via deposition from the atmosphere, irrigation, application of pesticides, or uptake from groundwater. Once in the plant, pollutants behave in different ways. Some elements (e.g., arsenic, beryllium, chromium, lead, nickel, and vanadium) accumulate normally in the roots, whereas others (e.g., cadmium, copper, and zinc) move freely to leaves and other edible portions of the plant (Kabata-Pendias and Pendias, 1984).

In general, the transfer of toxic pollutants through food chains is poorly understood. Consequently, most food-chain models use a simplified approach based on empirically derived concentration or bioaccumulation factors and on estimates of consumption rates for the contaminated food product. For example, estimates of exposures from a contaminated aquatic species are generally based on bioaccumulation factors that relate the pollutant concentration in the organisms to that of the surrounding water. These factors may be derived from experimental data for the pollutant of interest or inferred from data obtained for materials that are expected to behave similarly. When no bioaccumulation factor is available from direct measurement, it is often estimated based on parameters called *octanol/water partition coefficients*, denoted K_{ow}. This coefficient measures the tendency of a chemical to remain in water versus partition to octanol, which is used as a surrogate for lipids (fat). Through a regression equation, the K_{ow} value may be used to predict bioconcentration in aquatic organisms.

Likewise, the concentration of a pollutant in animal products such as meat, milk, or eggs is often calculated from the animal's feed and water consumption rates, the pollutant concentration in the animal's feed and water, and the transfer

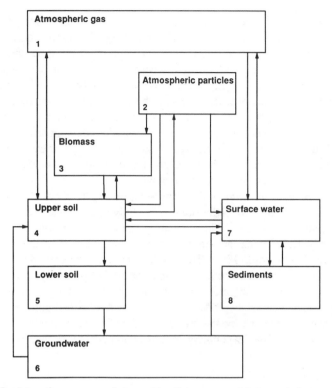

FIGURE 17.   Interactions among media in a multimedia transport model. Arrows indicate contaminant transfer. (Based on McKone and Layton, 1986.)

coefficients that give the fractional transfer of contaminants between food and water and the animal's products. To translate estimated pollutant concentrations in animals and plants to the concentrations in the food products that people actually ingest, food-chain models must account for any changes in concentration that occur during processing of the product by the producer or preparation by the consumer.

3.3.6. Multimedia Models

If the transport of a pollutant through the environment involves significant transfers and interactions among various media (e.g., air to land to groundwater), the pollutant transport and fate model may require coupling individual media models. Solvents buried in landfills, for example, often move from soil to the air or from soil to groundwater and surface water. *Multimedia models* simulate the transport and transformation of chemicals or other pollutants in multiple environmental media.

An example of a multimedia transport model is that described by McKone and Layton (1986). As illustrated in Fig. 17, this model views the environment as composed of eight interacting compartments. The compartments represent major components of the environmental system (including air, water, and soil) that exchange physical quantities such as thermal energy, chemical contaminants, or nutrients. Each compartment contains matter in one of three phases: solid, liquid, or gas. A chemical is assumed to be in chemical equilibrium among the phases of a single compartment; however, there is no requirement for equilibrium between adjacent compartments. Physicochemical and transfer properties are used to estimate the interphase transport rates, and a computer program is used to obtain the transient mass balance of a chemical contaminant in the multicompartment environment.

In general, multimedia models can be based on a fully coupled approach in which submodels for each media pathway are fully integrated as shown in Fig. 17, or on a composite approach wherein appropriate models are selected and loosely combined by transferring the output files of one pathway model to the input files of the next (Bolton et al., 1983). The development of fully coupled, computerized multimedia models is a considerable undertaking that generally requires a large amount of input data, computer core size, and run time; however, interconnecting existing media models to produce a composite is also difficult because most individual environmental models are not designed for interaction with other models. (Basic issues of model coupling are discussed in detail in Chapter 5.)

3.3.7. Exposure-Route Models

Exposure-route models are used to address a basic problem in risk assessment: how to convert the output of pollutant transport and fate models into the doses

TABLE 12.   Measures and Units Typically Used for Expressing Pollutant Concentrations in Various Media

Medium	Measures	Typical units
Air	Weight of pollutant per unit volume or mass of air	$\mu g/m^3$ — micrograms per cubic meter ppm — parts per million (by weight)
Air	Volume of pollutant per unit volume of air	ppm — parts per million (by volume)
Water	Weight of pollutant per unit volume or mass of water	mg/l — milligrams per liter ppm — parts per million (by weight)
Food	Weight of pollutant per unit weight of food	mg/kg — milligrams per kilogram ppm — parts per million (by weight)
Soil	Weight of pollutant per unit weight of soil	mg/kg — milligram per kilogram ppm — parts per million (by weight)

TABLE 13.   General Equation for Estimating Chemical Intake[a]

$$I = \frac{C \times CR \times EF \times EP}{BW}$$

I	=	Intake (mg/kg-body weight)
C	=	Average concentration in the media during the exposure period
CR	=	Contact rate, the amount of contaminated medium contacted per unit time or event
EF	=	Exposure frequency (days/year)
EP	=	Exposure period (years)[b]
BW	=	Body weight, the average body weight over the exposure period (kg)[c]

---

[a]Adapted from EPA (1989a).
[b]Typical values for exposure period (EP) are 70 years for lifetime exposures and 9 years at one residence.
[c]Typical body weight (BW) values are 70 kg for adults (70kg for men, 60 kg for women) and 20 kg for children (16 kg for children under 6 years). Situation-specific values should be used in actual risk assessments.

actually received by individuals.[*] The measures and scales by which such models represent exposure depend on the route of exposure, which might be inhalation, ingestion, or dermal contact. For example, *inhalation exposure* is often expressed in terms of an average inhaled concentration over a given time period. Ingestion exposure is often expressed as an average pollutant concentration in total food consumption. *Dermal exposure*, a less standard measure, might be expressed in terms of pollutant concentration in the contact medium averaged for continuous, whole-body exposure.

In general, exposure-route models estimate an individual's pollutant intake by multiplying the pollutant concentration in the medium (provided by a pollutant transport and fate model) by an estimated intake rate for that medium times the duration or period over which the individual is exposed to the contaminated medium. Table 12 lists the units typically used to express pollutant concentrations in various media. Table 13 presents the general equation used for computing an intake rate for chronic exposures to chemicals, and Table 14 provides some

---

[*] It is not always clear when a given model dealing with aspects of pollutant intake should be regarded as an exposure-route model (and therefore part of an overall exposure model) or as part of a dose-response model (and therefore part of an overall consequence model). The choice depends in part on whether the exposed entity is an individual, or a target organ (e.g., the lung or liver). In applying the taxonomic framework for categorizing risk assessment methods described in Chapter 1, we have chosen to treat the individual as the exposed entity. Therefore, models describing the activities of pollutants once they have entered the body are discussed in terms of consequence assessment (see Chapter 4). In some situations (see below) it may be more convenient to treat the target organ as the exposed entity and include aspects of pollutant transport through the body as part of an exposure-route model.

TABLE 14. Some Typical Parameter Values and Assumptions for Estimating Chemical Intake[a]

Pathway	C (concentration)	CR (contact rate)		EF (exposure frequency)
Ingestion of drinking water	Chemical in drinking water (mg/liter)	1.4 liter/day (adult); 2.0 liter/day (man)—1.4 liter/day (woman); 1.4 liter/day (child)		365 days/yr
Ingestion of surface water while swimming	Chemical in recreational surface water (mg/liter)	$CR = IR \times SD$	IR = Ingestion rate = .05 l/hr SD = Swim duration = 2.6 hrs/swim	7 swims/yr
Dermal absorption through contact with water while swimming	Chemical in recreational surface water (mg/liter)	$CR = SA \times PC \times SD \times CF$	SA = Skin surface area = 1.8 m² (adult), 1.94 m² (man), 1.69 m² (woman) PC = Chemical dermal permeability constant (e.g., 8.4×10^{-6} m/hr for water) SD = Swim duration = 2.6 hrs/swim CF = Conversion factor 1000 liter/m³	7 swims/yr
Ingestion of chemicals in soil	Chemical in soil (mg/kg)	$CR = IR \times CF$	IR = Ingestion rate = 200 mg/day (child ≤ 6 yrs) 100 mg/day (child > 6 yrs) CF = Conversion factor = 10^{-6} kg/mg	Depends on context (days/yr)

Dermal absorption through contact with soil	Chemical in soil (mg/kg)	$CR = SA \times AF \times ABS \times CF$	SA = Exposed skin surface area (m²/contact): = Adults: arms—.23, hands—.082, = Children (≤ 6 yrs): arms—.11, hands—.041, legs—.24	Depends on context; children 3 contacts/wk during school yr, 5 contacts/wk summer
			AF = Soil adherence factor = 1.45 mg/cm² (potting soil) = 2.77 mg/cm² (clay)	
			ABS = Chemical absorption factor (unitless)	
			CF = Conversion factor = 10^{-6} kg/mg $\times 10^4$ cm²/m²	
Inhalation of airborne (vapor phase) chemicals	Contaminant in air (mg/m³)	Inhalation rate = 20 m³/day (adult); 15 m³/day (child); .07 m³/shower		365 days/yr; 365 showers/yr
Ingestion of fish and shellfish	Contaminant in fish (mg/kg)	$CR = IR \times FI$	IR = Ingestion rate = .113 kg/meal (fin fish), FI = Fraction ingested from contaminated source	48 meals/yr (fish, shellfish)
Ingestion of contaminated fruits and vegetables	Contaminant in food (mg/kg)	$CR = IR \times FI$	IR = Ingestion rate (kg/meal - depends on fruit and vegetable type) FI = Fraction ingested from contaminated source = homegrown fruit—.20, homegrown vegetables—.25	Depends on context (meals/yr)

[a] Adapted from ICRP (1975), EPA (1989a)

common numeric assumptions. As indicated, intake is typically expressed per unit of time and per unit of exposed individual body weight. Thus, in the case of exposures through the food chain, the basic elements of the model for ingestion are: the concentration of the contaminant in each item of the diet (obtained from a food-chain model), the amount consumed (portion size) of each item that contains the contaminant, the frequency with which each item is consumed, and the average body weight over the exposure period.

Average consumption rates are generally used in estimating food intake. For example, *market basket analysis* typically produces an average or representative intake. Estimates of per capita food intake are typically calculated by dividing the sum of annual production plus imports of a given food item by the number of people in the country. Bolton *et al.* (1983) provide default consumption rates for various regional population groups for a number of animal and vegetable products, aquatic organisms, and drinking water. To obtain intake estimates for special groups with high intake rates, analysts often rely on dietary surveys in which consumers are asked to recall what foods they ate with what frequency and in what amounts over a defined period of time (Food Safety Council, 1980).

In the case of dermal contact, "intake" is estimated through an analogous process. For example, if the concern is dermal exposure at a polluted water recreational facility, exposure rates would be calculated using data on the length of the exposure period, the concentration of the pollutant in the recreational water, and the fraction of the body area exposed (which would depend on the recreational activity). If the concern is dermal contact through domestic water supplies, on the other hand, the efficiency of domestic water treatment processes would have to be accounted for by the model because such processes can remove significant fractions of dissolved and suspended pollutants. If the concern is dermal exposure to radiation, the body is typically regarded as being "immersed" in a radioactive field. As described in Chapter 2, the standard units of exposure measurement are the sievert and the rem.

If the pollutant is present in multiple media or if multiple exposure routes exist, each must be modeled separately. For example, to obtain the total dose originating from the concentration of a substance in water, it may be necessary to estimate the dose due to (1) direct ingestion through drinking, (2) skin absorption (from water during washing and bathing), (3) inhalation (from contaminants in the air resulting from showering, bathing, and other uses of water), (4) ingestion of plants and animals exposed to the water, and (5) skin absorption from contact with soil exposed to the water. It may be appropriate to sum the doses received by each individual route; however, this is seldom the case, since the toxic effects of many substances depend on the route of exposure. For example, inhaled chromium is carcinogenic to the lung, but it appears that ingested chromium is not. The extent to which exposures from different routes must be dealt with separately depends on how the pollutant behaves once it enters the body, a subject that is addressed more thoroughly in Chapter 4.

3.3.8. Population Models

For a model to estimate populations at risk from a given pathway of exposure, at least two aspects of the exposed populations must be accounted for: demographics and activity. Other characteristics of the population such as the presence of hypersensitive individuals may also need to be considered. For example, to estimate human populations at risk, one must determine who works or lives at various sites and who breathes the air, drinks the water, eats the food, or uses the products affected by a particular risk source. *Population models* provide this information by describing the population at risk.

Typically, population models disaggregate the exposed population into distinct population groups based on characteristics that increase the probability or severity of health effects occurring to members of the group. The characteristics used to define population groups are called risk factors and fall into two basic categories: lifestyle and genetic. *Lifestyle risk factors* include age, socioeconomic status, and behavioral traits or factors influencing exposure levels. *Genetic risk factors* are inherited characteristics, such as sex, that determine an individual's ability to deal with environmental insults. Hypersusceptible groups might be identified on the basis of capacity for enzymatic detoxification or elimination of harmful chemicals, immunologic competence, and developmental or metabolic abnormalities and predispositions to specific diseases. For example, the populations most susceptible to microorganisms are those whose immune systems have been compromised or are less effective, such as persons undergoing drug therapy for cancer, those with nutritional deficiencies, and those with diseases such as AIDS.

In its simplest form, a population model computes an integrated exposure for an individual within a population group by summing the products of the concentrations encountered by the individual in each microenvironment and the time spent in that microenvironment. Average exposures for any averaging period can be computed by dividing the integrated exposure by the time duration of the average period. At a minimum, a population model must include data on the distinct microenvironments visited by a representative individual from each population group, the concentration of the risk agent in each of those microenvironments, and the average time spent in each microenvironment. Population models typically include submodels for the population distribution within a geographic area surrounding the source of risk (e.g., a dam, power plant, aircraft flight path), submodels of the age distribution of a given population over time, and submodels of mobility and activity patterns of sensitive population groups.

An example of a detailed population model is the National Ambient Air Quality Standard Exposure Model, which is designed for estimating exposures of urban populations to carbon monoxide (Johnson and Paul, 1982). The model generates data on hour-by-hour movements of representative population groups through districts of a city and through selected microenvironments within each district over a period of one year. Another example, the Simulation of Human Air Pollution Exposures (SHAPE) model, combines data on activity patterns of the population with statistical descriptions of pollutant concentrations in specified microenvironments (Ott, 1984). SHAPE uses fourteen microenvironments, and exposures are computed on a person-by-person basis with a time resolution of one minute. The resulting 24-hour exposure profile is then computed for each person, and the frequency distribution of exposures for the population is generated.

If the entities of concern are plants and wildlife rather than humans, population models are needed to estimate the numbers and characteristics of the species that may be exposed. The difficulties associated with human population models are also present here, as well as several additional complicating factors. Most significantly, aquatic and terrestrial wildlife are composed of numerous species with different sensitivities and habits. At a minimum, this complication means that the population model must account individually for each important species or ecosystem exposed; in some cases, this is relatively straightforward. Population models for exposures of many types of aquatic species, for example, are a case in point. When pollutants are fairly evenly distributed in water, there is little need to account for the movement of aquatic species from location to location. With most wildlife, however, modeling the geographical location and behavior of each species is often critical. A population model for a critical species may need to account for feeding behavior, range patterns, and the extent to which individuals of the species are attracted to or repelled by a risk agent. As is the case with humans, some individuals within an animal population may be exposed to greater amounts of a risk agent than the average because of group status, habitat choice, specialized feeding habits, or other factors. Variations may also be related to sex and age, or to individual differences within a sex or age class.

The basic input for most population models is detailed, current demographic data. Compiling such data is often difficult but usually straightforward. Important sources for demographic data include census data, atlases, and environmental or safety reports. Data necessary for characterizing sensitive populations are particularly important, yet often difficult to obtain. Examples include the numbers and characteristics of people living in areas served by a particular drinking water supply, participating in specific recreational activities (e.g., swimmers, fishermen, joggers, and boaters), having particular dietary habits (consumers of seafood or home garden produce), or living in specific subregions (e.g., near sources). Sensitive subpopulations that might be identified include those that are particularly susceptible to specific health effects because of their age or health characteristics (such as asthmatics exposed to airborne toxic chemicals, cigarette smokers exposed to asbestos, pregnant women exposed to methylmercury, or the elderly exposed to influenza). Often the geographic location of certain public facilities such as hospitals, schools, nursing homes, recreational areas, and private wells provides useful information on important subpopulations. Detailed population data are especially needed for regional exposure assessments that use site-specific data on pollutant releases, environmental fate, and ambient levels.

Ideally, a population model should account for all important characteristics that might influence the effects produced by the exposure of concern, including variations by sex, health status, age, food consumption, distance from the source, and other exposures (e.g., medicines, cigarettes, or occupational risk agents). Thus, it may be necessary to subdivide the population into a relatively large number of population subgroups. For example, an EPA risk assessment for formaldehyde delineated more than 25 potentially exposed subgroups and estimated exposure levels for each (EPA, 1984a). Often, however, the data necessary for defining the characteristics of subgroups are not available and are simply assumed or estimated. As a result, little attention may be given to the variability in the exposed population. For instance, in national exposure assessments, it is still common to use an average population density for the total United States or to distinguish only between rural and urban densities.

3.3.9. Strengths

The major strength of modeling methods for exposure assessment is that they provide a means for estimating exposures in the absence of comprehensive monitoring data. Models generally provide the only formal means for estimating exposures that might result from future actions. Although the complexity and uniqueness of exposure processes generally require that exposure models be tailored to specific applications, the fundamental principles on which the models are based are nearly universal. Consequently, the basic equations that govern many exposure models are identical or very similar. Thus a broad range of exposure problems are addressed by advancements in representing basic physical phenomena such as the transport of groundwater or the diffusion of gases in the atmosphere.

3.3.10. Limitations

Most uncertainties in modeling exposures are not caused by inherent deficiencies in modeling techniques. Instead, they arise from lack of understanding and lack of data on transport and fate processes and from difficulties in predicting population behaviors that may contribute to or result in exposures. For example, in the case of atmospheric transport models, major uncertainties surround estimates of the dry deposition rates of particulate matter, which in turn affect estimates of the average level of pollution at various distances from an emissions source. Similarly, major uncertainties also surround estimates of the wet deposition caused by rainfall, which in turn may affect the low-probability, high-consequence tails of the distributions of exposures.

In the case of food-chain models, some pathways by which chemicals enter the food chain are often omitted due to a lack of knowledge. For instance, foliar uptake may be omitted from the model but may nonetheless be as crucial as root uptake in the transport of volatile chemicals deposited on soil. Similarly, metabolic transformation of chemicals by plants and their subsequent incorporation into the food chain may be difficult to estimate due to lack of knowledge and the complexity of the processes involved. The regression equation approach to estimating bioaccumulation factors based on octanol/water partition coefficients can overstate concentrations in fish tissue depending upon the chemical of concern and the studies used to develop the regression equations. For example, polycyclic aromatic hydrocarbons (PAHs), found in mixtures in fossil fuels and by-products of fossil fuels, can cause cancer in humans. PAHs with high molecular weights and high K_{ow} values, such as benzo(a)pyrene, lead to the prediction of high fish-tissue residues; however, PAHs are rapidly metabolized and do not appear to accumulate significantly in fish. Regression equations using K_{ow} cannot take into account such pharmacokinetics, and thus may overestimate bioconcentration (EPA, 1989a).

In the case of aquatic transport models, major uncertainties often surround estimates of groundwater transport and sedimentation in rivers. Even if the transport portion of a fate-and-transport model is appropriate for a risk assessment, the fate portion may not be. In the case of surface water models, the effects of biodegradation and the removal of pollutants from soils, sediments, and muds are often poorly represented. For example, the effect of temperature on biodegradation is not well understood. More generally, very little is known about how enzymes break down molecules or about structural characteristics of molecules that inhibit breakdown (SETAC, 1987). The problems are particularly significant if the risk agent is a microorganism. In exposure assessments of microorganisms, a common practice is to couple a transport model developed for particles to a simple fate-model describing the growth or death of the organisms; however, simple fate-models such as a first-order rate equation or the Monad equation represent steady-state conditions only and fail to account for transient conditions likely to be found after a microorganism is introduced into a new environmental setting. Also, if the microorganism is a genetically engineered organism in which DNA has been introduced, then the fate of the DNA rather than the organisms is what is important. As noted in Chapter 2, DNA may remain in the introduced microorganism, be lost from the introduced microorganism and degraded, and/or be transferred from the introduced microorganism into other microbes. Furthermore, because both the DNA and microorganism can replicate, conservation of mass, which lies at the heart of the transport equation, may not necessarily hold.

Exposure-route modeling can also be highly uncertain. Even when ample information is available for computing average exposure rates, the use of such averages can obscure population variations. For example, to estimate ingestion of contaminants in drinking water, risk assessors often assume a lifetime average ingestion rate of 0.03 liters of drinking water for each kilogram of body weight. Some sensitive population groups may, however, have a much higher (or lower) intake rate. Formula-fed infants and young children, for instance, have average intake rates that are as much as eight times greater than those of average adults (Cothern *et al.*, 1986).

CHAPTER 4

CONSEQUENCE ASSESSMENT

Consequence assessment is the process of describing and quantifying the relationship between exposures to a risk agent and the adverse health and/or environmental consequences that result from such exposures. Performing a consequence assessment typically means determining, as a function of the various possible exposure conditions, (a) the adverse human health effects, including fatalities, illnesses, or injuries, and/or (b) the adverse environmental effects, including ecological damage and the resulting losses to human welfare.

This chapter describes the major health and environmental effects produced by exposures to risk agents and evaluates the various methods used in consequence assessment. So far, most research has focused on human health effects rather than environmental effects, and our discussion reflects this emphasis. Similar to the other steps in risk assessment, the methods for consequence assessment include methods based on monitoring, testing, statistical analysis, and modeling.

4.1. EFFECTS OF RISK AGENTS ON HUMAN HEALTH

A wide variety of adverse health effects can be produced by exposures to risk agents. Table 15, for example, lists human health effects recognized by the EPA (EPA, 1987b). The nature of an effect can be minor and temporary (such as a minor infection, rash, or injury) or severe and permanent (such as irreversible organ damage and death). The spectrum of possibilities includes (Whyte and Burton, 1980):

- Minor physiological change
- Temporary emotional effects
- Behavioral changes
- Discomfort
- Temporary minor illness
- Minor disability

127

TABLE 15. Human Health Effects Identified by the U.S. Environmental Protection Agency[a]

Cancer	Noncancer
Lung	Cardiovascular (e.g., increased heart attacks)
Colon	Developmental (e.g., birth defects)
Breast	Hematopoietic (e.g., impaired heme [blood] synthesis)
Pancreas	Immunological (e.g., increased infections)
Prostate	Kidney (e.g., dysfunction)
Stomach	Liver (e.g., Hepatitis A)
Leukemia	Mutagenic (e.g., hereditary disorders)
Other cancers	Neurotoxic/Behavioral (e.g., retardation)
	Reproductive (e.g., increased spontaneous abortions)
	Respiratory (e.g., emphysema)
	Other (e.g., gastrointestinal)

[a]EPA (1987b).

• Chronic debilitating disease

• Severe acute illness or major disability

• Premature death of one individual

• Premature death of many individuals

The nature and the severity of a health effect depend on several factors. In addition to the amount of the risk agent to which the individual is exposed, the potency or toxicity of the agent is important. Arsenic, for example, is more toxic than table salt; however, a sufficiently large dose of even table salt can be lethal. Another important factor is the frequency and/or duration of exposure. Exposures at low doses for long durations can sometimes produce effects similar to a single, short-term exposure at a high dosage. The environmental conditions of exposure are also important, including the presence or absence of other risk agents. Factors specific to the exposed individual that influence the effect of exposure include the individual's genetic inheritance, age, sex, health status, lifestyle, diet, and the effectiveness of the exposed person's natural defense mechanisms. Finally, most chemicals will undergo metabolic changes in the body. As noted previously, metabolic changes can convert chemicals with minor toxicity to more toxic forms. Metabolic processes can also detoxify chemicals and expedite excretion of potentially harmful substances from the body.

Although these considerations may seem especially relevant when the risk agent is a toxic substance, they are applicable regardless of the risk agent. Thus, Fiksel and Covello (1986) note that the health effects caused by exposure to genetically engineered pathogenic microorganisms are likely to depend on (a) the number of infecting microorganisms, (b) the intrinsic characteristics of the microorganisms, such as invasiveness, toxin production, and resistance to the body's defense mechanisms, (c) the general health status of the exposed individual, and (d) the effectiveness of the individual's natural defense mechanisms and barriers including skin, microflora, local antibodies, and the immune system.

Additional considerations are relevant when the risk agent is a toxic chemical. The adverse health effects of chemicals depend on (a) the route by which the chemical enters the body, and (b) changes in the chemical as it moves through the body. For example, if a chemical is ingested through food or drinking water, the primary route of entry is the gastrointestinal tract. If the chemical is present in the air (e.g., as a gas, aerosol, or particle) the primary route of entry is the lungs. If the concentration is high enough, the risk agent may cause irritation at the point of initial contact (e.g., irritation of the skin, gastrointestinal tract, lungs, or eyes). Most often, however, toxicity occurs after the chemical (a) passes through a natural protective barrier (e.g., the wall of the gastrointestinal tract or the skin), and (b) enters the blood or lymph. Once a toxic substance is circulating in the bloodstream, it has access to almost all of the body's internal organs. Toxic substances, however, are not equally damaging to all the organ systems with which they come into contact. The organs that are most susceptible to damage are called *target organs*. The target organ is often not the site of the chemical's highest concentration, but rather the site of the highest damage potential.

In general, adverse health effects may be *acute* (short-term) or *chronic* (long-term). Acute adverse health effects occur within seconds or days. Examples of acute adverse health effects include skin burns and poisonings. Chronic adverse health effects, by comparison, last longer and develop over a longer period of time. Examples of chronic adverse health effects include cancer, birth defects, genetic damage, and degenerative illnesses. Acute and chronic adverse health effects may be produced by exposures that are acute and/or chronic. For example, a chronic adverse health effect can be caused by an acute exposure. Acute exposure can result from either a single exposure or multiple exposures within a short period of time.

The health effect most frequently considered in consequence assessment is death. Other types of health effects that are often estimated fall into four general categories: cancer, reproductive and developmental effects, clinical effects, and subclinical effects.

4.1.1. Cancer

Cancer is a disease (more accurately, a group of diseases) characterized by the malignant, uncontrolled growth of cells. Cancer may be exhibited at various sites within the body and through the development of various kinds of tumors. Carcinogenesis—the induction and formation of cancerous tumors—is a multistep process involving at least three distinct stages. In the first stage, *initiation*, a change occurs in the genetic material (DNA) of a cell. The change primes the cell for the next stage, called *promotion*. With promotion, the cell begins to multiply, forming a tumor. The third and final stage is called *proliferation*. In this stage, some cells break away from the tumor, enter the bloodstream or lymphatic system, and colonize other tissues. This process is called *metastasis*; and when this occurs, the original tumor is referred to as being malignant (benign tumors do not metastasize). Cancer becomes fatal only after metastasis has occurred. Since progression between stages can be slow, the time (*latency period*) between a cancer-causing event and malignancy can be long.

How carcinogens alter cells to produce the various stages of cancer is not fully known. Some risk agents, such as radiation, are capable of causing both initiation and promotion (*complete carcinogens*), whereas other agents only initiate, and a second agent called a promoter must act in order for a tumor to form. The cause of metastasis is even less well understood (OSTP, 1985; Health and Welfare Canada, 1992a).

Various classification systems are used by government agencies and international institutions to specify a "weight of evidence" for inferring whether or not specific substances should be considered carcinogenic. The EPA, for example, classifies substances into five basic groups (carcinogen, probable carcinogen, possible carcinogen, not yet classified, and evidence of noncarcinogenicity in humans). In most such systems, human data are needed before a substance is considered a proven carcinogen. Although hundreds of substances have been associated with cancer, there is sufficient direct evidence of carcinogenicity in humans for only about 30 chemicals and industrial processes (IARC, 1982; 1987). For reference, Table 16 provides one list of chemicals and physical risk agents regarded to be proven carcinogens.

4.1.2. Reproductive and Developmental Effects

The male and female reproductive systems and the developing fetus are particularly sensitive to many risk agents. Examples of adverse reproductive effects induced by chemical or physical agents include infertility, miscarriages, and defects in the fetus. Heritable genetic effects are a special class of reproductive effects that occur when a risk agent damages the DNA structure of the chromosomes and alters the behavior of the genes of the affected cells. Risk agents that cause birth defects are termed *teratogens*. The effects of teratogens on offspring range from subtle malfunctions to abnormal skeletal or muscle structure and mental retardation. Heritable reproductive or developmental effects are of special concern because they may be cumulative over many generations. Substances that have been associated

TABLE 16. Chemical and Physical Risk Agents for Which There Is Sufficient Evidence of Carcinogenicity in Humans[a]

4-aminobiphenyl	diethylstilbestrol (DES)
arsenic and certain arsenic compounds	ionizing radiation
asbestos	melphalan
azathioprine	methoxsalen with ultraviolet A therapy (PUVA)
benzene	mineral oils
benzidene	mustard gas
betel quid	myleran
bis(chloromethyl) ether	2-naphythlamine
chemotherapy for lymphomas (MOPP)	shale oils
chlorambucil	soots
chlornaphazine	tobacco smoke and smokeless tobacco
chromium and certain chromium compounds	treosulphan
coal tars and coal-tar pitches	ultraviolet radiation
conjugated estrogens	vinyl chloride
cyclophosphamide	

[a]Wilbourne *et al.*, (1986).

with reproductive and developmental effects include toxic metals and metallic compounds (e.g., lead and methylmercury), pesticides and herbicides (e.g., Agent Orange and dibromochloropropane), and drugs (e.g., thalidomide, DES, and alcohol).

4.1.3. Clinical Effects

Specific target tissues and organs including the lungs, heart, liver, kidneys, eyes, nervous system, and skin can be physiologically damaged by exposures to risk agents. Adverse health consequences range in severity from total loss of function (e.g., kidney failure due to heavy-metal intoxification) to less severe effects such as chloracne resulting from exposure to PCBs. Included within this category are adverse effects on neurological functions such as perception, memory, motor skills, reflexes, balance, intelligence, problem solving, and sleep.

4.1.4. Subclinical Effects

Some health consequences produced by exposures to risk agents are subtle, or not easily detectable, upon physiological examination. Examples include changes in enzyme systems, irritation of sensory tissue, and changes in psychological states. Such effects are generally referred to as *subclinical*. The health significance of many subclinical effects is unclear. For example, an association between levels of lead in blood and clinical anemia has been observed at concentrations of lead as low as 1 microgram per milliliter of whole blood (1 µg/ml); below this level, a direct association has not been observed. However, even very low levels of lead in blood have been shown to affect the activity of one of the enzymes in the hemoglobin chain. Whether this is significant for human health is unclear (Whyte and Burton, 1980). Other subclinical effects are unquestionably important. For example, victims of disasters and catastrophes often experience severe mental stress, anxiety, and emotional disturbances subsequent to the event. Fear of potential disasters and catastrophes can also induce high levels of stress and anxiety (Robinson *et al.*, 1983). Data on adverse subclinical effects are limited, since there are few administrative or legally mandated reporting requirements.

4.2. MONITORING METHODS FOR ASSESSING HEALTH CONSEQUENCES

When used to assess health consequences, monitoring consists mainly of health surveillance, that is, the collection, collation, and interpretation of health data. Much health surveillance occurs as part of our basic medical care system; for example, various kinds of routine health information are collected by clinicians, company and union officials, and government agencies.

The types of data collected through health surveillance are necessarily limited, so health surveillance methods are typically used more for hazard identification (the process that precedes risk assessment) than for risk assessment itself. Health surveillance has been very effective for hazard identification. For example, neurological hazards such as Kepone and methyl-*n*-butyl ketone (MBK) were first identified by alert physicians who had observed an unusual cluster of diseases in persons found subsequently to have been exposed to these agents (Cone *et al.*, 1987). Many of the known human carcinogens were identified in a similar manner (Miller, 1978).

In addition to its use in hazard identification, however, health surveillance can sometimes provide estimates of the frequency of specific health effects within populations that may be exposed to risk agents. Health surveillance has been most successful in recording causes of death, documenting cases of particular diseases, and compiling instances of injuries from different types of accidents. The most extensive health surveillance system is the collection of mortality data via the death certificate, a statistical as well as legal document. According to established procedures, information on conditions at the time of death and the causal sequence of conditions culminating in death are recorded by an attending physician, medical examiner, or coroner. Subsequently, this information is coded according to a standardized classification system for causes of death. To facilitate statistical tabulation and analysis, the standard operating practice is to select from among the conditions at the time of death a single underlying cause believed to have set in motion the sequence of conditions culminating in death. The resulting mortality statistics provide an important source of quantitative data on conditions that produce death quickly and that result in high mortality rates (e.g., cardiac arrest). The data are less useful for diseases, however, that are long in duration, that are amenable to treatment, or that have variable mortality rates.

Health surveillance systems are also in place to gather morbidity data. For example, data are routinely collected on such medical concerns as infectious diseases, abortions, congenital abnormalities, and school absences. Occupational accidents are also well-documented under the workers' compensation system. Methods for collecting morbidity data range from self-administered health questionnaires to professional recording of events using well-defined measurements and independent checks. In some cases, specialized tests are used to monitor the health status of high-risk populations. For instance, people suspected to be at high risk for cancer have been monitored using techniques that are sensitive to key steps in the carcinogenic process. Such techniques include the analysis of alkylation of macromolecules to measure adduct formation and analysis of body fluids to measure the induction of gene mutations.

Most health surveillance is designed to describe the distribution of disease as it exists in a given community at a given point in time. Only rarely has health surveillance been aimed at measuring exposures to risk agents. Thus, health surveillance data can seldom be used directly for estimating dose-response relationships; however, the data can be used to calculate mortality or morbidity rates. For example, mortality data are often collected according to occupation. These data, in turn, provide the denominator for calculations of occupational mortality rates. Detailed information on the size, sex, and age structure of the population at risk is generally required for the interpretation of mortality and morbidity statistics. However, in some situations (as in the analysis of rare health effects such as lead poisoning, silicosis, asbestosis, and coal workers' pneumoconiosis), the absolute number of cases of death or disease can be used to establish relationships with environmental factors (WHO, 1983).

4.2.1. Strengths

The main use of health surveillance and other health-monitoring methods is to provide a data base for epidemiology studies. The data also provide information needed to apply or evaluate models. For example, health surveillance data are sometimes used as inputs to dose-response models that are based on human or animal testing. Although health surveillance can be expensive, the costs are typically borne by the medical care system itself. Thus, the risk assessor or epidemiologist usually can obtain health surveillance data at low cost. Another advantage is the generally short time lag between observation of a case by the health surveillance system and its documentation within the data base.

4.2.2. Limitations

Monitoring for health-consequence assessment suffers from many of the same limitations as monitoring for release assessment and exposure assessment. The need for skilled personnel, effective reporting systems, and centralized data facilities creates substantial difficulties for the establishment of health-consequence monitoring systems. Errors can be introduced through (a) random sampling, (b) bias from incomplete or partial data, (c) inappropriate or unsuccessful attempts to quantify vague or imprecise information, (d) deliberate distortions, or (e) imprecision in the methods used to record, code, analyze, and retrieve results.

The principal limitation of the use of health surveillance data in epidemiological studies is the lack of information on exposures. Death certificates, for example, report only the cause of death, the place of residence and the place of occurrence of death, as well as basic demographic variables such as age, race, and sex. They do not contain information on other health factors such as diet, lifestyle, smoking habits, or occupational exposures. Consequently, they cannot be used to estimate exposures, which are critical to the study of chronic diseases. Furthermore, mortality statistics based on death certificates list only a single cause of death. Such data can be misleading, since death commonly results from a complex of diseases.

Another limitation of many routine health surveillance systems is their inflexibility. For example, routine health surveillance systems seldom allow for new items to be added to the coding system and for the processing of these data alongside the original data. In most cases, new data can be collected only through special studies that are conducted independently from the routine health surveillance system.

4.3. SCREENING METHODS FOR ASSESSING HEALTH CONSEQUENCES

Screening methods, conducted through laboratory analysis and tests, are designed to provide a qualitative determination of whether exposure to a risk agent causes harm. As such, they play a crucial role in hazard identification. However, like health surveillance, screening methods can sometimes be used to help quantify the intensity of exposure or the probability that exposure will produce harm. When applied in this way, screening methods may be used to support consequence assessment.

Two widely used screening methods for assessing health consequences are *molecular structure analysis* and *short-term tests*; each is designed to identify carcinogens. Molecular structure analysis is based on empirical data indicating that certain common molecular structures appear in many chemicals known to cause cancer. Thus, a chemical whose molecular structure is similar to that of a known carcinogen may itself be a carcinogen. More generally, molecular structure analysis involves comparing the molecular structure of a suspect substance with that of substances whose toxicity and metabolic pathways are known. The purpose of the comparison is to infer the toxic characteristics of the suspect substance.

The EPA relies heavily on structural analysis for estimating the likelihood that chemicals described in manufacturers' premarketing notices present health or environmental risks. Structural analysis is based on two assumptions: (1) that chemicals with similar structures tend to interact similarly with DNA, and (2) that measurements of chemical and physical properties such as solubility, stability, sensitivity to pH, and chemical reactivity can be used to infer a chemical's carcinogenic potential (EPA, 1986g; Auer and Gould, 1987; Auer, 1988). Because manufacturers already generate the relevant chemical structure information, regulatory agencies and others can quickly and inexpensively conduct molecular structure analysis.

Short-term laboratory tests involve observing the effects of exposing bacteria, mammalian cell cultures, or small organisms to chemicals. The tests are designed to detect mutations of genetic material (DNA). Any agent that causes such a mutation is called a mutagen. Because cancer is thought to originate as a change in DNA, mutagens may be the primary cause of cancer. While not every mutation causes cancer (other diseases can result instead), a substance that is a mutagen is a suspected carcinogen.

Different types of short-term tests are designed to examine different mechanisms of action. For example, the widely used *Ames test* (salmonella mutagenicity assay), named for its developer Bruce Ames (Ames, 1979), measures whether the introduction of a chemical to a genetically engineered strain of salmonella bacteria causes mutation in the bacteria. Other tests examine DNA damage and repair, chromosomal aberrations, or cell transformations. The tests may be conducted *in vitro* (outside the animal, as in a test tube or petri dish) using, for example, bacterial cells as in the Ames test, or *in vivo* (within the animal), making assays for chromosomal mutations in animals' cells.

In addition, several tests of intermediate duration involving whole animals have been developed. These include the induction of skin and lung tumors in mice, breast cancer in female rats, and anatomical changes in the livers of rodents (EPA, 1985a). Batteries of short-term tests, in which the tests are applied in a tiered or phased approach, have been designed to explore efficiently the mechanisms of action (e.g., Weisberger and Williams, 1981; Purchase, 1982; Williams *et al.*, 1982).

Various studies demonstrate how short-term tests can be used in consequence assessment. In one study, Lave and Omenn (1986) estimated the probabilities that various chemicals are carcinogens, using data from an international collaborative program on short-term tests. The analysis consisted of fitting a logit distribution (1 corresponding to a definite carcinogen and 0 corresponding to a definite noncarcinogen) to the spectrum of test results (1 corresponding to a positive test result and 0 corresponding to a negative test result). In another study, researchers applied an approach based on cluster analysis and Bayesian methods to derive probability estimates from short-term test results (Chankong *et al.*, 1985).

Quantitative estimates of carcinogenic potency do not have to be derived solely from qualitative short-term test results. Because quantitative data may be available from a short-term test (e.g., the number of bacterial colonies in a revertant salmonella test), quantitative results might be used to infer potency. Lewtas (1985), for example, has proposed a comparative approach for estimating carcinogenic potency from the relative potencies exhibited in short-term tests.

4.3.1. Strengths

The primary strength of screening methods is that they can be conducted quickly and with relatively little expense. Short-term tests, for example, can sometimes be conducted in less than one day. However, most require a few days to a few weeks, and the longest, involving mice, require eight to nine months. The cost of conducting short-term tests usually ranges from about $100 to several thousand dollars. Short-term tests assist in understanding the biological processes underlying the production of tumors. Comparison of the results of short-term tests with those from much costlier animal research shows that, for carcinogenic risks at least, a high degree of correlation exists.

Another strength of screening methods such as short-term tests and structural analysis is that they provide a feasible and intelligent way of dealing with the very large and increasing number of chemicals in current use. Since it is impossible to test immediately all of the chemicals to which people might be exposed, sequential testing represents a feasible and practical course of action. Structural analysis and short-term tests provide a relatively rapid and inexpensive means for collecting information that can be used to guide the allocation of testing resources, focusing them on the most suspect substances.

4.3.2. Limitations

A major limitation of structural analysis and short-term tests is their limited applicability to the assessment of human health risks. Cellular research is essentially limited to examining risks that have impacts at the cellular level. Although this includes the whole spectrum of cancer risks, it does not provide direct information about diseases or conditions that do not alter or otherwise impair individual cells (e.g., pulmonary or respiratory ailments).

Furthermore, many risk agents that have an effect on higher organisms are not reflected at the single-cell level. Thus, short-term tests are less useful, for example, with chemicals that produce health effects through metabolic activation by cellular enzymes, since cells in culture may or may not retain their enzymatic activity. Consequently, a finding of no effect in a cell culture test does not necessarily indicate that the agent will show no effect in multicellular organisms. Conversely, there may be risk agents that have no apparent effect on higher organisms but that show evidence of morphological transformations in cellular cultures. In some cases, biological processes in multicellular organisms can partially or completely counteract effects on single cells; for example, higher organisms may be able to compensate for impaired functions or defend themselves from invasive agents.

Several additional factors limit the usefulness of short-term tests for risk assessment. First, it is rare for researchers to record or publish quantitative results concerning potency. Second, test results are often ambiguous. Many short-term tests are relatively new and have not been standardized; results may be inconclusive and often vary from researcher to researcher. Third, tests that work well on some chemicals may not be appropriate for others. Also, tests have not been developed for many chemicals.

4.4. ANIMAL RESEARCH FOR ASSESSING HEALTH CONSEQUENCES

Since ethical considerations generally preclude the deliberate exposure of humans to risk agents, animal tests represent the most important alternative source of experimental data for health consequence assessment. A basic assumption underlying animal studies is that adverse health effects in humans can be inferred from adverse health effects observed in experimental animals (OSTP, 1985).

The most common species used in animal studies are rodents, especially rats and mice. Other rodents, such as hamsters and guinea pigs, are also used, as are rabbits, dogs, monkeys, and baboons. The appropriate animal depends on the objectives of the study. Ideally, species are chosen because their sensitivity to the risk agent under investigation is expected to be similar to that experienced by most human beings. For example, monkeys and other primates are often used for studying reproductive effects because their reproductive systems are most similar to that of humans. Rabbits are often used for dermal testing (e.g., tests of cosmetics) because the sensitivity of their skin is comparable to that of humans.

In general, the principal objective of animal studies is to determine (a) the nature of adverse health effects produced by exposure to a risk agent, and (b) the relationship between dose level and the magnitude of adverse health responses. The magnitude of adverse health responses can be measured by a variety of means, including measuring the level of severity of adverse effects or the number of animals that exhibit a particular adverse effect. If there is reason to believe that a dose level exists below which adverse effects do not normally occur, i.e., a *threshold*, then a principal objective of animal studies is to find the *NOEL* (no observed effects level).

Acute animal studies examine the results of a single dose or an exposure of short duration (e.g., 8 h of inhalation). Chronic animal studies examine the results of exposure for nearly the full lifetime of the experimental animals (e.g., 2 to 3 years for rats and mice). Exposures of varying duration between these extremes are referred to as subchronic.

Many of the main principles of animal testing are illustrated by the procedures commonly used to test the effects of exposures to toxic chemicals. First, the test population of animals is divided on a random basis into one or more treatment groups and a control group. Each group is maintained under identical conditions throughout the experiment. A relatively high dose is administered to one treatment group, and lower doses (e.g., half, one-quarter, etc., of the high dose) are administered to the other treatment groups. Animals in the control group are not exposed. The route of administration is selected to be as close as possible to the route through which humans are exposed. For example, the chemical may be administered through either ingestion, inhalation, skin absorption, or skin and/or eye contact (dermal contact). In some cases, however, administration must be by stomach tube (gavage) or by injection under the skin, into the blood, or into body cavities.

Data collected while the animals are still alive include size, weight, condition of external features (e.g., skin, hair, and eyes), gross evidence of internal abnormalities (such as bone deformation), reproductive capacity (including fertility, reproductive frequency, litter size, and changes in frequency of spontaneous abortions or live births), life span, behavior (e.g., food intake, sleep habits, aggressiveness, problem-solving ability), body functions, and genetic changes as evidenced in subsequent generations (Marcus, 1983). As the animals die or are killed during the study, additional information is obtained through pathological examinations conducted to determine the cause of death and the nature and extent of any morphological abnormalities (such as tumors) in internal organs or tissue samples. The measurements obtained for the test group are then compared and contrasted with that of the control group using statistical methods similar to those discussed in Chapter 2. Haseman and Kupper (1979) provide a review of the most common statistical methods used in animal toxicological experiments.

Although many animal toxicity tests use specialized experimental procedures, most elements in the design of experiments are well-established. For example, most of the basic principles of good laboratory practice (i.e., quality standards to be maintained in laboratory testing of chemicals) are standardized. Most of the principles for carcinogenicity bioassays are also standardized (OSTP, 1984). Study designs for carcinogenicity animal bioassays, for example, generally advocate including 50 males and 50 females in each dose group and two to four treatment groups in addition to the control group. The highest exposure level is generally the *maximum tolerated dose* (MTD), which is defined as the maximum dose that the animal species can tolerate for a major portion of its lifetime without significant impairment of growth, significant weight loss, or observable toxic effects other than carcinogenicity (e.g., not so high as to produce death by poisoning). At the end of the experiment, the incidence of cancer, expressed as a function of dose, is tabulated by the examining pathologists. Statistical methods, such as Fisher's exact test (Gart *et al.*, 1979) and the Cochran–Armitage trend test (Armitage, 1955), are then applied to examine the relationship between observed tumor incidence (the fraction of animals having a tumor of a certain type) and dose. If the administered risk agent produces a significant life-shortening effect, more complex "survival-adjusted" methods of statistical analysis (e.g., Cox, 1972) may be needed to account for the shortened latency period. The minimum duration of animal carcinogenicity tests is generally recommended to be 2 years in rats and 18 months in mice.

Similar testing procedures have been developed for investigating other forms of toxicity, such as birth anomalies, reproductive dysfunctions, mutation, skin sensitization, and behavioral modification (NAS–NRC, 1977; FDA, 1982). In addition to tests involving the exposure of animals to chemicals, procedures have also been established for studying the pathogenicity of microbes.

The strength of evidence provided from animal studies is generally considered to be enhanced if (1) results are replicated in more than one sex, strain, species, and experimental setting, (2) greater exposure is associated with greater response, (3) the route of exposure and dosing regimen are similar to those for humans, (4) the animal is known to process (e.g., absorb, metabolize, detoxify, and excrete) the chemical in the same manner as humans, and (5) the study sample size is large enough to ensure a high likelihood of detecting relevant adverse health effects. For example, the International Agency for Research on Cancer regards evidence of carcinogenicity in animals as "sufficient" only when studies show an increased incidence of malignant tumors (1) in multiple species or strains, and/or (2) in multiple experiments (routes and/or doses), and/or (3) to an unusual degree (as regards incidence, site, type, and/or precocity of onset) (IARC, 1982). Inevitably, there is a strong element of judgment in applying these evidentiary criteria in specific cases, particularly when judgments must be made about the significance of observed abnormalities.

4.4.1. Strengths

The principal strength of animal tests is that they allow the potential hazards of risk agents to be evaluated before they are released into the environment. The assumption that effects on animals will be similar to effects on humans is persuasive. Laboratory animals and humans have much in common. For example, humans and most animals possess natural defense mechanisms that allow them to tolerate exposure to many risk agents. These defense mechanisms include metabolic detoxification, chemical neutralization of ions and radicals, tissue regeneration, and immunological surveillance. For the most part, animal tests work rather well. In cancer testing, for example, all of the compounds or mixtures that have been judged by the International Agency for Research on Cancer to be carcinogenic in humans have also produced cancer in at least one species of laboratory animal. Seven substances were found to be carcinogenic in animals before they were also discovered to be carcinogenic in humans.

Another strength of animal studies is that they offer the researcher considerable experimental control. Critical experimental factors such as dose can be varied in a systematic way to perform scientifically rigorous studies. Animal studies can be used to assess a wide variety of substances and conditions such as microbes, nutrients, stress, and trauma. The controlled laboratory setting also permits the researcher to isolate effects caused by specific substances or conditions. Because animals may be allowed to die, the full effects of the substance can be examined, including the presence of various forms of biological injury and pathological change that cannot be detected clinically. In rats and mice, the effects of lifetime exposures to an agent can be detected in 2 or 3 years, the normal lifespan of these species. Furthermore, experimental results can be replicated to confirm their validity or ensure the elimination of extraneous factors.

4.4.2. Limitations

Differences between animals and humans in physiology and the functioning of sensitive organs place important limits on the usefulness of results of animal research. For example:

- Although the liver is the primary organ for detoxifying hazardous substances in both humans and rats, specific metabolic reactions can differ considerably between the two species.

- The kidneys remove and excrete hazardous substances from the blood-stream. Although the basis of action is similar for rats and humans, the relative rates of excretion can be quite different.

- The lungs of both humans and rats provide some detoxification of inhaled hazardous substances; however, depending on the hazardous substance in question, the efficiency of the lungs in humans and rats may be different because rats breathe much faster than humans and their lungs have a somewhat different structure.

- The spleen stores red blood cells and acts as a source of immunological defense.; however, the response of the spleen to hazardous substances can be quite different for humans and rats. For example, rats incorporate arsenic into their red blood cells differently than humans.

Other factors that can create interspecies differences include (a) differences in genetic inheritance, (b) enzymes that activate or inactivate toxic substances, (c) intercellular pathways of toxicity, (d) membrane biochemistry and receptors, (e) absorption, distribution, storage, and excretion, and (f) physiology. Because of such differences, exposures to the same hazardous substance may produce different effects in different species or a significant effect in one species and no apparent effect in another. For example, one of the most widely studied animal carcinogens, acetylaminofluorene (AAF), is not carcinogenic in the guinea pig (Park and Snee, 1983). This insensitivity is due to the guinea pig's inability to metabolize AAF to its active carcinogenic form 2-hydroxy-AAF$_\infty$. More generally, a study of interspecies variability by Ames $et\ al.$ (1987) found that for 226 chemicals tested in both rats and mice, 130 were carcinogens in both rats and mice, but 96 chemicals were positive in the mouse and negative in the rat or vice versa. This discrepancy occurs despite the fact that rats and mice are very closely related and both have short lifespans.

Other interspecies risk comparisons have uncovered additional anomalies (Crouch and Wilson, 1979; Calabrese, 1983; Brown et al., 1987). For example, a National Academy of Sciences study of six chemical compounds found that the estimates of cancer risks in animals (based on studies of the most sensitive species of laboratory animal) were about the same as estimates of cancer risks in humans (based on epidemiological studies) for three of the chemical compounds (benzidine, chlornaphazine, and cigarette smoke). The estimates of cancer risks in animals, however, exceeded the estimates of cancer risks in humans for the three remaining chemical compounds (aflatoxin, DES, and vinyl chloride) by a factor of 10 for aflatoxin, a factor of 50 for DES, and a factor of 500 for vinyl chloride (NAS, 1975). Sometimes, the differences between animals and humans are so great as to severely limit the applicability of animal tests. For example, one of the real handicaps to AIDS research at present is the shortage of animal species susceptible to the virus.

A related limitation concerns the choice of a test animal. Scientists generally agree that the most reliable information for assessing health consequences comes from tests using animals that are the most biologically similar to humans. It is often difficult, however, to identify which similarities are important, especially if the concern is the development of chronic diseases such as cancer (NAS–NRC, 1986a; OSTP, 1985). Moreover, in many cases, the choice of animal species is influenced by a variety of practical and financial factors including cost, ease of care, shortness of lifespan, ease of breeding, ease of handling in large numbers, and genetic homogeneity (i.e., inbred strains). Maintaining large animals such as monkeys for their lifetime (let alone several generations) is costly and time-consuming. Consequently, small rodents such as rats, mice, and hamsters are the animals most typically used in animal testing.

Even when the relevance of animal results to humans has been clearly established, interpreting the significance of the results can be difficult. In carcinogenicity studies, for example, one major area of uncertainty and debate is the interpretation of benign tumors. In establishing total tumor incidence, a common practice is to combine animals having malignant tumors with animals having particular kinds of benign tumors. The basic arguments for this practice are (a) that benign tumors can, in some cases, progress to malignant tumors, and (b) that the distinction between benign and malignant tumors is not always clear. The legitimacy of these arguments has, however, been questioned by numerous critics (e.g., Nichols and Zeckhauser, 1986).

A second major area of uncertainty is derived from the different physical dimensions (e.g., body size) and lifespans of laboratory animals and humans. Because of these differences, laboratory animals and humans can be expected to respond differently to the same dose of a hazardous substance. Although doses are scaled in an attempt to achieve comparability between laboratory animals and humans, scaling is more difficult than simply accounting for differences in relative body size. Differences in metabolism, ingestion rates, respiration rates, organ uptake, storage, elimination, and other biological processes also influence the *effective dose*—the portion of the administered dose that affects the animal in ways thought to be similar in humans. When the biological mechanisms of effect of exposures to hazardous substances are poorly understood (as they are at present), it can be extremely difficult to determine appropriate scaling factors for obtaining comparable dose levels.

A third major area of uncertainty is dose level. The dose given to test animals is often different from the level at which humans are normally exposed in the environment, even after dose scaling is taken into account. In most cases, the dose to animals must be artificially high in order to obtain a statistically significant effect among the small number of animals used in most animal studies (typically, about 200 rodents). If lower doses were given to this small sample of animals, the adverse effects of the toxic substance might escape detection. One problem associated with this practice is that artificially high doses may interfere with the ability of the animal to neutralize and excrete toxic substances before adverse health effects can occur. A variety of factors affect this ability including normal repair mechanisms, metabolic mechanisms of inactivation, and barriers to penetration.

An example of the significance of the problem of setting dose levels is provided by animal studies involving Alar, an agricultural chemical used to slow the ripening of apples. Rodent studies conducted in the 1970s showed a significant increase of tumors in animals exposed to the chemical's active by-product at doses of 29 milligrams per kilogram of body weight (29 mg/kg). Citing cancer potency estimates based on this study, the EPA succeeded in removing the product from the market. Meanwhile, the tests were repeated because it was recognized that the original study utilized doses that exceeded the MTD. New tests utilizing doses of 13 mg/kg implied that the cancer potency estimate should be decreased by a factor of 10. Still, many toxicologists continued to believe that the dosages used produced cancer in ways that would not occur at lower doses in the range experienced by people. The most recent EPA tests have implied that the potency estimate should be further reduced by another factor of 2. The reduction in the potency estimate of a combined factor of 20 has led some to question whether the original decision to ban the product was premature (Marshall, 1991).

Occasionally, the dose given to test animals may be lower than the level at which humans are normally exposed. This would be necessary, for example, if the risk agent in the administered form is toxic to the test animal in ways not directly relevant to the study. The dose level may also have to be reduced if a higher dose level would prevent the adequate uptake of food or would cause the animal to reject the food due to alteration in taste. Doses that are too low can, of course, miss effects that would occur in similarly exposed humans.

Finally, animal tests for even a single chemical can be extremely time-consuming and expensive. Long-term bioassays, for example, can take 3 to 14 years and cost more than $1 million per chemical. As of 1991, the average time needed to complete testing on the 16 chemicals evaluated under EPA's Toxic Substances Control Act was 8 years (GAO, 1991). This expense, as well as the complexity of the study, increases substantially when chemical mixtures and interactions between two or more chemicals are studied. Partly due to this expense, and partly due to the large number of man-made chemicals in commercial use (approximately 70,000 with about 1,000 new chemicals being introduced each year), less than 10 percent of man-made chemicals have been screened and tested for human health risks (NAS–NRC, 1984). Moreover, due to the limited availability of trained toxicologists, laboratory facilities, and test animals, it has been estimated that no more than 500 chemicals could be tested each year in the United States (Majone, 1982).

4.5. EPIDEMIOLOGICAL METHODS FOR ASSESSING HEALTH CONSEQUENCES

Analytic epidemiology is the study of the distribution and determinants of disease and other adverse health effects in human populations. The studies may be longitudinal, meaning that they are designed to collect data on health effects for specific individuals or communities over time; or cross-sectional, meaning that they are designed to collect data on health effects for different communities at one point in time. For risk assessment purposes, the primary objective of epidemiological studies is to establish a statistically significant association between adverse human health effects and exposures to risk agents (Krewski *et al.*, 1990). Epidemiology is also a powerful method for risk identification; for example, 20 out of the roughly 30 agents confirmed to cause cancer in humans were first identified using epidemiological evidence (Tomatis *et al.*, 1978).

Epidemiological methods have been used successfully to analyze (a) relationships between adverse health effects and the duration and level of exposure, (b) disease incidence rates and mortality differences between geographic regions, and (c) time trends in disease incidence rates and mortality differences associated with the introduction or removal of a specific risk agent. Two types of epidemiological studies are especially important for assessing health consequences: *prospective* studies and *case-control* studies.

Prospective (cohort) studies typically compare groups of persons who have been exposed to a suspected risk agent with a control group that has not been exposed. Exposure is measured at the start of the study and periodically afterwards. After each group is identified, any changes in the health status of either group are observed. Such changes may develop over an extended period of time. Data can be collected for each group on disease incidence rates (the number of new cases of disease per unit of population per unit of time) or on mortality rates (the number of deaths per unit of population per unit of time). Any excess incidence of disease or increase in mortality or morbidity rates is regarded as potential evidence of an adverse effect of the risk agent. Examples of major prospective studies include the Framingham Heart Study in Massachusetts and the Atomic Bomb Casualty Commission's study of the survivors of the atomic explosions at Hiroshima and Nagasaki (WHO, 1983).

Case-control studies are generally retrospective in nature and attempt to compare a group of persons who have a given disease or illness with a control group of persons who do not have the disease or illness. The people with the disease or illness are the *cases*, and the people without the disease are the *controls*. The primary objective in case-control studies is to identify factors such as lifestyle characteristics or exposure to a toxic substance that may be responsible for the disease or health impairment. Case-control studies are particularly useful for studying rare diseases and for investigating potential associations between a disease and several different risk agents. Case-control studies typically require less time and smaller population samples than prospective studies; however, case-control studies depend heavily on (a) the ability of subjects to recall information on past habits and exposures, and (b) the availability of historical records.

Through the use of prospective or case-control studies epidemiologists are able to investigate human responses to general environmental conditions or to specific risk factors such as diet and lifestyle. Epidemiological studies can be narrowly restricted to clinical observations on relatively small populations of hospital patients or they can encompass retrospective and prospective observations of much larger populations. Both types of study have proved useful in understanding dose-response relationships.

The results of epidemiological studies typically are analyzed using conventional biostatistical methods similar to those used in animal studies. These methods are used to assess the nature and significance of the observed relationships. The level of statistical significance, usually measured in terms of a "p value," indicates whether the observed difference could be the result of chance. If the p value is small (traditionally, less than .05) chance is generally ruled out as an explanation for the results.

In epidemiological studies, research design protocols require that the groups be comparable in all respects except for exposure to the particular risk factor of interest. In prospective epidemiological studies, care must be taken that all relevant factors are controlled or randomized (i.e., that they do not vary in a systematic way and thereby bias the results). In case-control epidemiological studies, statistical controls are used, that is, selection procedures are used to match individual cases and controls for comparability. Sociodemographic variables, including age, sex, ethnicity, race, education, income, occupation, and place of residence are commonly used for matching.

Molecular epidemiology is a relatively new approach within epidemiology designed to incorporate human molecular dosimetry data into epidemiological studies (Hattis, 1986). For risk assessment purposes, one of the primary objectives of molecular epidemiology is to identify, at the biochemical or molecular level, specific exogenous agents and/or host factors that play a role in causing human disease (Perera, 1987). Molecular epidemiological methods include (1) techniques to assess host factors that influence susceptibility, (2) assays that detect toxic chemicals in human tissues, cells, or fluids, (3) cellular-level assays of the biologically effective dose (the amount of the toxic substance or risk agent that reacts with critical cellular targets, such as DNA), and (4) methods to measure early preclinical or subclinical biological and biochemical responses to toxic substances.

An important contribution of the field to date has been the identification of molecular indicators that serve as *biomarkers* for quantifying human exposures to carcinogens. These molecular biomarkers include carcinogen-DNA and carcinogen-protein adducts (chemical products resulting from the addition of the carcinogen), somatic cell mutations, and other biological responses that have been linked to exposures to carcinogens and tumor formation. Biomarkers increase the power of epidemiological studies by providing a means for more accurately estimating dose (i.e., through measurement of the biomarker). An example of a molecular epidemiological study is a case-control study in which levels of polycyclic aromatic hydrocarbon-DNA (PAH-DNA) adducts in peripheral blood cells were compared for patients with and without lung cancer, taking into account the potentially confounding effects of age and cigarette smoking, a major source of PAH (Perera et al., 1988). Another example is a study in which excised aflatoxin DNA adducts in urine were found to be moderately correlated with liver cancer incidence rates experienced by an ethnic group (Autrup *et al.*, 1987).

Although most molecular epidemiological studies conducted to date have focused on cancer, virtually all health effects are, at least in theory, amenable to study via molecular epidemiological. By changing the unit of analysis from whole organisms to the cellular or molecular level, molecular epidemiology methods can be used to more effectively quantify dose-response relationships. For example, measurements involving hemoglobin have been used to more clearly identify the low-dose relationships between dose and response (Hattis, 1986). Furthermore, since many of the same indicators of biologically effective dose can be applied across different species, molecular epidemiological methods can be used to provide a more rational basis for interspecies extrapolation.

4.5.1. Strengths

The principal strength of epidemiological studies is that they yield data for humans, the species typically of most concern in risk assessment. Incidences of death, disease, illness, or injury in humans can be directly related to the actual levels of exposure in humans. Since the data are for human beings, the results of epidemiological studies are more readily accepted as evidence than are the results from animal studies. Especially convincing are the well-designed and well-conducted epidemiological studies that show a positive, statistically significant association between a risk agent and an adverse health effect.

Epidemiological studies also eliminate many of the problems encountered in conducting animal studies, especially those arising from the need to extrapolate from one species to another. Since exposure is already in the human dose-response range, the choice of an extrapolation model is often less crucial than for animal studies. In addition, molecular epidemiological methods are emerging as a means for clarifying the form of dose-response relationships at low doses and for improving understanding of human variability.

4.5.2. Limitations

An important limitation of epidemiological studies is the difficulty of detecting adverse health effects at low exposure levels. As in laboratory animal studies, observed associations are usually less pronounced at low levels of exposure, making it difficult to assess alternative explanations such as chance, errors, biases, or confounding factors. To provide a valid basis for assessing health consequences where the exposure is low, or where the excess risk is small compared with that of the baseline incidence rate, very large numbers of human subjects are needed. This makes epidemiological studies, especially prospective studies, expensive.

Another limitation of epidemiological studies is the difficulty of measuring lifetime risks from partial lifetime data. In many epidemiological studies of chronic health risks, the exposure duration is short relative to the latency period of chronic illnesses and diseases. Thus in the case of cancer, for example, people who have been exposed to a risk agent for a comparatively short period of time (e.g., a few weeks, months, or years) must be tracked for periods of up to 30 or 40 years. Because cancer incidence generally increases with the duration of exposure and with age, epidemiological studies usually detect only a fraction of the lifetime risks resulting from exposure. This complicates the detection of a relationship and makes it difficult to identify the chronic risks of newly introduced risk agents.

Also important is the difficulty of measuring exposure (e.g., level, frequency, duration, and route). Unlike animal laboratory studies, epidemiological studies are not controlled laboratory experiments, with exposure to the risk agent under the control of the epidemiologist. Rather, the epidemiologist is generally limited to the study of exposures and diseases that occur naturally or accidentally. Precise measurements of exposure are difficult to obtain for several reasons:

1. The exposure of interest often cannot be measured directly. As a result, surrogate measures of uncertain reliability are typically used (e.g., measures based on occupation or place of residence).
2. Exposure to a given hazardous substance can originate in different sources (e.g., consumer goods, food, or the workplace) and at varying rates (e.g., short-term or long-term, intermittent or continuous). People can also be exposed at different times in their lives and with differing frequency.
3. Exposure data are usually derived from historical records generated for other purposes or from the subjects' recollections. As a result, personal bias or misclassification of exposures may be introduced. In case-control studies, for example, a subject's ability to recall exposure to a carcinogen might be biased by the knowledge that he has cancer.
4. Appropriate study populations are often unavailable or difficult to identify; for example, it is often difficult to locate suitable control popula-

tions. In prospective studies of worker populations, for instance, the use of the general population as a control group introduces a bias known as the "healthy worker effect"—that is, effects caused by the fact that employed persons are generally healthier than the general population.

Errors in estimating exposure can introduce bias into the statistical analyses of data. For example, errors in exposure measurements can cause the estimated effect of exposure on health to be underestimated in bivariate linear or logistic regression analysis (Cochran, 1968; Burr-Doss, 1985). In analyses with more than one independent variable, the magnitude of the effect of the exposure may be under- or overestimated, depending on the error in the independent variables and the correlation among the independent variables (Cochran, 1970; Kamlet et al., 1985).

Another limitation of epidemiological studies is the difficulty of identifying and excluding confounding factors; adverse health effects can often be traced to complex exposures involving a variety of risk factors. Disentangling the effects of confounding factors such as cigarette smoking, alcohol consumption, exercise patterns, and diet can be a formidable task. The problem of confounding factors can sometimes be dealt with through the careful selection of controls; however, this is not always possible. In contrast to animal testing, variables such as lifestyle, diet, use of medication, or cigarette smoking cannot easily be controlled or matched in study populations. Furthermore, controls can be introduced only when confounding risk factors are already recognized.

A final limitation of epidemiological studies is that their primary use has typically been in identifying adverse health effects after the fact, that is, after humans have been exposed to toxic substances. The primary use of risk assessment, however, is in identifying adverse effects before they occur. Since the latency period of diseases such as cancer and birth defects may be as long as 20 to 40 years after exposure, irreversible damage may have been done to large numbers of people by the time that adverse effects are evident to the epidemiologist. Even after exposure is recognized and stopped, cancers may continue to occur for many years (Doll and Peto, 1981).

While some of these limitations may be overcome by developments in molecular epidemiology, substantial resources are needed to develop and validate the necessary laboratory methods. Much of this work is currently in the experimental stage. Furthermore, the lack of background data such as data on the normal variability in populations creates serious difficulties in the design of studies using biomarkers. Biomarkers are still somewhat crude indicators of dose; for example, immunoassays, the method commonly used to detect carcinogen-DNA adducts, are not a precise means of measurement. Moreover, there are as yet no known markers for detecting human exposures to nongenotoxic carcinogens such as promoters (Perera, 1988). It is still unclear whether methods can be developed that are sensitive enough for specific applications, such as detecting and measuring low-level occupational exposures. Additionally, generalizing about the sensitivity of a given method is difficult, since the level of exposure necessary to induce a particular effect varies by chemical (Lohman *et al.*, 1983).

4.6. CONTROLLED HUMAN EXPOSURE STUDIES

A well-designed controlled study involving humans provides the most convincing evidence of a relationship between exposure to a risk agent and an adverse health effect. The methods used in controlled human exposure studies are similar to those used in epidemiology. Subjects may be selected from the general population or from a specific subpopulation, such as a particular age cohort or occupational group. Exposures, however, usually take place in a controlled laboratory setting, as with animal tests. Responses to one or more levels of exposure are compared with the responses obtained under controlled conditions. Typically, the investigator controls both the level and conditions of exposure. Alternatively, human exposure studies can be conducted in a field setting, such as a neighborhood or a workplace. Although the level of exposure may not in this case be under the investigator's direct control, the exposure conditions can be carefully documented, together with the responses of exposed subjects. The control case is often a similar environment in which the risk agent has been removed or does not exist.

Due to ethical and practical problems associated with experimenting with human subjects, controlled human exposure studies typically have been limited to the study of mild and reversible health effects (e.g., allergic skin reactions). In the past, studies of more severe adverse health effects were sometimes conducted using prisoners; however, studies of this type are no longer conducted. Most current studies focus on exposures to mild air pollutants and on adverse side effects of drugs designed to treat or to prevent disease or illness. For example, the health effects of sulfur dioxide and ozone have been investigated in chamber studies in which human volunteers breathe varying concentrations of either agent, and the resulting changes in lung performance are measured. Certain food preservatives known as sulfites have been given to asthmatics to evaluate allergic reactions.

4.6.1. Strengths

Controlled human exposure studies provide the strongest possible scientific evidence of risk to humans. Direct cause-effect relationships can be determined by comparing control groups to exposed groups. Controlled human exposure studies also provide opportunities for rigorous analysis of the relationship between dose and response. Relatively precise biological and environmental measurements can be obtained from such studies, and confounding variables can be systematically identified and controlled. Since the studies are often simple in design, the results are relatively easy to understand and enjoy a high degree of scientific and public credibility. Although controlled human exposure studies can be costly, it is sometimes possible to conduct small studies without excessive commitments of time and resources.

4.6.2. Limitations

The major limitations of controlled human exposure studies are the ethical, practical, and legal restrictions associated with experiments involving humans. Exposures must produce minimal discomfort and no lasting adverse health effects. Furthermore, the experimenter must obtain the informed consent of the subjects; informed consent usually requires that the subjects fully understand the risks and implications of the study. Because of these limitations, controlled human exposure studies are relatively rare. Moreover, subjects with the desired characteristics are difficult to find, and the dropout rate is often high.

Another typical shortcoming of human laboratory studies is the difficulty of simulating the real world. In air pollution studies, for example, the exposure levels, air mixtures, psychological stresses, and behavior patterns observed in the laboratory are likely to differ from those existing outside the laboratory. Also, interpretation of the results is often difficult. Due to cost, (1) experiments rarely involve more than about 20 subjects, (2) histological follow-up is limited, and (3) laboratory subjects may be exposed to risk agents via different routes than is common in real-life settings.

As with other testing methods, combining evidence from multiple studies poses computation problems, and simplifying assumptions are necessary to keep the mathematics tractable. For example, it is typical to assume that the treatments studied and effects observed in multiple trials of a new drug are comparable despite differences among the experimental conditions (e.g., different patient populations). Assumptions about the probabilistic independence of evidence from separate trials and the conditional independence of study results are often made but difficult to support. Furthermore, the significance of the likely violation of such assumptions is generally difficult to assess.

4.7. MODELING METHODS FOR ASSESSING HEALTH CONSEQUENCES

The primary purpose of a *health-consequence model* is to translate exposures to a specified risk agent into adverse health consequences. The principal type of health-consequence model is the dose-response model. A *dose-response model* is a functional relationship between the dose (i.e., measure of exposure) and an adverse health response (the measure of health impact).

Another type of health-consequence model is the *health end-point model*, which translates physiological effects estimated by a dose-response relationship (such as reduced pulmonary function) into the health effects of greatest concern to people (e.g., chest pain). Health-consequence models may also contain submodels for relating exposure levels estimated by exposure assessment to the specific measure of dose needed for analyzing the dose-response model.

4.7.1. Dose-Response Models

Dose-response models are frequently used to assess the adverse health effects of exposure to toxic chemicals, biological substances, and ionizing radiation. The vast majority of research on dose-response modeling, and most of the literature on the subject, deals with models for estimating the risk of cancer from exposures to carcinogens. However, dose-response models have also been used for estimating the adverse health effects from other kinds of risk agents including toxic chemicals, injuries from accidents, and noise.

The relationship between exposures and health effects is typically more complex than the simple term "dose-response" suggests; neither dose nor response is easily quantified. Exposures vary over time and, in principle, must be specified by a time-varying dose rate. Health effects vary in terms of both frequency and severity. There may also be a time delay between exposure and the onset of the adverse health effect, as with cancer. In addition, the type of adverse effect may change with dose. For example, anesthetic gases may cause death at high doses, sleep at lower doses, headaches or lethargy at still lower doses, and no detectable effects at very low doses (Environ Corp., 1986). Some chemicals produce a biphasic response wherein a beneficial effect is shown at low doses and an adverse effect appears at higher levels. Selenium, for example, is required at very low levels by every living thing, is protective against carcinogens at a higher range, is a possible carcinogen or tumor promoter at still higher levels, and finally, is chronically and acutely lethal at still higher concentrations (Gillett, 1987).

Ingeneral, the response exhibited by a large population exposed to increasing levels of a risk agent varies as follows (see Fig. 18):

1. At sufficiently low exposures, no effects will be detected regardless of the duration of exposure.
2. At slightly higher doses, subtle effects may be detected in a very small proportion of exposed individuals who are particularly sensitive to the risk agent.
3. As the dose increases, a greater proportion of the population will respond with subtle effects, and a small proportion will experience more severe adverse effects.

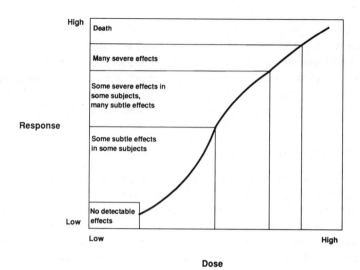

FIGURE 18.   A general dose–response relationship.

4. As the dose is increased still further, the incidence of adverse effects in the population will increase and the severity of those effects will also increase.
5. At a high enough dose of sufficient duration, nearly the entire population will experience severe adverse effects, with some individuals responding with more severe effects than others.
6. Nearly any risk agent, if delivered at a high enough dose, will cause death.

   Available dose-response models typically provide only a limited and highly simplified representation of this progression. For example, many models estimate only the incidence of a specified response without accounting for differences in severity. Alternatively, a dose-response model may estimate the severity of response experienced by a specified exposed individual without accounting for the fraction of such individuals who would experience such responses.

   The dosage scale selected for a dose-response model depends on the risk agent and the route of intake. Typically, dose is expressed in terms of a cumulative exposure or rate per unit of time. The response scale depends on the specific nature of the response and might measure severity, the probability of a given effect occurring, or the time until the occurrence of an effect. Dose-response models often estimate "excess" risk, that is, the increase in the incidence of some effect above the normal background level.

If sufficient data are available, a dose-response relationship can sometimes be derived directly from the statistical analysis of empirical observations. In such cases, regression analysis is typically used to estimate a quantitative relationship. Even when appropriate empirical data are available, however, extrapolations based on theoretical models and expert judgment are often needed to derive dose-response relationships. For example, adjustments may be necessary to account for the greater diversity in the sensitivity of the potentially exposed population compared with the sample population. Pregnant women, the elderly, and infants less than a few months old, for instance, may not be adequately represented in the sample and yet may be especially sensitive to exposures.

When the data for a dose-response model are derived from animal studies, additional extrapolations are needed before the data can be used to set model parameters in a way that is applicable to humans. As already indicated, laboratory animals differ from humans in various respects, including different physical dimensions, rates of intake (e.g., ingestion and inhalation), life spans, and pharmacokinetics. Consequently, they can be expected to respond differently to a specified level of exposure to toxic substances or other risk agents. One approach to extrapolation is to develop human and animal versions of the dose-response model using analogous assumptions and then to verify the animal model through animal tests. For example, to understand the responses of humans to high levels of microwave radiation, analogous computer models have been developed to simulate the flow of heat into and out of the bodies of both humans and squirrel monkeys. In both cases, the models accounted for internal heat generation, cooling and distribution of heat by blood, thermal conduction throughout the body, evaporative heat loss from heating and respiration, and radiation and convection from the outer surface of the body. Partial verification for the human model was provided when the predictions from the animal model were found to be in close agreement with the results of tests performed using squirrel monkeys (EPA, 1985b).

For exposures to toxic substances through ingestion and inhalation, extrapolation from animal data is typically accomplished by converting animal doses and responses to levels that would be equivalent for humans. Conversion factors are usually based on surface area or body weight. The extrapolation is generally based on standardized dosage scales for interspecies comparisons, such as milligrams per kilogram of body weight per day (mg/kg/day) milligrams per square meter of body surface area (mg/m^2 BSA), or milligrams per kilogram of body weight per lifetime. The choice of a conversion factor is highly significant. For example, when surface area is used to scale dose rates from experimental animals to humans, the estimated equivalent rates for humans are substantially higher than rates derived from body weight (OTA, 1981).

Extrapolation from animals to humans must also take into account differences in absorption rates and in the duration, nature, and route of exposure.

Absorption rates for toxic substances depend on the medium in which the hazardous substance is present; for example, a hazardous substance present in water might be absorbed differently than the same hazardous substance present in food. Absorption rates may also vary among animal species and among individuals within a species.

In the absence of data to the contrary, absorption rates are usually assumed to be equal when experimental animals receive the chemical by the same route as humans. If humans are exposed by a route different than that used in animal testing, differences in absorption rates may be extremely important. For example, if a chemical has been administered orally to a test animal but human exposure is by inhalation, it is crucial that data be obtained on the amount absorbed orally by the animal and on the amount absorbed through inhalation by humans. Direct measures of absorption are rarely available, however, and human data can seldom be obtained without controlled human exposure studies. Consequently, absorption is often assumed to be complete, or measures of absorption are obtained from studies of compounds with similar chemical and physical characteristics (Nisbet, 1980; Calabrese, 1983).

Most of the literature on dose-response models focuses on chemical risk agents; however, dose-response models can also be developed for other risk agents, including physical risk agents. For example, researchers have developed simulation models for predicting injuries to individuals involved in automobile accidents. The models are generally based on accident monitoring data or performance testing. Performance testing data are derived from tests using anthropometric dummies, animals, or (rarely) human cadavers (Schneider and Beier, 1974). Using such data, analysts have been able to establish systematic relationships between the characteristics of an accident and the injuries sustained by the automobile occupants. In one study, severity of injury was represented by an injury scale. A multiple regression analysis was then conducted to find a best-fit equation relating injury to vehicle damage, impact velocity, windshield bond separation, and occupant ejection. The results of the analysis permitted researchers to predict expected injuries to occupants using different safety devices, such as occupant restraint systems (Oday, 1974).

The following subsections describe various categories of dose-response models ranging from simple dose-response curves to complex pharmacokinetic models.

4.7.1.1. Simple Dose-Response Models. The simplest dose-response models are merely curves relating some single measure of dose (e.g., cumulative exposure) to some single measure of health response (e.g., number of fatalities). A dose-response curve is a graphic representation of the quantitative relationship between the level of exposure and the intensity or occurrence of a resulting adverse health effect. The curves may be linear, linear-with-threshold, quadratic, or sigmoidal (S-shaped).

Simple dose-response curves are widely used for estimating the number of cases of cancer caused by exposures to low-level radiation. The most frequently used models are the linear and quadratic curves (NAS, 1980; Rall *et al.*, 1985). With such models, the frequency of additional carcinogenic effects in a population increases as a linear function of the radiation dose in the low-dose domain. Thus, for low-dose applications, the slope of the curve (i.e., the number of additional health effects per unit increase in dose) and the baseline incidence rate are sufficient to define the models. The appropriate slope, of course, depends on the cancer type or site. In addition, the slope is also typically assumed to be a function of the age of the exposed individual at the time of irradiation. For illustration, Table 17 presents estimates of the incremental increases in the incidence of various cancers derived from epidemiological studies involving A-bomb survivors, together with the corresponding baseline incidences.

For applications involving toxic substances, dose-response relationships are often represented by curves with thresholds. According to the *threshold theory* of toxicity, a toxic substance must be present in an organism at some threshold concentration before any toxic effects are evident. Virtually all chemicals act at the cellular or molecular levels to cause damage. If a large enough number of cells are damaged or killed, vital tissue may be destroyed and death or serious disorder may result. Conversely, if only a few cells are damaged, an organism may be able to repair the damage or scar it over and survive without any noticeable effect.

Dose-response curves that assume the existence of a toxicity threshold are often based on the observation that many biological responses vary linearly with the logarithm of dose. The specification of such models requires stipulating (1) the threshold below which the constant (background) level of response is assumed to occur, and (2) the slope of the log dose-response curve, which specifies the rate at which response increases with the log of the dose.

4.7.1.2. Tolerance Distribution Models. Tolerance (or threshold) distribution models are based on the assumption that each person in the population has an individual threshold tolerance for a specific risk agent. For this class of models, the probability that a particular individual will experience an adverse effect when exposed at a dose level d is the same as the probability that the tolerance level of the individual is less than d. Depending on formulation, dose d may be a daily dosage rate or total accumulated dose. The specification of a functional form for the distribution of tolerances determines the shape of the dose-response curve.

The most commonly used tolerance model is the *log-probit model* (Finney, 1952, 1971). This model assumes that the logarithms of tolerances (the doses at which responses are first observed) have a normal or Gaussian distribution. The

TABLE 17.   Estimated Health Effects of Radiation-Induced Cancers of Different Organs in Relation to Age at Exposure and Corresponding Baseline Incidence[a]

	Age at exposure (years)			Spontaneous baseline incidence (per 10^6/yr)
	20–34	35–49	50+	
Cancer type or site	(Excess cancers per million per year per Sv)[b]			
Leukemia[c]				
(males)	80	110	160	80
(females)	50	70	100	60
Esophagus (both sexes)	5	8	22	35
Stomach (both sexes)	300	50	130	95
Colon (both sexes)	20	30	90	325
Liver (both sexes)	30	30	30	50
Pancreas (both sexes)	20	30	80	95
Lung (both sexes)	60	90	120	500
Breast (females)	490	310[d]	80	900
Urinary (both sexes)	20	40	60	220
Thyroid[e]				
(males)	50	50	50	20
(females)	150	150	150	60

[a]From Upton (1988). The author notes that the estimates (originally obtained by Rall et al., 1985) may need to be revised upward somewhat pending revision of the dosimetry for the A-bomb survivors; [b]Excess cancers (values rounded) expressed from 10th to 30th year after exposure unless otherwise specified (1 Sv [sievert] = 100 rem); [c]Excess cancers expressed from 5th to 26th year after exposure (CLL excluded); [d]Value interpolated from figures in original report; [e]Excess cancers expressed from 10th to 34th year after exposure.

implication of this assumption is that the proportion of positive responses in an exposed population increases with the logarithm of doses in such a way that a plot would have the sigmoidal S shape shown in Fig. 19. Superimposed on the plot are the same data plotted as a frequency distribution in which the y-axis represents the increment in responses as the dose is increased. For the log-probit model, this frequency distribution is a Gaussian distribution.

The log-probit model is popular because the results of toxicity tests often fit the shape assumed in that model. As a check, the proportion of observed responses may be expressed in terms of the number of standard deviations on either side of the median response. Since a proportion of responses less than the median would

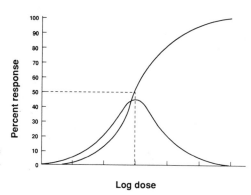

FIGURE 19. Log dose-response curve for the log-probit model and the corresponding frequency distribution.

result in a negative number, a convention has been adopted wherein the number 5 is added to each value and the result is called the *probit value of responses*. If the log-probit model is to provide a good approximation of the dose-response relationship, then a plot of log dose versus the probit of responses must be approximately a straight line, as illustrated in Fig. 20. By picking an appropriate measure of dose (e.g., volume or mass, concentration in food, proportion of the animal's body weight) the plot of probit response versus log dose can often be made to fall approximately along a straight line.

One area in which the log-probit model has been used is in modeling the dose-response relationship for exposures to toxic gases (AIChE/CCPS, 1989). As illustration, Table 18 provides the log-probit equation and the suggested parameter values for estimating the probability of fatality from human exposures to various gases. The parameter values were obtained by fitting the model to animal data, with the extrapolation based on differences in air intake and body weight. Dose in the model is measured in terms of the concentration raised to a power, multiplied by the duration of exposure. The probit value Pr may be converted to an estimate of the percentage of fatalities in the exposed population using standard probit tables, such as the simplified version given in Table 19.

In addition to applications to chemical risk agents, the log-probit model is a common model for estimating infections from disease-causing organisms. Each individual in the potentially exposed population is assumed to have a minimum infective dose, which is distributed log-normally. In this context, the log-probit model is sometimes referred to as the *log-normal model* (Levin and Strauss, 1991). A similar approach has been used in automobile safety. For example, one application assumed that each automobile has a tolerance level for impacts that produce little or no fuel leakage (and, therefore, minimum risk of fire danger). The tolerance level was expressed as the threshold impact velocity representing the maximum

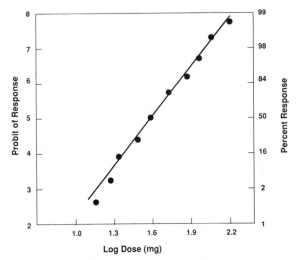

FIGURE 20.   A typical log dose-probit plot.

collision severity that the vehicle could withstand without rupture of the fuel tank (Carnahan and Krishnan, 1989).

Although the log-probit model frequently provides a good fit to data, it is used primarily for deriving estimates within the range of empirically observed responses (interpolation) rather than for deriving estimates outside the range (extrapolation). For extrapolating responses to low doses based on experimentally observed responses at medium to high doses, the log-probit model is often modified. One modification of this model, the Mantel–Bryan equation, assumes a slope of 1.0 on the log dose–probit plot, which means that each tenfold reduction in dose decreases the incidence of effects by one standard deviation of the Gaussian distribution. This slope is considered conservative for low-dose extrapolation because it is shallower than what is normally observed in experimental data. The assumption is used to correct for the steeper dose-response relationships that homogeneous strains of laboratory animals exhibit compared with heterogeneous human populations.

Two other common tolerance distribution models are the log logistic, or *logit model* (Berkson, 1944) and the *Weibull* model (Krewski and Van Ryzin, 1981). The logit model assumes that the logarithm of tolerances is distributed according to the logit distribution. The logit distribution is similar to the normal distribution in that it is bell-shaped and centered about its mean; however, it allows for a higher fraction of values at a fixed distance away from its mean than does the corresponding normal distribution with the same mean and standard deviation. Thus, like the Mantel–Bryan equation, the logit model may allow for a better fit to data derived

TABLE 18. Constants for Lethal Toxicity Probit Equation[a]

$$Pr = a + b \log_e (c^n t)$$

where c = concentration (ppm) and t = exposure time (minutes)

Substance	a	b	n
Acrolein	−9.931	2.049	1
Acrylonitrile	−29.42	3.008	1.43
Ammonia	−35.90	1.85	2
Benzene	−109.78	5.3	2
Bromine	−9.04	0.92	2
Carbon monoxide	−37.98	3.7	1
Carbon tetrachloride	−6.29	0.408	2.50
Chlorine	−8.29	0.92	2
Formaldehyde	−12.24	1.3	2
Hydrogen chloride	−16.85	2.00	1.00
Hydrogen cyanide	−29.42	3.008	1.43
Hydrogen fluoride	−35.87	3.354	1.00
Hydrogen sulfide	−31.42	3.008	1.43
Methyl bromide	−56.81	5.27	1.00
Methyl isocyanate	−5.642	1.637	0.653
Nitrogen dioxide	−13.79	1.4	2
Phosgene	−19.27	3.686	1
Propylene oxide	−7.415	0.509	2.00
Sulfur dioxide	−15.67	2.10	1.00
Toluene	−6.794	0.408	2.50

[a]Adapted from AIChE/CCPS (1989).

Note: Parameter values assume log to the base e; i.e., $\log_e$ = ln.

from heterogeneous populations because tolerances (more precisely, log tolerances) for such populations tend to exhibit more biological variability than could be captured through the corresponding normal distribution. Like the log-probit model, the logit model reflects an assumption that the proportion of responses increases with dose and exhibits a symmetric, sigmoidal shape, but it approaches the extreme levels (0 and 100 percent response) more gradually than the probit.

TABLE 19.   Transformation of Probits to Percentages

| % | \multicolumn{5}{c}{Probit value, Pr} | | | | |
	0	2	4	6	8
0	–	2.95	3.25	3.45	3.59
10	3.72	3.82	3.92	4.01	4.08
20	4.16	4.23	4.29	4.36	4.42
30	4.48	4.53	4.59	4.64	4.69
40	4.75	4.80	4.85	4.90	4.95
50	5.00	5.05	5.10	5.15	5.20
60	5.25	5.31	5.36	5.41	5.47
70	5.52	5.58	5.64	5.71	5.77
80	5.84	5.92	5.99	6.08	6.18
90	6.28	6.41	6.55	6.75	7.05
99	7.33	7.41	7.46	7.65	7.88

The Weibull model assumes a Weibull probability distribution for the tolerances (not log tolerances in this case) for exposures to the risk agent. The Weibull distribution (discussed in Chapter 2) is slightly skewed about its mean so that smaller log tolerances (values a given number of standard deviations below the log of the mean) are less likely than corresponding larger log tolerances. Although the Weibull model was originally proposed for use in engineering reliability risk assessment, it has also proved useful for describing many biological data sets.

Within the typical range of observed toxic responses (10 percent to 90 percent response levels of the dose-response curve), the probit, logit, and Weibull models are often so similar that it is nearly impossible to distinguish between them. In the low dose range, however, the logit and Weibull models may predict doses producing no observable effects that are more than an order of magnitude lower than those produced by the log-probit model.

4.7.1.3. Mechanistic Models. Depending on the level of scientific knowledge, more sophisticated dose-response models may be developed based on theoretical assumptions concerning biological processes. A description of several such mechanistic dose-response models is provided below. Most of these models were originally developed for cancer risk assessment; however, the same or similar models may be applicable to reproductive, genetic, and other effects.

Mechanistic models typically represent the biological processes leading to an adverse effect as a series of events evolving over time. These events are assumed to follow stochastic (random) process that is affected by the dose level. Included among these events are known or suspected processes that control uptake or residence time of the toxic substance, mechanisms of cellular or organ damage or dysfunction, and mechanisms of repair.

One class of mechanistic dose-response models is based on the premise that specific biological events (referred to as "hits") trigger the response. The *one-hit model* (Iverson and Arley, 1950), also known as the linear model, was first developed to estimate the incidences of tumors from exposures to radiation. The model assumes that only one molecular interaction between the risk agent and the target site is sufficient to produce an adverse effect. The model also assumes that the probability of an interaction is directly proportional to the level of exposure and is independent of the age of the exposed organism or the pattern of the exposure. The dose-response curve implied by the one-hit model is nearly linear at low doses, but it actually has a concave slope over the entire dose range.

In addition to its use as a cancer dose-response model, the one-hit model has also been used to represent the effects of exposures to organisms causing disease (Zanetos, 1984). In this context, the model represents two key steps in the disease process: (1) the probability of exposure to one or more organisms capable of causing disease, and (2) the fraction of the original dose of disease-causing organisms that actually reaches the target tissue in a viable form. Assuming that the exposure to even one organism may result in disease, the one-hit equation gives the probability that an individual exposed to a specified number of organisms will become infected.

The one-hit model is computationally simple and insensitive to minor fluctuations in the data, but ignores thresholds and *no-effect levels* (dose levels low enough to assume a negligible probability of an adverse effect in the lifetime of a population). Neither the one-hit model nor variations of the model using upper statistical limits (Gaylor and Kodell, 1980) are good predictors of tumor production at very low exposure levels. For example, in various cases involving carcinogens, low-dose estimates provided by the model have been invalidated by human epidemiological data (Gehring *et al.*, 1979; Ramsey *et al.*, 1979; Reitz *et al.*, 1978) and by animal data, as in the National Center for Toxicological Research's ED_{01} Study, which used over 24,000 mice and was designed specifically to clarify the shape of the dose-response curve at the low end (Carlborg, 1981a).

The *multihit model*, also called the gamma multihit model (Cornfield and Mantel, 1977; Rai and Van Ryzin, 1981), assumes that two or more hits of a substance are required to induce a response and that the number of hits over time follows a Poisson distribution. As with the one-hit model, the multihit model does not always provide a good fit in the low-dose region. The dose-response curve predicted by the multihit model at low doses may, in some cases, be essentially linear, depending on the values selected for its parameters. The multihit model has, in some applications, been found to predict doses producing no observable effects that are either higher or lower than the doses that produce an observed effect in laboratory experiments. For example, the no-effects level predicted by the multihit model appears too high for nitrilotriacetic acid and too low for vinyl chloride (Food Safety Council, 1980). Furthermore, even when no evidence of a confounding background level of exposure is present, the model may estimate a background rate.

The *multistage model*, also called the Armitage–Doll function (Armitage and Doll, 1954; Guess and Crump, 1976), is a mechanistic model based on the assumption that a tumor originates as a predisposed cell that goes through a series of stages until it becomes malignant; a carcinogen is assumed to influence the rate of progression through the various stages. The exact nature of each stage, however, is not clearly defined by the model. The analyst has the flexibility to hypothesize, for example, that cancer is a five-stage process, with the carcinogen affecting the first and fourth stages. Timing of the transitions from the impacted stages is expressed by a probability function defined by a rate that is proportional to the dose.

The multistage model is widely used in cancer risk assessment. It is attractive not only because of its great flexibility in curve fitting, but also because of some supporting empirical evidence. For example, the multistage model correctly predicts that the incidence of many kinds of cancer within populations of different ages is approximately proportional to the age of the population raised to a power p (incidence at age t = a constant multiplied by t raised to the power p). Armitage and Doll, in fact, developed the multistage model to explain this power law. In the model, the power p is related to the number of stages (usually between 4 and 6) that are assumed (Peto, 1978).

The physiological basis for the multistage model also has some support. As mentioned at the beginning of this chapter, research suggests that some substances are cancer *initiators* (primary-stage carcinogens) and/or cancer *promoters* (late-stage carcinogens). According to this theory, an initiator causes a cell to change from its normal state to a premalignant state, in which it could remain indefinitely; a promoter causes an initiated cell to proliferate. Dimethylbenzanthracene (DMBA) is considered an initiator. Croton oil (more specifically, its phorbol ester constituent) is considered a promoter. *Complete* carcinogens (e.g., tobacco smoke) are thought to be both promoters and initiators. The multistage model allows initiators to be handled through effects on the early stages of the model, and promoters through effects on the later stages (Freedman and Zeisel, 1987).

Similar to the one-hit model, the multistage model is considered a conservative extrapolation model because the curve approaches linearity at low dose levels; however, its greater flexibility permits nonlinearities of data at higher doses. For some sets of data, the multistage model reduces to the one-hit model; in other cases, the resulting slope is much shallower than that produced by the one-hit model. The multistage model tends to work well in the experimental dose range, but, like the other models, at low doses it ignores changes in kinetics, metabolism, and other potentially confounding or modifying processes and mechanisms. The multistage model also has the disadvantage of being relatively sensitive to small changes in the data to which it is fit. For example, the dose-response relationship implied by the model may change significantly if fit to data showing a few tumors more or less at the lowest experimental dose.

The *linearized multistage model* (Crump, 1981, 1985) is a variation of the multistage model that is designed to provide an upper confidence limit on the level of risk. Similar to the standard multistage model, this model employs a sufficient number of parameters to be able to fit almost any monotonically increasing dose-response data. At the higher doses, where experimental data generally exist, the model behaves like the multistage model and accommodates the nonlinearities often observed in data. At the lower doses to which the data are extrapolated, the model constrains the results to be linear. In this regard, the model resembles the more conservative one-hit model.

The basic form of the linearized model is identical to the multistage model. The low-dose behavior of the model is "linearized" through the statistical methods used to estimate the values of the parameters. Specifically, the model incorporates a procedure for estimating at low extrapolated doses the largest possible linear slope (the 95 percent statistical confidence limit) that is consistent with the available data. Since the model relies on the upper confidence level for the linear term in the model and ignores the best estimate for this term (as well as the lower confidence limit), the model can produce a high estimate of risk even when exposure levels are well below the NOEL (Park and Snee, 1983). Use of the linearized model typically increases the risk estimates by a factor of two or three over what they would be with the standard model, although in some instances the approach can increase the estimates by several orders of magnitude.

The various mechanistic models described above all assume that the risk agent affects the carcinogenic process through cellular transformations—a steeper curve means that exposure produces more cellular transformations but does not necessarily affect cell proliferation. Some scientists believe that cell proliferation is also crucial to the carcinogenic process. Accordingly, Moolgavkar and Venzon (1979) and Moolgavkar and Knudson (1981) have proposed a model (the *MVK model* or two-stage model) that attempts to account for risk agent-induced cell proliferation. The key assumptions of the MVK model are that (1) a malignant transformation of a single cell is sufficient to produce a tumor, (2) cells progress through the transformation process irreversibly and independently of one another, and (3) once a fully malignant cell has been generated, the time to tumor detection is approximately constant. Mathematically, the MVK model is a mixture of stochastic and deterministic components. The numbers of neoplastic and fully malignant cells at any given time are assumed to be random variables with constant rates of occurrences. The number of normal cells at risk of transformation at time t is assumed to be deterministic and known, due to the large number of cells involved and to well-established, age-dependent organ growth rates. Under these assumptions, the model of the carcinogenic process is a mathematical form known as a *filtered Poisson process*. Thorslund *et al.* (1987) have extended the MVK model to allow time-dependent rates for transition, birth, and death of preneoplastic cells; this extension allows the model to be used in situations with time-dependent dosing patterns. The parameters of the model can be interpreted in biological terms and therefore can potentially be estimated from data obtained from sources other than carcinogenesis bioassays.

The usual formulations of mechanistic models assume chronic lifetime exposures; however, various assumptions enable the models to be applied in cases where exposures are brief or intermittent. For example, Crump and Howe (1984) have extended the multistage model to allow for variable dosing regimens. In addition, some variations of the models have been proposed to better represent the mechanisms of the cancer process under short-term exposures. For example, Whittemore and Keller (1978) provide a version of the multistage model that can be applied in cases of intermittent exposures. The risk estimates depend on the number of stages in the carcinogenic process, the particular stages that are affected by the exposure, and the age at exposure. Similarly, Chen *et al.* (1988) provide a version of the MVK model that produces age-specific estimates for exposures that occur during a single period or as a single instantaneous dose.

4.7.1.4. Time-to-Response Models. Time-to-response models are used for assessing the risks of carcinogens and other agents for which a significant time delay exists between the exposure and the adverse response. Such models are based on the observation that the median time to occurrence of an adverse effect (e.g., cancer) generally decreases as dose increases. Rather than simply predicting the incidence of latent health effects, time-to-response models account for both the probability of effect and the length of the latency period. Accounting for latency can be important, especially if the dose level is so low that the latency period is beyond the life expectancy of most exposed individuals. It may also be important if significance is attached to the age at which a person experiences an adverse health effect; for example, cancers related to a woman's reproductive cycle.

Various types of time-to-response models have been reviewed by Kalbfleisch *et al.* (1983). One type, called a *log-linear model*, assumes a lognormal distribution for the time to response with a median time that is dependent on dose and a standard deviation that is independent of dose (Albert and Altschuler, 1973). Specifically, the relationship between dose and median time to response is assumed to be such that the dose is inversely proportional to the median time to response raised to some power. Another model type assumes a Weibull distribution for the time to response (Whittemore and Altschuler, 1976). Other time-to-response models have been proposed by Hartley and Sielken (1977).

Compared with other mechanistic models, time-to-response models provide a more realistic representation of latent health effects, but they also typically require a greater amount of data. For example, to obtain animal cancer data for a time-to-response model, animals must be serially sacrificed. This is required because internal tumors and related health effects are difficult to observe in live animals. Such experiments are, however, quite costly. As a result, the quality and quantity of available data are seldom sufficient for specifying the models, or may be insufficient for discriminating among alternative model forms using a goodness-of-fit criterion.

4.7.1.5. Differences among Dose-Response Models. Table 20 shows the mathematical expressions for some of the more common dose-response models. As with other models, application of any of these models requires its parameters to be set to specific values. These values may be established through reliance on expert judgment or by fitting the model to data obtained from animal tests, epidemiological studies, or controlled tests on humans. Krewski and Van Ryzin (1981) provide a general discussion of the methods for fitting dose-response models to data. Crump *et al.* (1977) and Rai and Van Ryzin (1981) provide details for the multistage and multihit models, respectively.

Depending on the model selected and the values of the parameters, the curve relating dose and response will be sublinear, linear, or supralinear in the low-dose range. As shown in Fig. 21, for a specified low level of dose, the supralinear dose-response curve will typically estimate the largest probability of response, while the sublinear dose-response curve will typically estimate the smallest probability of response. Table 21 summarizes the possibilities for each model.

If data are limited, or if most of the experimental data are for dose levels far above those of concern, statistical methods for model fitting will be inadequate for choosing among the various model forms. Consequently, independent information on mechanisms is needed to direct the selection of an appropriate dose-response model. For example, if the test compound is known to act in a manner that is additive to an ongoing process, then the dose-response curve can be shown to be linear in the low-dose region (Crump *et al.*, 1976). In such situations, a model that produces a linear, nonthreshold curve at low doses (e.g., the multistage model) would be more appropriate than one with a threshold or threshold-like shape (e.g., the log-probit model, which has a steep, threshold-like curvature).

In their simplest forms, the log-probit, one-hit, multihit, multistage, and related models are not formulated to account for time-dependent dosing. If dose

TABLE 20. Mathematical Expressions of Several Dose-Response Models Used in Cancer Risk Assessment[a]

Model	Equation for the probability of a response (proportion of population affected at dose d)[b]	Parameter constraints
Log-Probit[c]	$\phi\,(a + b \log d)$	$(b > 0)$
Logit	$[1 + e^{-(a + b \log d)}]^{-1}$	$(b > 0)$
Weibull	$1 - e^{-(a + bd^m)}$	$(a \geq 0)$ $(b > 0)$ $(m > 0)$
One-hit	$1 - e^{-(a + bd)}$	$(a \geq 0)$ $(b > 0)$
Multihit[d]	$[\Gamma(k)]^{-1} \displaystyle\int_0^{\lambda d} u^{k-1}\, e^{-u}\, du$	$\lambda \geq 0$ $k > 0$
Multistage	$1 - e^{-(c_0 + c_1 d^2 + \ldots + c_k d^k)}$	$(c_i \geq 0)$

[a] Adapted from Munro and Krewski (1981).
[b] The equations assume zero incidence of response in the control population. If an independent background incidence is assumed, $P^*(d) = \tau + (1 - \tau)\, P(d)$, where τ $(0 < \tau < 1)$ denotes the background tumor incidence. If an additive background incidence is assumed, $P^*(d) = P(d + \sigma)$, where $\sigma > 0$ denotes the "background" dose.

[c] $\phi\,(\ )$ denotes the standard cumulative Gaussian (normal) distribution: $\phi(x) = \dfrac{1}{\sqrt{2\pi}} \displaystyle\int_{-\infty}^{x} e^{-u^2/2}\, du$

[d] $\Gamma\,(\ )$ denotes the standard gamma function: $\Gamma(t) = \displaystyle\int_0^{\infty} x^{t-1}\, e^{-x}\, dx$

varies over time, the usual approach is to use the constant-dose form of the models, taking the time-average dose as the constant dose. The dose-response model that is chosen is the primary factor in determining whether the failure to take the time-varying behavior of dose into account will produce significant error in estimating the prevalence of toxic response. For example, prevalences predicted by the one-hit and multihit models depend only on the time-averaged dose, so the use of a time-averaged concentration in the one-hit and Weibull models provides no additional modeling error. For the multistage model, on the other hand, prevalences predicted by the constant-dose model (with dose set equal to the time-averaged

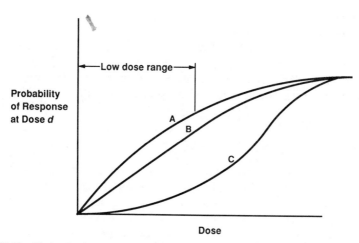

FIGURE 21. Variously shaped dose-response curves at low dose. A = supralinear; B = linear; C = sublinear.

TABLE 21.   Low-Dose Behavior of Various Dose-Response Models[a]

Model	Low-dose behavior		
	Supralinear	Linear	Sublinear
Log-probit	Never	Never	Always
Logit (b = shape parameter)	$b < 1$	$b = 1$	$b > 1$
Weibull (m = shape parameter)	$m < 1$	$m = 1$	$m > 1$
One-hit	Never	Always	Never
Multihit (k = number of hits)	$k < 1$	$k = 1$	$k > 1$
Multistage (c_1 = linear coefficient)	Never	$c_1 > 0$	$c_1 = 0$

[a] Adapted from Munro and Krewski (1981) and Rai and Van Ryzin (1981).

dose) may differ considerably from the prevalences predicted by a fully time-dependent model. Kodell *et al.* (1987), for example, show that the use of a time-averaged dose in a multistage model can underestimate the actual health effects by a factor equal to at most the number of stages in the model. Order-of-magnitude errors or greater may occur if short, intense exposures are treated as time-averaged quantities, particularly when these models have parameter values that strongly prevent their reexpression in terms of time-averaged concentrations (Bolton *et al.*, 1985).

4.7.2. Pharmacokinetic Models

Pharmacokinetics is the study of the absorption, distribution, metabolism, and elimination of chemicals in humans and animals. Pharmacokinetic understanding provides a means for evaluating the assumptions underlying dose-response models. The result is a basis for developing more realistic and accurate models (Hoel *et al.*, 1983; Hoel *et al.*, 1985; NAS–NRC, 1986a; Krewski *et al.*, 1991). For example, the discussion of models thus far has implicitly assumed that the dose in a dose-response model is the exposure level or, in the case of animal or human tests, the administered dose. However, many toxic substances exhibit toxic effects only after they have been absorbed into the body and delivered to specific organs. The dose actually reaching organs of the body is called the effective dose or target dose. If the administered dose is strictly proportional to the effective dose, then the administered dose is a useful surrogate for fitting dose-response models. Frequently, however, the relationship between administered and effective doses is markedly nonlinear.

Figure 22 indicates how chemicals are transferred and distributed within the body. First, after entering the body, some chemicals are metabolized, that is, chemically altered within the body to form metabolites. Toxic effects may be produced by the chemical itself or by one or more of the chemical's metabolites. Second, chemicals vary widely in the degree to which they or their metabolites are stored in the body. For example, many toxic chemicals circulating in the bloodstream can become temporarily attached to protein molecules in the blood; this reduces the amount of toxic chemical free to damage the target organ, but also prolongs the time that a toxic substance circulates in the body. The net result is a chronic rather than an acute dose of the chemical to the target organ. Also, some substances can be stored for long periods of time in fat or bone; for instance, lead binds to calcium in the bones. Most toxic substances do little harm when so sequestered. Third, chemicals differ in their absorption rates and the degree to which they or their metabolites are excreted (e.g., through urine or feces). Compounds such as DDT and PCBs are known to accumulate in mothers' milk, while substances that are both fat-soluble and easily vaporized, such as acetone and alcohol, may be exhaled. Finally, chemicals produce varying effects on different animal species and on individuals within a species. For example, it has been estimated that about 20 percent of all people are at special risk from certain chemicals because of a particular sensitivity or allergy (Harte *et al.*, 1991).

High doses of substances in the amounts typically utilized in animal studies can saturate the normal detoxification and excretory mechanisms of animals, resulting in highly nonlinear relationships between administered and effective doses. To illustrate, Krewski and Murdoch (1988) analyzed a simple two-compartment model wherein it was assumed that an administered toxicant may be either eliminated from the body or activated to a reactive metabolite. The reactive metabolite, in turn, was also assumed to be eliminated or detoxified. Figure 23 shows how the relationship between the administered dose d and the effective dose $d*$ can vary, depending on which processes are assumed to saturate. When both activation and detoxification are linear, the relationship between d and $d*$ is linear. If the detoxification process is assumed to saturate, $d*$ is proportional to d at low doses, but increases more rapidly once saturation of the detoxification process occurs. Conversely, if only the activation step is saturable, then the relationship

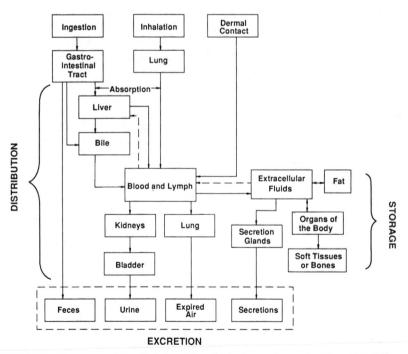

FIGURE 22. Key routes of chemical absorption, distribution, and excretion [from U.S. Office of Technology Assessment (OTA, 1981)].

levels off as saturation occurs. If both activation and detoxification are assumed to be saturable, more complicated, nonlinear relationships are produced. The results clearly demonstrate how the use of models that ignore nonlinear kinetics can either greatly overestimate or greatly underestimate potential health effects.

Pharmacokinetics is an important source of information in developing dose-response models that account for the nonlinear relationship between administered and effective doses (Hoel *et al.*, 1985; Perera, 1986). A *pharmacokinetic model* is a set of equations used to describe the time course of a parent chemical or metabolite in an animal system. The key feature of such models is the attempt to relate, and thereby translate an administered dose to an effective dose as a function of exposure level. Depending on the circumstances, a pharmacokinetic model may express effective dose in a number of ways, such as the percentage of dose absorbed from the gastrointestinal tract, the movement of micrograms of chemical across a given area of skin over a specified time period, or the percentage of inhaled material absorbed in the respiratory tract.

Clewell and Andersen (1985) group pharmacokinetic models for toxic chemicals into two categories: *compartmental* and *physiological*. Compartmental models typically relate the concentration of the chemical or active metabolite in blood or tissue to the administered dose of the chemical, using a set of mathematical equations based on the concept of connected compartments. The compartments do not necessarily represent any real anatomic regions of the body. A simple two-compartment model has been used to study the effects of inhalation of styrene (a volatile liquid) by rats (Ramsey and Young, 1978; Ramsey *et al.*, 1980). The model consists

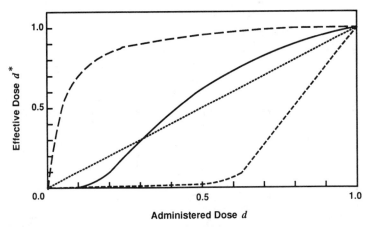

FIGURE 23. The relationship between the effective dose d^* delivered to the target organ and the administered dose d with saturable activation and detoxification. (———) = both saturable; (— —) = activation saturable; (– –) = detoxification saturable; (- -) = both linear.

of a central compartment that is in equilibrium with the blood and a peripheral compartment whose concentration is related to the central compartment by rate constants describing transport to and from the central compartment.

The parameters for the equations describing compartmental models (e.g., compartment volumes and rate constants) are determined by fitting the model to empirical data from experiments that measure the concentration of the chemical in body fluids or specific tissues over time. This process amounts to adjusting the values of the rate constants and the volumes of the compartments to fit the experimental data. Since the parameters of compartmental models generally do not correspond to physiologically identifiable entities, the models do not allow for extrapolation across animal species. Consequently, the models are used primarily for interpolation and limited extrapolation within an animal species.

Physiologically based pharmacokinetic (PBPK) models differ from conventional compartmental models in that they are based on the physiology of the exposed subjects (Bischoff, 1987). Instead of using abstract compartments with composite rate constants determined from fits to experimental data, PBPK models represent the actual organs or groups of organs involved, defined in terms of their volumes, weights, blood flows, and other factors. The physicochemical and biochemical constants of the compound are used to specify transformation rates. By modifying the initial model to incorporate insights gained from comparisons with experimental data, one can produce a refined model that can be used for quantitative extrapolation well beyond the range of experimental conditions. Ramsey and Andersen (1984), for example, have developed a PBPK model for styrene inhalation.

The construction of PBPK models generally requires considerable knowledge. For example, to construct a model for estimating the concentration of an active carcinogen at a target tissue as a function of the administered dose, the following information is needed: (1) absorption, distribution, and excretion patterns as a function of the administered dose; (2) identification of metabolic products as a function of administered dose; (3) blood levels (or other relevant measures of effective dose) as a function of administered dose; (4) DNA binding or alkylation as a function of administered dose; and (5) effects of the exposure regimen, including duration, frequency, level, and route, on blood levels. For most toxic substances, this kind of information is not available. For well-studied substances such as radionuclides, methods for calculating effective target doses have been developed for bone marrow, lungs, endosteal cells, stomach wall, lower intestine wall, thyroid, liver, kidney, testes, and ovaries, as well as for the total body (Fiksel and Scow, 1983). In the case of noncarcinogenic toxicants, only a few chemicals have been intensively investigated in terms of their pharmacokinetic characteristics. Examples include the solvent tetrachloroethylene and the paint stripper methylene chloride (Travis *et al.*, 1987; Andersen *et al.*, 1987).

4.7.3. Strengths

The strength of dose-response models is that they provide a means of estimating adverse effects in the absence of direct data. Since the relationships on which the model is based are described explicitly through mathematical equations or computer codes, the logic is open to review and criticism. Pharmacokinetic models, especially physiologically based ones, possess a high degree of predictive power for estimating the adverse effects of exposures to toxic chemicals. Since these models represent fundamental metabolic processes, they permit dose extrapolation over ranges where saturation of metabolism occurs. Different species and exposure regimens can also often be represented by adjusting the appropriate parameters or developing additional equations to the model.

4.7.4. Limitations

Dose-response models have many limitations, including the availability of the data or the knowledge and understanding needed to set their parameters and verify their accuracy. For the overwhelming majority of risk agents, knowledge is insufficient to permit confidence in the selection of a dose-response function. Few dose-response models are available for estimating effects other than cancer or acute lethal toxicity. Yet, nonfatal effects not addressed by dose-response models may be important, even if they are less important from a health perspective. For a risk assessment of a possible toxic chemical spill, nonfatal acute effects such as eye irritation, lacrimation (secretion of tears), and dizziness may be of crucial importance if these effects impede escape from an area of contamination.

Several fundamental questions related to dose-response models are not fully resolved. These include: (1) how to extrapolate results to doses outside the range of observation in laboratory experiments, (2) how to choose an appropriate dose-response model for extrapolating from high doses given to experimental animals in laboratories to the low doses normally received by humans, and (3) how to select appropriate conversion factors for translating data from laboratory animals to humans (e.g., because of differences in body size, life span, and metabolic processes).

A second major limitation of available dose-response models is the uncertain accuracy of their predictions. To the extent that such models represent underlying causal mechanisms, confidence in their predictions might be warranted; however, dose-response models are generally gross oversimplifications of complex processes. There are many reasons underlying these shortcomings.

First, with the exception of some pharmacokinetic models, most dose-response models currently in use represent oversimplifications of complex biological and biochemical processes. The general approach to the development of a dose-response relationship is statistical curve fitting, and the simple functional forms that are assumed are often not completely consistent with available knowledge. For instance, although a simple linear, age-dependent, nonthreshold model is often assumed for radiation-induced cancers, the relationship between dose and cancer incidence is more complicated than this. Upton (1988) lists the complexities that are not captured by the simple model: (1) for a given neoplasm, the dose-incidence curve generally rises more steeply and is less dependent on the dose rate with high-LET radiation (alpha rays and other radiation involving particles that release a relatively large amount of energy per unit length of path when passing through a substance) than with low-LET radiation; (2) with many types of neoplasms, the incidence passes through a maximum at some intermediate dose and decreases with further increases in dose; (3) the dose-incidence curve may reflect initiating effects, promoting effects, anticarcinogenic effects, or a combination of all three, depending on the type of radiation, the dose, and the dose rate; (4) the effects of radiation may be additive, synergistic, or antagonistic with those of other physical or chemical agents, depending on the agents in question and the conditions of exposure; and (5) susceptibility to radiation carcinogenesis varies among individuals as a result of factors in addition to age, such as genetic background, DNA repair capacity, and other characteristics. Also, some effects of radiation exposure such as erythema of the skin, cataract of the lens, depression of hematopoiesis, and impairment of immunity, are known to have distinct thresholds (ICRP, 1977).

In the case of mechanistic models, only limited progress has been made to date in relating the mathematical forms of the models to the underlying causal mechanisms and to biological and biochemical processes. The justifications that have been provided are not fully consistent with experimental evidence. Freedman and Zeisel (1987) list some questionable assumptions underlying the purported physiological basis of the multistage model, including the following: (1) that the order of progression through the stages of the cancer process is fixed and irreversible, (2) that the waiting times spent in the various stages are statistically independent, and described by the exponential distribution, and (3) that cells progress through the various stages independently of one another.

Recent research has also shed doubt on the simple distinction made between cancer initiators and promoters (Freedman and Zeisel, 1987). The original animal research supporting the distinction between initiators and promoters demonstrated that the order in which agents are administered affects tumor yield (mainly, nonmalignant papillomas). When an initiator (such as DMBA) is administered first, and a promoter (such as croton oil) is administered second, the yield is much higher than if the agents are administered in reverse order. However, the experimental data relate to the progression of tumors while the mathematical model relates to the progression of an individual cell. Cells within a tumor become remarkably heterogeneous in their genetic makeup, so progression of the tumor is not necessarily evidence about the progression of individual cells. Furthermore, experiments have shown that for some initiators and promoters the sequence initiator-promoter-initiator produces a much larger yield of malignancies than the sequence initiator–promoter. Likewise, the sequence promoter–initiator–promoter increases the tumor yield. Finally, there is now evidence for the reversibility of some lesions, including certain kinds of tumors. The fixed-order progression through stages and the irreversibility of the common multistage model do not appear to be consistent with these results.

Mechanistic models frequently involve approximations that do not hold in certain applications. Moolgavkar (1978) points out that the multistage model depends critically on there being a low probability that any individual will develop a tumor. Such models break down when applied to carcinogens and exposure scenarios where this low probability assumption does not hold. Moolgavkar and Dewanji (1988) note that the time-dependent extension of the MVK model provided by Thorslund et al. (1987) similarly requires an assumption that only a small proportion of the exposed population will develop tumors.

The underlying assumption of greatest practical importance for most cancer risk assessments—the assumption of low-dose linearity—also appears inconsistent with growing scientific understanding. Ames et al. (1987) summarize the evidence. According to the predominant current view, the multistep cancer process includes stages of initiation, promotion, and proliferation (invasiveness and metastases). While a linear relationship may be plausible for initiation, promotion appears to involve a threshold, possibly because of the association of cell proliferation with the killing of neighboring cells. Proliferation is poorly understood, but may be accelerated by oxygen radicals, which may be produced through chronic cell killing. Proliferation, however, seems to involve dose-response relationships with apparent thresholds. Thus, the dose-response relationship logically depends on the particular stages of the cancer process that it accelerates. Furthermore, if the carcinogen affects several stages, multiplicative effects would be expected. Indeed, there is growing evidence to support the idea that a nonlinear dose-response relationship applies for some genotoxic carcinogens (agents that initiate cancer through a direct effect on genetic material) and most nongenotoxic carcinogens. Dose-response curves for saccharin, butylated hydroxyanisole, and a variety of other nongenotoxic carcinogens appear to be nonlinear (Carlborg, 1982). Formaldehyde, a genotoxic carcinogen, also has a nonlinear dose-response (Starr and Gibson, 1985).

Only rarely have attempts been made to evaluate and compare, through animal or human studies, the ability of the available dose-response models to provide reasonably accurate estimates. As a result, it is difficult—at least in the case of carcinogens—to determine precisely which model is appropriate for representing the low-dose region of the dose-response relationship. The question is of considerable practical importance. For example, as illustrated in Fig. 24, at responses above 2 percent, the probit, logit, multihit, and similar models produce dose-response curves that are highly similar in shape. Thus, all five of the models provide essentially identical fits to the observed data. At low doses, however, the doses estimated by the various models can differ by 3 to 4 orders of magnitude (IPC, 1984). When the data suggest convexity, estimates of the NOEL produced by the various tolerance distribution and mechanistic models increase in the following order: one-hit < multistage < Weibull < logit < multihit < log probit. When the data suggest concavity, however, the order of the NOEL estimates is reversed (Park and Snee, 1983). For more complicated data sets, other orders may result.

The few cases in which model results and animal data have been directly compared show chemical-specific differences. In one study, predictions for the one-hit model were compared to animal data for 308 different chemicals and 1,212 animal tests (Bailar *et al.*, 1988). Differences larger than expected by chance were found in about 10 percent of the cases. The model overestimated risk in about 5 to 7 percent of the cases and underestimated risk in about 2.5 to 4 percent of the cases. The large amount of animal test data for vinyl chloride made it possible to make the comparison at low as well as moderate doses. Despite the reputation of the one-hit model for being overly conservative in the low-dose range, it was found to underestimate risk by a factor of nine.

Pharmacokinetic models can provide a firmer biological basis for extrapolation, but they do so at the expense of requiring more complicated models with more equations and parameters. No single pharmacokinetic model can be used for all chemicals, since the number of compartments and the way they are connected must vary depending upon the chemical's metabolic behavior and the nature of the available animal test data. Moreover, for any given chemical, there is typically not enough pharmacokinetic information available to allow development of a pharma-

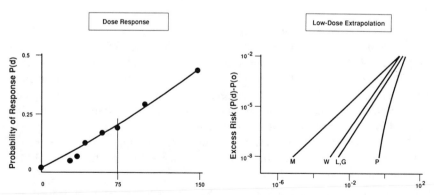

FIGURE 24. Five dose-response models fit to data—indistinguishable in the range of data but very different when extrapolated to low doses. M = multistage model; W = Wiebull model; L = logit model; G = multihit model; P = log-probit model. [Adapted from Krewski *et al.* (1984).]

cokinetic model. Since the behaviors of most toxic substances are not well understood, it is difficult to generalize from existing pharmacokinetic studies.

Given the current lack of pharmacokinetic information and the wide variations in the low-dose results of various tolerance distribution and mechanistic models, it is crucial that a dose-response model be chosen on the basis of all relevant quantitative and qualitative data. To this end, various statistical methods have been proposed for combining the results of different studies and thereby obtaining a more comprehensive use of available data. For example, one proposed procedure is to compute a weighted average of the estimates produced by each study, where the weights are selected to be inversely proportional to the variances of each estimate (St. John *et al.*, 1982). Another approach is to incorporate parameters in the model to account for differences between studies, including the use of animals of different sexes or different strains (Carlborg, 1981b). Such methods allow for the computation of statistical error estimators, such as confidence intervals, that provide a measure of residual uncertainty. Such estimators, however, will be statistically correct only if the model used to compute them is an accurate representation of the underlying dose-response function. In any case, statistical confidence intervals and similar estimators do not provide a measure of modeling error.

A third major limitation of dose-response models is that the models developed for a single hazardous substance may misrepresent situations involving concurrent or sequential exposures to multiple hazardous substances (e.g., product mixtures, toxic wastes, tobacco smoke, and pollutants in the air, water, and the workplace). This deficiency in current modeling efforts is most evident in risk assessments of hazardous waste, which usually contains mixtures of several chemicals. Little information is currently available on the joint action of mixtures of chemicals, which can produce additive, synergistic, or antagonistic effects (NAS–NRC, 1977; NAS–NRC, 1984). Available dose-response models are generally based on studies involving exposure to a single, relatively pure chemical.

In the absence of information to the contrary, the usual approach to the problem of chemical mixtures is to assume that the effects of the risk agents are separate and noninteractive. As a result, additivity in either dose or response is assumed. With dose additivity, the toxic substances in a mixture are assumed to behave as if they were dilutions or concentrations of each other. Predicted response can be obtained from the model by summing the individual doses after adjusting for differences in potency. Response additivity assumes that toxicants act on different receptors and that observed effects are the sum of effects estimated individually (after accounting for possible correlations among tolerances to different toxic substances within individuals).

Although the assumption of additivity is mathematically convenient, the literature contains numerous examples of synergistic and antagonistic interactions. For example, a chemical in a mixture may exhibit greater toxicity if other toxic substances in the mixture enhance the ability of the chemical to penetrate body membranes such as the skin, the stomach lining, or the placenta. Numerous examples of antagonistic effects based on direct chemical-to-chemical interactions have also been observed. One example is the use of ammonia as an antidote for the ingestion of formaldehyde (Goldstein *et al.*, 1974). Since most, but not all, examples of nonadditivity involve relatively high exposures to toxic substances that act rapidly and cause acute effects, additivity is generally regarded to be the most reasonable assumption for assessing mixtures of similar chemicals that induce the same effect by the same mechanism (Stara and Erdreich, 1984).

When the additivity assumption cannot be justified, few viable alternatives exist. Several models for interactions among toxic substances have been proposed (Finney, 1971; Durkin, 1981); however, the available data typically are insufficient for estimating the necessary parameters, let alone for testing the hypothesis of additivity. Using the additivity assumption in cases where interactions occur can introduce numerous errors (NAS–NRC, 1980). For example, the degree of interaction may be a function of dose, the adverse effects may differ from species to species, the response variance may be greater between individuals for exposures to mixtures than for exposures to a single chemical, and the adverse effects of sequential and simultaneous exposures may differ. In addition, different permutations of sequential exposure may have different effects.

A fourth limitation of dose-response models is that applications often fail to take into account important qualitative information relevant to the selection of a dose-response model. An example of qualitative information that may be important to the choice of a dose-response model is genotoxicity. Current theory suggests that a threshold is unlikely for genotoxic chemicals, but that a threshold may exist for chemicals that operate through mechanisms other than direct genotoxicity. Consequently, it has been proposed that effects assessment should include dose-response models that produce threshold-like responses (e.g., loglinear or log-probit models) when (a) sufficient data exist to demonstrate that a particular chemical does not interact with DNA, and (b) the likely mechanism of action is a simple expression of localized toxicity (Park and Snee, 1983).

The choice between linear and threshold models, however, is not easy and may have significant consequences. An illustration is provided by the example of dioxin. Key data for dioxin consequence assessment come from a 1978 animal study. In this study, 50 female and 50 male rats fed 100,000 picograms of dioxin per kilogram of body weight per day (pg/kg/day) were found to have significantly more liver cancers than controls. A similar group of rats fed dioxin at 10,000 pg/kg/day was found to have a slightly elevated cancer rate. No excess tumors were found in animals fed dioxin at 1,000 pg/kg/day. Reasoning that the study was too insensitive to identify the linear response that would be anticipated at the lowest dose rate, researchers at the U.S. EPA applied a linearized multistage model and standard animal-to-human extrapolation procedures. The conclusion was that human exposures to 0.006 pg/kg/day of dioxin would lead to no more than one excess cancer death for every million individuals exposed (Kociba, 1984).

Regulatory agencies in Canada, however, took a different approach (Finkel, 1988). Based on qualitative evidence, they adopted the premise that dioxin is a cancer promoter only; that is, it can only promote development of a tumor from a cell already initiated by some other stimulus. They then applied a threshold model consistent with the single data point from the animal study showing no excess tumors in animals fed dioxin 1,000 pg/kg/day. If the threshold model were used as the basis for U.S. regulations, current regulatory practices would lead to the conclusion that daily dioxin exposures in the range of 1 to 10 pg/kg/day are "virtually safe" for humans.

Although the concept of thresholds for nongenotoxic promoters may seem reasonable, there are two problems with using this assumption in dose-response models. First, due to the diversity of the human population, individuals are likely to have different thresholds. The presence of spontaneous disease in the population indicates that the threshold dose for the population, if one exists, has already been exceeded due, perhaps, to endogenous and/or exogenous factors. The addition of a risk agent for this process produces an incremental risk no matter how small the effective dose. This reasoning has been used to argue that threshold models are inappropriate for any cancer (OSTP, 1984). Second, recent *in vivo* research (Reynolds *et al.*, 1988) suggests that some promoters can directly cause subtle mutations in the genetic material within mouse liver cells, casting doubt on the general applicability of a threshold model.

A final limitation of human health dose-response models is the limited generalizability of models developed for carcinogens to other risk agents. For example, most models developed for assessing carcinogenic risk are quantal, that is, they predict whether or not a specific effect, such as the occurrence of a tumor or death, is elicited. For noncarcinogens, however, the severity of the effect, rather than its frequency, may be the desired response measure. In such cases, a model capable of predicting a continuous or graded response may be needed. A *continuous response* is a change in some measurable biological indicator, such as weight loss or the concentration of a toxic substance in a sample of blood following exposure, while a *graded response* specifies the form or severity of adverse effects as a function of dose. An example of a sequence of graded severity responses is fatty infiltration of the liver, single-cell liver necrosis, and liver necrosis. Continuous and graded response data do not lend themselves easily to statistical testing nor to the construction of dose-response curves. Thus, dose-response models for continuous or graded effects are not highly developed. Furthermore, because of the significance of the biological distinction between quantal effects and graded/continuous effects, the use of graded or continuous data in models designed for quantal effects may be inappropriate.

4.8. EFFECTS OF RISK AGENTS ON THE ENVIRONMENT

While most risk assessment has focused on effects to people, the importance of risks to the environment is increasingly being recognized (Health and Welfare Canada, 1992b). The quality of human existence crucially depends on the benefits we derive from a healthy natural ecosystem. For example, forests purify the air, reduce the risk of flooding, and moderate our climate; insects pollinate many of our crops; and tropical plants are the source of many modern medicines. For many risk agents, especially toxic chemicals, plants and animals are more vulnerable than are people; for example, pesticides are more lethal to insects and, often, to birds of prey than to people. Certain trace metals such as aluminum or selenium can kill fish or birds in concentrations far lower than those that would harm people.

A wide variety of adverse environmental effects can be produced by exposures to risk agents, and generalizing about them is difficult for three reasons. First, many diverse elements of the environment may be affected by exposures to risk agents, and these elements may react in very different ways. Second, environmental response is often determined by complex ecological interactions. Thus, the effect of exposure on a plant, animal, or other organism generally requires understanding the response of the overall ecological system to which that organism belongs. Third, few generally accepted measures of ecological response have been developed. Unlike the human health situation, where simple measures such as white blood cell counts are available for quantifying a person's health status, end points for describing the health of an ecosystem are much more complicated.

Risk assessors have studied adverse environmental effects of risk agents in a variety of ecosystems including lakes, streams, wetlands, estuaries, near-coastal and open-ocean systems, coniferous and deciduous forests, grasslands, desert and semi-arid systems, and alpine/tundra systems (Harwell and Kelly, 1986). In such ecosystems, risk agents produce effects that vary in scope, nature, intensity, and duration. The scope of an effect may be highly localized (e.g., local environmental damage from an abandoned hazardous waste site), regional (e.g., loss of forest yield due to acid rain), or global (e.g., alterations in climate resulting from the emission of greenhouse gases into the atmosphere). The nature of the effect may involve changes to (1) the population level or health status of important species, such as threatened and endangered species, (2) ecological processes, such as rates of growth, nutrient cycling, and decomposition, and (3) animal/plant community structure, such as alterations in the species diversity or richness. Effects can range from minor to irreversible destruction. In addition, adverse effects to ecosystems can trigger other types of adverse effects that are often losses to the public welfare. For example, damage to ecosystems can result in reduced commercial fishing yields, reduced property values, and lost opportunities for recreation.

Environmental consequences of exposures to risk agents depend crucially on exposure conditions, on the unique characteristics of individual ecological elements, and on the spatial distribution of risk agents. Ecosystems are composed of many populations of organisms that have differing sensitivities. Some fauna, for example, are immune to particular toxic substances while others are not. Thus, the exposures received by specific parts of the system (e.g., benthic organisms or predators) may be crucial to determining response. Even within a species, some members will be more susceptible than others, depending on age and genetic or health factors. Difficulties in performing environmental consequence assessment include (1) estimating the effects of pollutants at various concentrations on plant and animal species under different conditions, (2) extrapolating from localized or small case studies to larger aggregates, and (3) attributing adverse effects to particular risk agents when several risk agents are acting simultaneously.

Environmental effects that are often the target of risk assessments include effects on natural resources, effects on wildlife, effects on aesthetic values, material damage, effects on recreation, stratospheric ozone depletion, and CO_2 buildup and global warming.

- *Effects on natural resources.* Natural resources that may be threatened by risk agents include crops, livestock, commercial fisheries, forests, and other productive assets, sources of food, and raw materials. Major environmental problems that may cause damage to natural resources include the buildup of atmospheric ozone, acid precipitation, stratospheric ozone depletion, pollution of surface waters, and global warming. As described in Chapter 2, significant effects on natural resources could also occur from deliberate or unintentional releases of genetically engineered microorganisms (EPA, 1987a).

- *Effects on wildlife.* Wildlife resources that may be threatened include fish, birds, terrestrial and aquatic plants, and other living organisms. A wildlife resource may be regarded as injured by a risk agent if any of its members or their offspring experience death, disease, behavioral abnormalities, cancer, genetic mutations, physiological malfunctions, or deformations. Numerous risk agents pose a threat to wildlife. For example, acid precipitation can lead to declines in fish populations. Physical alterations of wildlife habitats, caused by agricultural activities, dredging and filling, highway construction, urbanization, damming, mining, shoreline stabilization, and other activities can also be destructive to wildlife (EPA, 1987c).

- *Effects on aesthetic values.* Effects on aesthetic values relate primarily to hearing, smell, taste, and sight. Adverse aesthetic effects include noise, unpleasant odors, foul-tasting drinking water, and reduced visibility. Air pollution can diminish visual experiences by reducing visual range and by discoloring and layering the atmosphere. Atmospheric sulfates are a principal contributor to reductions in visibility (EPA, 1987d).

- *Material damage.* Air and water pollutants can damage natural and man-made materials. For example, nitrogen dioxide and ozone can fade the dyes used in many types of fabrics. Acid precipitation and sulfur dioxide can accelerate the corrosion of metals, deteriorate paint, and damage cultural properties and other irreplaceable artifacts such as statues, monuments, and buildings with carved stone surfaces. Some types of stone, such as sandstone, are more affected by acid rain than others. Particulate matter can contribute to soiling. Corrosive water can break pipes and damage water meters and storage facilities (EPA, 1987d).

- *Effects on recreation.* Most of the losses to recreational opportunities associated with environmental degradation are due to water pollution. Effluent discharges from industrial and municipal sources and the runoff of pesticides, acid mine-drainage, and fertilizers from the land can seriously limit water-oriented recreational activities. For example, lakes and streams can become too degraded to support fishing, boating, and swimming. Polluted water in estuaries, coastal waters, and oceans can threaten swimming, boating, and sportfishing opportunities. Pollution of near-coastal waters can also affect the coastal tourist industry and waterfront development (EPA, 1987d).

- *Stratospheric ozone depletion.* Because the ozone layer shields the earth's surface from damaging ultraviolet radiation, ozone depletion can adversely affect basic ecologic processes. In many ecosystems, the effect could be extreme, as, for example, destruction of the phytoplankton that exist in the surface layer of the oceans (EPA, 1987c). Recent data from Antarctica indicate that an exceptionally intense hole developed in the stratospheric ozone layer in the spring of 1987 and spring of 1989.

- *CO_2 buildup and global warming.* combustion of fossil fuels and other releases of CO_2, coupled with deforestation, may cause an increase in global temperatures. Even small increases in global temperatures can adversely affect ecosystems. For example, global warming can raise the sea level, significantly alter the hydrological cycle, and have major impacts on coastal estuaries and tidal wetlands. Global warming also can significantly alter the composition of biomass, especially biomass produced in terrestrial systems (EPA, 1987c).

4.9. MONITORING METHODS FOR ASSESSING ENVIRONMENTAL CONSEQUENCES

Monitoring to assess environmental consequences consists of acquiring data on the status of elements of the natural environment. Examples include recording losses to commercial fisheries attributable to water pollution, estimating visibility (the distance at which a prominent object is just visible to the unaided eye) to detect reductions attributable to air pollution, measuring pollution levels in national parks and other protected areas, assessing levels of material damage and soiling due to air pollution, and quantifying the health status of wildlife communities (Bartell *et al.*, 1992).

Since it is not always practical to directly measure the environmental consequences of greatest concern to risk assessment, as it is in other monitoring applications, monitoring for environmental-consequence assessment focuses on more readily measured indices of environmental quality. For example, whether an endangered species will survive may be of greatest concern, but current population will be easier to monitor. In addition to predictive ability, key considerations for selecting measures for environmental monitoring are the natural variability of the measures and their sensitivity to risk agent exposures. Low natural variability and large sensitivity permit statistical inferences to be generated from smaller sample sizes.

In the simplest approach, ecosystem monitoring is limited to estimating population levels for important plants, animals, or other organisms. The reasoning is that if the introduction of a risk agent has not produced a change in population levels, then it has probably not significantly affected the ecosystem. Increasingly, though, environmental monitoring has focused on more descriptive measures of ecosystem status, rather than just the health status of specific species. To measure ecosystem status, environmental monitoring systems collect data on contamination levels, species mortality, reproduction rates, growth behavior, bioconcentration levels, ecosystem productivity and complexity, species diversity, and alterations of physical and chemical properties (SETAC, 1987).

For some well-understood ecosystems, their status can be conveniently assessed by monitoring a few basic ecosystem parameters. For example, for many freshwater ecosystems, acid-neutralizing capacity (buffering) is strongly correlated with levels of total alkalinity and important nutrients. The latter tend to determine the sensitivity of the ecosystem to different types of stress. Thus, the alkalinity of freshwater systems is monitored as a simple way of measuring ecosystem stress (SETAC, 1987). Ecosystem monitoring also often focuses on *indicator species*, that is, species whose health provides a reliable indicator of the health of the total ecosystem. In the case of water ecosystems, the health status of benthic organisms (organisms that live at the bottom of the water body) is often monitored. Benthic organisms are sensitive indicators of environmental conditions. As low-level links in the food chain, they play an important role in controlling the productivity of aquatic ecosystems. Benthic samples, for example, have been collected from the Chesapeake Bay since 1972 (Miller, 1987). Indicator species that are tolerant of, rather than sensitive to, contamination are also useful. The ratio of tolerant to sensitive species provides a measure of the level of impact on community structure. Such measures are often used to assess the effect of sewage discharges on aquatic habitats (Courtemanch and Davies, 1987).

When injuries rather than fatalities of plants and animals are of concern, direct measures of injury may be obtained through standard histopathological examination methods (Meyers and Hendricks, 1986). Such methods have been utilized to investigate the sublethal effects of cadmium on birds and the structural effects of air pollutants on plants (EPA, 1989c). Oftentimes, however, a less costly approach based on indicators is used. For example, eggshell thickness is an indirect indicator of injury to bird populations exposed to the insecticide DDT. Other biological indicators of injury or stress include changes in respiration rate and alterations of pigment content. Biomarkers also serve as indicators of sublethal stress. An example is the monitoring of readily observable skeletal deformities, such as in birds exposed to selenium-enriched drainage waters (Hoffman *et al.*, 1988). Other useful biomarkers include photosynthetic rates, enzyme activity changes, and ethylene and ethane production.

As with other applications of monitoring, interpreting the data obtained from environmental monitoring requires having a baseline for reference. Thus, environmental consequence monitoring often involves simultaneous monitoring of a site suspected to be exposed to a risk agent and a reference site that is not subject to such exposures. Selecting a reference site is particularly difficult because so many factors influence environmental quality. Important considerations for choosing a reference site include physical similarity (e.g., elevation, landscape shape, soils), environmental similarity (e.g., precipitation, temperature, wind patterns), and ecological similarity (e.g., habitat type, habitat disturbance).

Statistical analysis of monitoring data requires that the data be an unbiased, representative sample. The basic entities to be measured are called *population elements* (e.g., soil organisms or birds nesting within a given area). Measurements are typically taken in groups, called *sampling units*. For example, the sampling units may be subregions of the area to be monitored. With *random sampling*, every sampling unit has the same chance of being included in the sample. With *stratified sampling*, the target population is divided into several groups or strata, and then selected independent samples are obtained from each stratum. Stratified sampling is used to increase precision for measurements of greatest concern, for instance, by sampling more intensively the more variable portions of the target population. If measures of exposure are collected simultaneously with measures of consequence, dose-response relationships may be obtained from the data using regression analysis methods (e.g., Finney, 1978).

Environmental monitoring has long been used to study the impacts of pollution on trees. For example, growth rates of sensitive species such as the Ponderosa, Jeffrey, and Eastern white pine are often monitored by measuring annual growth rings (EPA, 1987c). One of the most thoroughly monitored ecosystems in the U.S. is the mixed-conifer forest ecosystem in the San Bernardino Mountains of southern California. Data collected through this monitoring program from 1968 to 1972 revealed high mortality rates for the Ponderosa pine (Miller, 1973; McLaughlin, 1985). Monitoring studies that began more than 20 years ago have also revealed declines and diebacks of red spruce in the northeastern United States and reduced growth rates of red spruce, balsam fir, and Fraser fir in central West Virginia and western Virginia (NAS–NRC, 1986b). More recently, remote sensing, using satellite imaging, has been used to monitor forest impacts. Such surveys have been used to define the geographic extent of environmental impacts and to make quantitative assessments of damage (EPA, 1986f).

In recent years, increased attention has been given to monitoring for material damage. For example, many studies have sought to determine the extent of material damage to water distribution and household plumbing systems caused by corrosive water. Corrosive water is a concern because it can break pipes, damage water meters and storage facilities, and create leaks that can cause water loss and water contamination. Consequences of such damage include excessive repair and replacement of equipment, increased pumping costs due to the reduced hydraulic efficiency of corroded or partly blocked pipes, loss of service pressure, and increased operating costs of providing water to customers. Rather than attempt to measure the corrosiveness of water directly, monitoring systems focus on measuring corrosion by-products such as lead. While most water leaving the public water treatment plants is relatively free of lead, corrosive water generally causes widespread leaching of lead, copper, and cadmium from pipes. Thus, monitoring increased concentrations of these corrosion by-products makes it possible to estimate material damage (EPA, 1987d).

4.9.1. Strengths

Monitoring to assess environmental consequences provides a knowledge base for developing environmental-consequence models and for validating those models. Monitoring is most directly useful for uncovering existing environmental risks, since it focuses on assessing the current situation. The information and understanding provided, however, are also essential for projecting risks that may occur in the future. For example, the monitoring of temperatures over the last 100 years has provided some of the evidence for global warming (Holdgate, 1991).

4.9.2. Limitations

In addition to the economic and logistical limitations of monitoring methods that have already been discussed, monitoring to assess environmental consequences suffers from several special difficulties. Ecosystem properties tend to be highly variable and are difficult to interpret. In many cases, basic indicators of ecological stress have not been identified or, if they have been, ways of monitoring them have not been developed. Indicator species for one pollutant, such as sewage, are often not appropriate for others, such as toxic chemicals. Sewage may stimulate certain species by increasing their food supply and altering interspecies competition, while toxic chemicals tend to affect all members of a community. With the exception of tissue damage, there are few quantitative models for relating biomarkers to higher-level effects. In addition, although numerous monitoring systems provide data on the health of ecological systems, few systems are designed to determine ecosystem exposures.

Using monitoring data to infer material damages caused by specific pollutants is often difficult, due to the need to separate out the effects of different risk agents. For example, nitrogen dioxide is believed to accelerate the corrosion of metals. However, levels of nitrogen dioxide are highly correlated with other causes of corrosion, such as sulfur dioxide and smog in general. As a result, monitoring data cannot easily delineate the proportion of observed material damage that might be attributed specifically to nitrogen dioxide (EPA, 1982).

Special problems also exist in the monitoring of wildlife; for example, it is often difficult to assess area-wide population levels. The movement of individuals or plant seeds offsite tends to obscure effects. Some species, such as birds, are especially difficult to monitor, due to their wide-ranging nature. Behavior patterns also create difficulties; for example, sick animals often seek out secluded locations. The extent to which this behavior tends to bias the results of the estimates of animal health based on sampling is unknown (SETAC, 1987).

Perhaps the most significant limitation is poor planning in the design of monitoring systems. For instance, large data-collection systems are often initiated without first identifying the risk assessment questions that the system is meant to answer. As a result, the data are often of little use for risk assessment (Braat and van Lierop, 1987a).

4.10. TESTING FOR ASSESSING ENVIRONMENTAL CONSEQUENCES

Tests conducted on elements of the natural environment represent an important class of methods for assessing environmental consequences. Such tests are analogous to controlled human exposure studies for assessing health consequences. Similar to human exposure studies, environmental tests may be acute or chronic and may be conducted in the laboratory or *in situ*, that is, in the field. Field and laboratory tests provide basic data on the environment's response to risk agents and thereby provide the information needed for constructing ecological dose-response models.

Laboratory tests are conducted using plants or animals relevant to the risk of concern. A relevant test species might be one that is particularly susceptible to a risk agent or one with economic or ecological significance. For example, in the case of pesticides, test species often include honeybees (because of their economic importance), birds, since they are likely to eat insect carcasses containing the pesticide, and fish, since they are less able to move away or avoid contamination.

The use of certain test species in laboratory studies has become relatively standardized. Standard laboratory test species usually have low individual-to-individual variability and easily measured sensitivity to risk agents. They are also usually small, easy to handle, and short-lived, so that researchers can observe effects throughout the animal's life cycle. Standard aquatic test species include microcrustaceans (e.g., *Daphnia*) and fish such as the fathead minnow, bluegill, and rainbow trout. Birds often used for testing include Bobwhite quail and mallards (Kendall, 1987). Green algae are often used in tests concerned with impacts on aquatic plants (algae are sensitive to chemicals that inhibit photosynthesis), and earthworms are frequently used in tests concerned with soil contaminants. Standardized testing protocols have been developed for many such species, for example, the 2-day Daphnid and fathead minnow acute toxicity tests, the 4-day algae (*Salneastrum capricornutum*) growth inhibition test, and the 14-day earthworm test (EPA, 1989c).

As an illustration, the 14-day earthworm test uses the species *Eisenia foetida*, which is easily cultured in the laboratory, reaches maturity in 7 to 8 weeks, and is responsive to a wide range of risk agents. Contaminated soil is mixed with artificial soil to yield homogeneous exposure media at various exposure concentrations (e.g., 80%, 40%, 20%, 10%, 5% and 0%). Three replicate exposure chambers are used at each concentration level. Ten adult earthworms are added to each chamber, and the chambers are then incubated at 20° C ($\pm 2\,^\circ$C) for 14 days. Mortality rates are measured at the end of the period (EPA, 1989c).

To enable exposure conditions to be controlled in the laboratory, special equipment may be required. Figure 25 illustrates an exposure chamber designed for testing the effects of exposures to pesticides on wild game birds. The pesticide may be introduced into the chamber in various ways (e.g., as an aerosol, spray, or pellet) to allow control over the pathways by which pesticide exposure can occur (e.g., inhalation of aerosols, absorption of sprays through the skin, ingestion of pesticide pellets). The many doors to the chamber are needed to allow for easy access to the birds.

Single-species laboratory tests may not capture interactions important to determining ecological impacts. Multispecies tests include tests with two species, such as predator-prey and competition tests and more complicated tests involving microcosms or larger ecosystem simulation models. Multispecies tests and tests designed to more accurately account for complex interactions generally require large-scale facilities. For example, the Aerosol Research Facility at Pacific Northwest Laboratories (Ligotke *et al.*, 1986) is a large facility designed to explore the environmental effects of air pollution. It includes a recirculating wind tunnel and controlled environmental chambers large enough to accommodate multiple biological systems including microcosms, complex plant canopies, soils, and animals. In addition to allowing the measurement of effects on plant and animal communities, the facility permits detailed study of visibility reduction as a function of the concentration of airborne material, aerosol particle size, temperature, humidity, and wind speed.

Most laboratory tests quantify health effects in terms of survivability of test organisms. A standard goal is to estimate the exposure to the risk agent that would cause various percentages of a population to die. Some studies use more complex

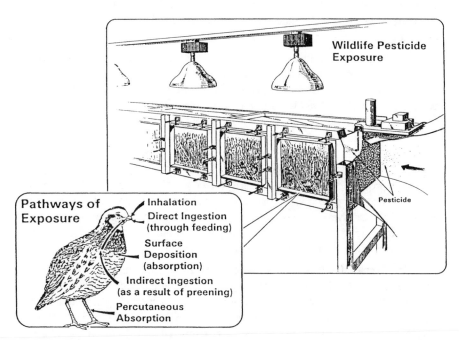

FIGURE 25. Types of exposure pathways investigated in a laboratory study of wild game birds (provided by Peter Van Voris).

biomarkers, such as detailed physiological and biochemical measurements coupled with whole-animal response evaluations (Canter and Knox, 1985). For most aquatic species, investigations are limited to acute lethality measurements, embryolarval tests, chronic toxicity tests, measurement of reproductive effects, and residue accumulation studies (Mehrle *et al.*, 1987). For mammals, many investigations include blood chemistry profiles, blood cell analyses, and pathological examinations of various organs and tissues. Bioassays have been used to assess the biological impacts of toxic air pollutants on different animal species (EPA, 1987b).

Field tests are utilized in place of laboratory tests when it is difficult or impossible to capture all factors within the laboratory setting. Although field tests usually allow the researcher less control, they provide more realistic exposure conditions. Field tests allow natural, indigenous populations to be studied in their natural environment while accounting for interspecies sensitivity, environmental variation, chemical interactions, and bioavailability. Field studies identify the flora and fauna at risk as well as provide data for quantifying environmental effects. Although conducted in the field rather than in the laboratory, field tests and laboratory tests are similar in many respects. The effects may be measured on indigenous plants or animals or standard test organisms may be brought to the site. To ensure access to test animals, animals may be contained in cages or marked for recapture after the test. In addition to the end points commonly measured in the laboratory setting, community effects are often quantified as well.

Testing for environmental consequences generally follows a logical progression, with acute tests conducted before chronic tests and laboratory tests conducted before field tests. The recommended regimen for pesticide testing illustrates the basic approach (EPA, 1989d). Initially, short-term, high-level exposures are investigated in the laboratory using standard pesticide test species. Such tests are relatively inexpensive and serve as a screener for detecting possible adverse effects. If adverse effects are found, then more detailed acute and chronic tests are conducted at exposures consistent with conditions actually expected under typical use of the product. Multispecies tests are utilized to help determine the species that may be affected and to investigate the potential for disruption of the food chain. For example, to investigate the impact on an aquatic system, representatives from all macroscopic trophic levels would be tested as a unit, including fish, aquatic insects, invertebrates, and aquatic plants.

If adverse effects are suspected on the basis of the laboratory test results, more expensive field tests are performed. A field site is selected for the test and divided into segments or "blocks." Each block is further subdivided into plots of sufficient size for practical and accurate application of the pesticide. For example, each block may contain two plots, one that is sprayed with the pesticide and one that is not. Measurements are taken to assess the health status of specific plants and animals within each plot both before and after application of the pesticide. The selected species may be either indigenous to the site or placed there for the purposes of the test. The measurements may include ecological, behavioral, biochemical, and histological effects. For simple measurements such as plant yield, the entire plot is measured. For measuring effects such as chemical or microbial contamination, selected samples are collected (Bunyan *et al.*, 1981).

Statistical methods such as those discussed in Chapter 2 are utilized to help choose the number of blocks, the number, location, and size of samples to be collected, and to analyze the results. Treatment of plots is randomized to help eliminate bias in statistical estimates and to ensure that environmental and treatment effects can be separated. For example, in a study comparing the frequency of colony-forming units of indigenous microorganisms, if treatment were routinely introduced on one side of the block, it would not be possible to determine whether any differences between treated and untreated blocks were due to characteristics of the species or to differences in the environment (McIntosh, 1991).

In addition to their use for assessing consequences of pesticide application, field tests have also been used to investigate the impact of air pollution on forests. Stewart *et al.* (1973), for example, fumigated 70 plant species with ozone to determine the concentration of ozone necessary to cause foliar injury to various species prevalent in intermountain grassland, oak, aspen, and conifer communities. Even a slight level of pollution-induced stress can be significant to forest production, since weakened trees are more susceptible to attack by predators such as bark beetles and pathogens such as root rot fungi (Stark and Cobb, 1969).

Recent research on pollutant–insect–plant interactions has shown how effective field and laboratory tests can be for clarifying cause-effect mechanisms important to assessing environmental consequences. For example, it is well-known that exposures of many plant species to high levels of air pollution, especially ozone and sulfur dioxide, are often followed by accelerated rates of insect damage (Alstad *et al.*, 1982). Chappelka and Kraemer (1988) offer a partial explanation based on a review and analysis of roughly two dozen relevant field and laboratory tests. First, field tests indicate that insects are attracted to and prefer to feed on plants that have been exposed to ozone and sulfur dioxides. This is probably due to changes in plant metabolism caused by exposures to the air pollution, since laboratory tests show that insect plant selection is influenced by leaf sugar concentrations and the release of volatile chemicals, which are determined by plant metabolism. Second, tests have shown that rates of insect growth and development are stimulated by plant exposure to ozone and sulfur dioxide. Other tests suggest that this may be due in part to the fact that exposures of plants to air pollutants often cause increases in levels of free amino acids, proteins, sugars, phenolics, and other metabolites that can be utilized by insects as a source of food. Third, tests have shown that insect reproduction is stimulated by plant exposure to ozone and sulfur dioxide. Again, it is suspected that metabolic changes involved in the stimulation of insect growth and development rates are probably responsible. Finally, tests have shown that in at least some cases, the survival of insects feeding on plants can be enhanced by exposure of the plants to ozone or sulfur dioxide, although no mechanism for this last effect has yet been proposed.

4.10.1. Strengths

Tests conducted on the environment provide a means for experimentally investigating how elements of the environment respond to risk agents. The basic processes by which individual animals and ecosystems respond to pollution can be studied directly. If the environmental conditions of concern can be accurately represented in the test, the results give an easily understood and highly credible prediction of what might actually happen under real-world conditions. Testing can also provide knowledge and data needed to develop and verify ecological models.

4.10.2. Limitations

Field and laboratory tests are often cost prohibitive and difficult due to the number of observations needed and the amount of time required to show statistically significant differences between treated and nontreated populations. In the case of field tests, finding appropriate control or reference sites is another major difficulty. Full tests can also be time-consuming due to the need to conduct studies over several seasons. In practice, most field tests investigate the responses of only a few species to a single risk agent under a limited number of exposure scenarios. As a result, field tests often provide equivocal data (Walton, 1987).

Many of these difficulties are encountered in pesticide field tests. Pesticide field tests usually focus on short-term effects on wildlife, that is, effects occurring immediately after pesticide application or within the same season. Although such tests may show little short-term impact, some of the species present might exhibit greater impacts if they were to encounter similar exposures over a longer period of time. Such repeated exposures might well occur through common agricultural practice (e.g., the routine use of pesticides on a crop grown in one place for several years). Even a single application of a pesticide might produce long-term effects that could be missed by a field test. For example, a single application of a highly persistent chemical, such as an organochlorine insecticide, can adversely affect wildlife many years after its application.

Another limitation of field tests involving wildlife is the emphasis on wildlife deaths as the measure of effect. Tests that measure deaths only are not well suited for studying chemicals that may produce important behavioral and physiological effects at sublethal doses. If natural selection is severe enough to penalize even minor debilitation, behavioral and physiological effects too minimal to measure could produce severe long-term consequences.

In the case of laboratory tests, it is often unclear whether the laboratory strains used to predict environmental effects are good models for their wildlife counterparts. In the field, exposures to risk agents occur through ingestion of contaminated foodstuffs, inhalation of airborne chemicals, and direct skin contact. In the laboratory, exposure usually occurs only through feeding. In addition, animals in the wild are often able to alter their contact with chemicals by modifying their behavior, an option less available to captive animals.

Another limitation of laboratory tests is their failure to consider the role of stress. For example, organisms in the field may be under greater stress, at least during certain periods of the year, than organisms in the laboratory. This may make them more susceptible to risk agents than laboratory organisms. Other errors and biases may be introduced by the laboratory setting. For example, changes in blood chemistry and nutritional needs can have a large impact on an animal's uptake of chemicals through food. In the case of birds the dynamics of flight—which is usually highly restricted in laboratory settings—can produce large biochemical changes (Kendall, 1987).

Laboratory studies involving plants produce similar problems. For instance, experiments designed to explore the effects of air pollution on trees frequently use more sensitive, easy-to-handle seedlings or saplings rather than full-grown trees. They also frequently use short-term exposures at relatively high concentrations in place of long-term, low-concentration exposures. Interpretation requires translating the results of experiments conducted on seedlings or saplings to impacts on large trees and stands. It also involves determining the effects of forest insects and disease, elucidating the effects of pollutants on competitive relationships among species, and translating the impacts of high pollutant concentrations over short periods to the impacts of low concentrations over long periods.

Although microcosms and mesocosms (larger versions of microcosms) would appear to allow for more accurate and comprehensive tests, the limitations of microcosms in assessing exposure (discussed in Chapter 3) also apply when assessing environmental consequences. Difficulties include a lack of realism, high costs and personnel requirements, and a lack of data indicating that microcosms are any more sensitive than single-species tests (van der Shalie, 1987). Many fundamental questions about microcosms have no answers. For aquatic microcosms, these include the following: (1) What fish species are most appropriate and/or necessary? (2) What size microcosm is required? (3) What are the most crucial end points for measurement? (4) How should changes in the end points be interpreted? (5) At what concentrations should microcosms be dosed and how should this dose be determined? (Graney, 1987). Similar questions can be asked for terrestrial microcosms. Moreover, methodologies developed for terrestrial microcosm studies are generally not applicable to investigations in aquatic regimes (Southworth et al., 1982).

Although most tests investigate exposures to a single risk agent, real-world exposures involve multiple agents. For example, pesticide field tests generally address a single pesticide. In commercial use, however, a variety of different chemicals are likely to be used simultaneously or in succession on the same plot of land. Wide-ranging species may be exposed to many pesticides applied to different fields within a locality. Little is known about whether these combinations affect animals in a purely additive way, or whether there may be potential synergisms among chemicals.

4.11. MODELING METHODS FOR ASSESSING ENVIRONMENTAL CONSEQUENCES

For several reasons, modeling for the assessment of environmental consequences lags behind the state of the art of modeling for human health consequences. First, and most important, comparatively little effort has been devoted to environmental-consequence models. Since risk assessment has tended to emphasize human health effects more than ecosystem effects, the development of the two fields has been unequal. Second, ecological systems often cannot be represented by simple models. Organisms interact with one another and with their environment in complicated ways; interactions often involve "feedback," that is, effects at subsequent stages may be fed back to earlier stages so as to reinforce or partially cancel the effects. Finally, basic knowledge about the workings of ecological systems is often lacking, and with it the understanding needed to select and quantify environmental-consequence models. Because of these problems, there are relatively few comprehensive environmental-consequence models.

Available environmental-consequence models differ according to the elements of the environment they are meant to represent and the types of risk agents and environmental end points they consider. For example, ecosystem models may address freshwater environments, marine environments, or terrestrial environments. They may deal with organisms according to whether they function as producers, decomposers, herbivores, carnivores, or omnivores. The models can be narrow in geographic scope (e.g., a small pond) or they can be regional, national, or global (e.g., a model for global climate warming due to the emission of greenhouse gases). Environmental-consequence models also differ in the time horizon over which consequences are estimated, ranging from instantaneous or immediate effects to effects developing over hundreds or even thousands of years. The models also differ in their size; small models may contain only a few variables, while large models may involve hundreds of variables. Model size and complexity are determined largely by the degree to which the elements of the environment considered to be at risk are interconnected with other elements of the environment.

For example, models designed to estimate material damage from air pollution may not require consideration of ecosystem interrelationships; however, models designed to estimate adverse effects of air pollution on plants and animals are often quite complex. The health of most plants and animals is highly dependent on interrelationships. The development of a useful model requires encompassing the complexity and variability of the many interrelated species contributing to the stability or resilience of the ecosystem.

Environmental dose-response models are often distinguished by the types of mathematics incorporated into the model. For example, a *static model* is one that does not consider changes in the environment over time. Such models compute steady-state conditions and do not include time as a variable. *Dynamic models* explicitly represent temporal dynamics. They are usually based on rate equations, specified in terms of ordinary or partial differential equations if time is treated continuously, or by difference equations if only discrete points in time are considered. *Deterministic models* implicitly assume that the elements of the environment behave in a predetermined and predictable fashion. *Stochastic (or probabilistic) models*, on the other hand, are based on probability theory. Such models assume that different elements of the environment act independently and unpredictably, but behavior is such that the population as a whole can be described by a probability distribution. A *simulation model* attempts to simulate each important environmental event, with cause-effect relationships represented by functional equations (e.g., deterministic or stochastic equations). *Empirical models* are statistical models; that is, they are formulated directly from data, rather than from underlying physical or other theoretical principles.

The types of models most widely used for assessing environmental consequences are *simple dose-response models, dynamic models, matrix models, stochastic models, and Markov models*. Less widely used types include *topographic models* based on catastrophe theory. The sections below describe the most popular model types. Special attention is given to two important areas of application: models for the impact of harvesting on biological populations and models for ecosystem responses to pollution.

4.11.1. Simple Environmental Dose-Response Models

The simplest environmental-consequence models are analogous to simple dose-response models for assessing health consequences. They are curves or simple mathematical functions that relate one or more measures of dose to a single measure of response. The choice of the mathematical form typically has little or no theoretical basis. For example, curve-fitting techniques have been used to describe the relationship between recreational activity and ecosystem properties (Hylgard and Liddle, 1981) and the relationship between groundwater extraction and vegetation (Reijnen and Van Wiertz, 1981). Polynomial equations are often used to represent population growth processes. Simple models have also been developed that relate concentrations of atmospheric particulates to the range at which objects are visible.

Most simple dose-response models are derived from statistical data such as that from monitoring or testing (Fries, 1974). Examples are the linear dose-response models used to estimate materials damage from various air pollutants. For instance, based on controlled laboratory and field experiments, damage to galvanized (zinc-coated) steel from exposures to sulfur oxides has been estimated as a function of sulfur dioxide exposure and precipitation acidity (Silvers and Hakkarinen, 1987). Alternatively, simple environmental dose-response models may be derived from theoretical considerations with little or no basis in empirical data. For example, it might be assumed that the relationship between the amount of food available to a predator and the amount eaten is linear. Simple dose-response models are easy to incorporate into a risk assessment; however, the conclusions from such models often leave much room for doubt.

4.11.2. Dynamic Models

While most simple environmental dose-response models are static (that is, they do not include time as a variable), most ecosystem models explicitly represent temporal dynamics. Dynamic ecosystem models typically consist of sets of differential or difference equations. The equations specify the changes that take place per unit of time. Differential equations represent the system as changing continuously, with all rates of change being instantaneous functions of the current state of the system. Difference equations express the model in terms of the discrete changes that take place over unit intervals of time. Models based on difference equations are more common, for two reasons. First, many ecological processes do in fact happen more or less discretely (e.g., in many species, reproduction and mortality happen annually over a fairly short period of time). Second, even when the process is inherently continuous (e.g., plant growth), the data to which the model is calibrated are usually collected on a discrete basis (e.g., daily), so that it is reasonable to model the system using corresponding discrete time steps.

The variables represented in dynamic models consist of *input variables* (model parameters), *state variables*, or *output variables*. Input variables allow the model to be tailored to the specific situation under study. For example, input variables would include environmental attributes (such as temperature and rainfall), exposure characteristics (such as effluent volumes and pollutant characteristics), and control options (such as dam construction or pollution treatment). The state variables collectively represent that collection of quantities necessary to fully describe the environmental system under study, including such variables as pollutant concentrations, organism populations, energy levels, and supply of nutrients. The output variables are the relevant measures of ecosystem response, which typically include some of the state variables. The equations represent state transition functions or output functions. For example, a state transition function constructed of difference equations shows how to calculate the state at time $t + 1$ as a function of the state and inputs up to time t. Mass- and chemical-balance equations are typical examples of state transition equations.

An example of a simple dynamic model is a model developed by Clark (1987) for representing the depletion of large baleen whales (e.g., blue, fin, and humpback whales) in the Antarctic. The model consists of difference equations involving two state variables, one representing the number of blue whales at time t and the other representing the fleet capacity of whaling nations at time t. The model accounts for increases and decreases in whale stock through new births and harvesting, with the rate of harvesting depending on fleet capacity. A more complicated example is a dynamic model for estimating the impact of acid rain on a coniferous forest stand (Ingestad *et al.*, 1981; Ågren, 1983; Ågren and Kauppi, 1983). The model consists of a system of nonlinear differential equations involving three state variables and six input variables. The state variables measure the needle biomass, nitrogen in the needle biomass, and the nitrogen in the needle litter. The nonlinearity in the model is negative feedback from the needle biomass to the production rate of new needles. The model accounts for external forces that may influence the system state (e.g., fertilization) by controlling for the rate of nitrogen flow into the nitrogen needle-litter pool. By appropriately setting model input variables, it is possible to explore the effect of decreases in the mineralization rate of nutrients caused by acid precipitation damage to soil microorganisms.

Epidemic models represent an important subset of dynamic models. Epidemics are commonly characterized by population growth curves for either the pathogen or the symptom caused. The growth curve is called a *disease-progress curve* (DCP). The simplest epidemic models consist of a single differential equation describing the DCP. Examples include the *exponential model*, the *logistic model* (VanderPlank, 1963), the *Gompertz model* (Berger, 1989), and the *Richards model* (Levin and Strauss, 1991). More complicated epidemic models represent various interacting subsystems of the ecosystem in which the epidemic occurs. Epidemic models may be coupled with other models that translate the amount of disease present over time to other measures of interest. For example, epidemic models for disease in agricultural crops have been linked to yield loss models to translate the estimate of disease to dollar value of crop losses (Johnson *et al.*, 1987).

4.11.3. Matrix Models

Matrix models take advantage of special simplifying properties associated with matrix algebra. While the mathematical constraints inherent in matrix models limit their capabilities, these limitations may be balanced by the convenience of the computations and the relative ease of establishing the values of model parameters.

A matrix model widely used in ecosystem modeling is the *Leslie matrix,* a deterministic model used to predict the future age structure of a population of animals from the present known age structure and assumed rates of survival and fecundity. The population is divided into age groups and the resulting numbers in each group are used to form a vector for matrix algebra.The Leslie matrix contains information on the age-specific survival and reproduction probability from one time interval to the next. Multiplication of the vector by the matrix simulates the dynamics of the population. Mathematical analysis of such matrices determines the stable structure of the population without the necessity for time-consuming calculations (Braat and van Lierop, 1987b). Variations of this model have been explored and described by Usher (1972), Caswell (1989), and De Roos *et al.* (1992).

4.11.4. Stochastic Models

Stochastic models explicitly account for uncertainty in ecosystem response by incorporating probability theory into mathematical modeling. The simplest stochastic models are based on statistical distribution theory. They describe the variation in numbers, growth, or density of organisms in space and time. The modeling methods are the same as, or similar to, the statistical methods utilized for release assessment (see Chapter 2). For example, the same experimental testing and monitoring methods utilized in release assessment are frequently uutilized to determine variation in environmental effects on different parts of ecological systems. Regression analysis is the most widely used of all stochastic modeling procedures (van der Zande *et al.*, 1984).

Stochastic elements are often introduced into dynamic models to represent the impact of random environmental fluctuations. An example is a dynamic model developed to analyze the problem of spruce-budworm attacks on balsam fir and white spruce trees in Canada (Jones, 1977). The model uses a set of difference equations to represent growth and development. Trees are assumed to progress through 75 discrete age classes, and budworms are assumed to grow through five discrete stages of development: eggs, small larvae, large larvae, pupae, and adults. A stochastic submodel is utilized to account for randomly fluctuating weather conditions, which are assumed to affect outbreaks of the parasite through their impact on larvae survival. The model produces temporal-spatial maps of live-tree volumes and budworm egg densities.

4.11.5. Markov Models

Markov models are dynamic models that can be viewed as a hybrid of stochastic and matrix models. They are stochastic in that they explicitly represent uncertainty, but can be analyzed mathematically using matrix algebra. Depending on model inputs and the outcomes of random events, a Markov model assumes that the ecological system could be in any one of a finite number of possible states (e.g., bare ground, shrubs, mature forest). Uncertainty is quantified by specifying a matrix of probabilities describing the likelihood that the system will undergo a transition from one state to another. Development of the system is determined by its present state and the various forces that originate within or outside the system. Development does not depend on the sequence of events that led to the current state of the system, only on the current state and the probabilities for transitions to other states. Many ecological systems appear to exhibit this Markov property.

Like other matrix formulations, Markov models offer important computational advantages. For example, the models can be solved to determine ecosystem states that are transient, closed, or irreversible. With further analysis, the transition matrix can be partitioned into submatrices which can be analyzed separately, thereby simplifying the ecological system being investigated. Analysis of the transition matrix can provide estimates of the mean time it takes to move from one state to another and of the mean length of stay in a particular state once it has been entered. Finally, where irreversible or absorbing states exist, the probability of the system reaching those states, and the mean time to absorption, can be calculated (Jeffers, 1987).

4.11.6. Models of the Impact of Harvesting on Biological Populations

One of the earliest applications of environmental-consequence models has been to study the impact of harvesting on biological populations (Staley, 1987). *Harvest models* typically represent species populations either by numbers of individuals or by the weight or biomass of the living population. Populations are often disaggregated according to age or size to represent more realistically the biological processes of birth, death, growth, and aging. Stock expansion typically assumes that the recruitment of young animals into the harvestable population is significantly influenced by the stock of adults left to reproduce after harvesting.

Harvest models play a critical role in commercial fisheries management. One example is the model of baleen whale populations described earlier. Such models can be used to quantify the effects of open, unregulated access to a fishery, which can severely deplete the fish stock and can cause yields to be far below the maximum sustainable yield (Clark, 1987). The earliest fisheries models were simple deterministic models designed to estimate the impact of different fish harvesting rates on future fishery yields. More recent models have incorporated stochastic elements to represent random fluctuations in fish stocks and other uncertainties. Reed (1979), for example, has developed a stochastic stock-recruitment model. Although most stochastic models have adopted a classical interpretation of probability, Bayesian models have also been developed. Clark and Kirkwood (1979) have modified Reed's model by assuming a Bayesian prior distribution for annual recruitment of fish stock.

Harvest models have been extended to study ecosystems other than fisheries. For example, the *DYNAST-MB model* (for *dyn*amically *a*nalytic *s*ilviculture *tech*nique-*m*ultiple *b*enefits) is a dynamic model for forestry management. In this model, the forest is divided into seven habitats characterized by the average sizes of trees: seedling habitat, sapling habitat, 6-inch pole habitat, 8-inch pole habitat, 10-inch pole habitat, mature timber habitat, and old-growth habitat. The model assumes that the forest develops as a linear progression through the different habitats, each habitat type having its characteristic time constant (Boyce, 1978). In addition to timber production yield, the model estimates the suitability of the forest for wildlife (several species of game and nongame species), aesthetic values, and sediment flow.

4.11.7. Pollution-Response Models

Numerous ecological models have been developed to study ecosystem response to pollution and other habitat disturbances. For instance, ecological models have been developed to help assess the environmental consequences of major categories of environmental disturbance, for example, point sources and nonpoint sources of air and water pollution, estuary and wetlands development, water impoundment, entrainment, and land diversion (Staley, 1987). Other models have been developed to estimate the impacts of increased transportation activities on wildlife, of harbor-dredging on fish and other animals, and of oil spills and their cleanup on biological resources. In some cases, pollution-response and harvest models have been combined to estimate the direct and indirect effects of habitat disturbances on fish, birds, and marine animals during harvesting (Staley, 1987).

Water-resources models are an important subcategory of pollution-response models. As described in Chapter 3, there exists a wide range of mathematical modeling methods for predicting impacts on water quality (Orlob, 1983). These methods have been used to study fully mixed, steady-state, one-dimensional systems that receive wastes from a single point-source. They have also been used to help estimate impacts on three-dimensional, dynamic, multiconstituent systems that include aquatic ecosystem organisms that receive waste from nonpoint as well as point sources (Loucks, 1987; Bartell *et al.*, 1992).

4.11.8. Strengths

Nearly all of the strengths of modeling methods described in the sections on release assessment, exposure assessment, and health-consequence assessment are also present here. Most important, consequence models provide a means for estimating environmental impacts in situations where monitoring is ineffective (such as when releases of risk agents have not yet occurred) and testing is infeasible (e.g., because it might produce irreversible environmental damage). Models for assessing environmental consequences allow environmental impacts to be simulated mathematically without the need for costly or unacceptable experiments.

The explicitness of models is an important strength because of the complexity and controversy often surrounding environmental impact estimates. Models provide a logic for estimating impacts which is open to review by those not involved in model development. Although models invariably involve simplifying assumptions, their precision allows these assumptions to be clearly stated in a form that can be reviewed and questioned. Key assumptions become research questions that can be answered through additional experimentation or monitoring.

Many environmental models appear to be extremely complex, but this is not necessarily a deficiency of modeling. Environmental models are complex because environmental systems are complex. A good environmental model provides as simplified a representation of the environment as is possible. The symbolic logic of mathematics extracts those elements, and only those elements, that are important to the deductive logic needed for estimating environmental consequences. The model focuses on underlying processes, and the equations allow the model to mirror or mimic the behavior of the system.

Another strength is the flexibility of modeling methods to describe diverse system functioning, including nonlinear responses and both positive and negative feedback. Dynamic models offer the modeler almost complete freedom in expressing underlying relationships among the variables and entities. Stochastic models allow the modeler to represent the inherent randomness in nature. The usefulness and power of models has also been enhanced by the many general-purpose computer modeling languages that are now widely available, such as DYNAMO and CSMP (Jeffers, 1987) and PROLOG (Robertson et al., 1991).

4.11.9. Limitations

The most significant limitation on environmental-consequence models is the lack of data on how the environment is affected by risk agents. Exposures can have a direct adverse effect on individual plants and animals as well as indirect effects (e.g., the risk agent may upset a delicate equilibrium inherent in the ecosystem). However, because the molecular mechanisms by which risk agents are absorbed and distributed and affect the well-being of plants and animals are poorly understood, even the direct effects of many risk agents on many species are not known. Furthermore, there is little basis for extrapolating knowledge about a well-studied species to one not studied, since few comparative metabolic data currently exist. Knowledge about indirect effects is even less well developed, due to the uncertainty concerning interspecies interactions and the factors that control community structure. Lack of understanding is particularly acute in situations where models are needed most—when the risk assessment requires estimating consequences from exposures that have not yet occurred.

The significance of fundamental uncertainties is illustrated by an assessment of the ecological risks associated with offshore oil and gas development on the north coast of Alaska (Truett, 1980). The environmental-consequence model utilized in the risk assessment involved a large ecosystem model of a barrier island lagoon system. Monitoring indicated that fish and birds, the organisms considered to be at risk, were most abundant in shallow lagoons. These lagoons contained small, shrimp-like marine invertebrates that served as food for the fish and birds. These same invertebrates, however, were also abundant outside the lagoon. If it was assumed that the fish and birds were dependent on the lagoon for feeding, then drilling inside the lagoons would have created a serious environmental risk. On the other hand, if the fish and birds could feed outside the lagoon, as they were known to do elsewhere, then the option of drilling inside the lagoon posed the least risk. The reason for this was that any oil spill that might occur from drilling inside the lagoon would be naturally contained by the lagoon, thereby protecting the bulk of the invertebrate resource that lives and breeds offshore from the islands. Regardless of how well the lagoon ecosystem model was designed, it could not improve the accuracy of estimations due to the major uncertainties that existed about the habitat requirements of animals.

Success in modeling simplified environmental systems does not necessarily translate into success in representing more complicated, real-world systems. Results demonstrated for one point in time or space do not necessarily apply to wider populations or ecosystems. Although ecological models of simplified ecosystems may be useful for research, they are often of little use in risk assessment. For example, models of a single tree or of one square meter of tundra typically are of little value in resolving conflicts about the environmental impacts of different land uses.

Environmental-consequence models are necessarily simplifications, and these simplifications may well mask important processes. For example, many stock-recruitment models assume a constant environment. All of the processes related to the animals' physical habitat, food resources, competitors, and predators are embodied in a few parameters (growth, fecundity, and mortality), and these usually remain constant through time. Such models are incapable of taking into account any drastic changes in the structure of the system.

Ignoring ecosystem interrelationships can result in severe underestimates of an organism's vulnerability. Natural communities have evolved in intimate relationship with their abiotic environment—soils, water, and climate—and have developed complex structural and functional characteristics such as biogeochemical cycles and food webs, that both sustain and define them. Any changes in structure or function due to an external stress may upset a delicate equilibrium inherent in the ecosystem, leading either to increased vulnerability to other stresses or to a shift to a new equilibrium state, or both.

The failure to model ecosystem interactions fully does not necessarily mean that environmental consequences will be underestimated. As Graney (1987) has observed, more realistic, detailed, and complex models are not always more reliable. For example, field tests conducted to validate model predictions often produce no observable effects, even when adverse consequences are predicted. A commonly cited example is the field tests involving the botanical insecticide pyrethrum and its synthetic equivalent, pyrethrin. The failure of such predictions appears to be due to several factors, including conservatism in risk assessment procedures, a resiliency of ecosystems that is not captured by simple models, and ecosystem variability that makes it difficult for field studies to identify chemical-specific alterations in an ecosystem.

CHAPTER 5

RISK ESTIMATION

Risk estimation (also referred to as risk characterization) is the final step in risk assessment. Its goal is to produce measures of the health, safety, and environmental risks that are being assessed. As discussed in Chapter 1, risk is, at a minimum, a two-dimensional entity involving (1) a possibility of adverse consequences and (2) uncertainty. Ideally, the outputs of a risk assessment include explicit measures of both the magnitudes of possible adverse consequences, over time and the uncertainties involved. Summary statistics that collapse such estimates into a single number do not provide all of the information that may be necessary for decision making and risk management.

The most rigorous way to express uncertainty over consequences is through probability distributions (e.g., see Fig. 11). Probability distributions for risk outcomes, with outcomes specified in terms of type, severity, when they occur, and to whom they occur, represent a logical output of risk assessment. Summary statistics for the level of risk can be easily computed from probability distributions. Common summary statistics include the probability of damage, the probability of an individual death, and the expected number of deaths per year.

Often, a variety of probability distributions is needed to describe fully the different aspects of a given risk. To reflect total (aggregate) societal risk, for example, the analyst might estimate a probability distribution for the magnitudes of total adverse health and environmental effects (e.g., total number of fatalities). To represent individual risk the analyst might estimate the probabilities of consequences to representative individuals (e.g., the probability of a typical individual dying). Other probabilistic representations of risk might also be important in certain situations. For instance, to evaluate the equity of the distribution of risk, it might be necessary to compute measures of group risk, that is, probabilities and consequences to individuals grouped by occupation, geographic location, sex, or race. Developing useful measures of risk is a complicated problem for risk assessment; no single means captures all of the aspects of risk that may be of concern.

Although probability distributions over adverse consequences represent the logical outputs for risk assessment, surprisingly few risk assessments to date have provided outputs of this type. Notable exceptions include assessments of the safety of nuclear reactors (NRC, 1975; NRC, 1990), several assessments of the risks associated with common air pollutants (e.g., Richmond, 1987), and assessments of the risks of chlorofluorocarbon releases and the resulting depletion of stratospheric ozone (NAS, 1979a, 1979b). The reason that risk assessments producing probability distributions as output are relatively rare is the difficulty of the task. It requires having the resources and skill to develop or locate the data or other means for deriving probabilities as well as having adequate knowledge and computational capabilities to manipulate probabilities in a logically sound manner. Due to these difficulties, risk assessments have often not included explicit expressions of probability, either in the form of probability distributions or summary statistics. Given the existence of applicable methods for quantifying uncertainty, the majority of risk assessments do not conform to the available state of the art.

When explicit expressions of probabilities are not computed, risk analysts often compute quantitative estimates of health and environmental consequences as if uncertainty did not exist. For example, the risk analyst may compute "nominal" or "best-guess" estimates for the number or magnitude of health consequences that might occur. Another approach is to compute "worst-case" or "conservative" estimates of risk outcomes to provide upper bounds for the magnitudes of risk consequences. Such approaches are most reasonable for situations in which the magnitude of health effects can be estimated with considerable accuracy, as is the case with automobile deaths.

Another approach to risk assessment is comparative or relative. Such assessments do not attempt to estimate consequences or probabilities explicitly; instead, they provide a relative measure of the level of risk posed by various risk sources or agents. An example is the *Hagen index* method for estimating the relative risk of the failure of dams (NAS–NRC, 1983b). In this method, each dam is assigned a series of scores on scales that reflect the importance of various factors judged to influence risk. For example, such factors might include the number of homes endangered by a dam's failure, its capability to resist failure by overtopping, the potential for local seismic activity, and the evidence of structural distress. The scores are then combined through an equation to produce an overall "relative risk" score. The EPA's Hazard Ranking System (HRS) is another example of a relative measure of risk (Caldwell *et al.*, 1981). The HRS is used to rank hazardous waste sites, with the higher ranked sites assigned priority for cleanup.

Relative risk assessment systems such as the Hagen index and the HRS are useful when the goal is to rank health or environmental problems in order of severity or urgency; however, they are considerably less useful for deciding whether the level of concern should be sufficient to warrant some action or what that action ought to be. The weakness of relative risk assessments is that they produce measures that can be interpreted only in a relative sense, for example, a relative score of 80 is worse than a relative score of 50. Relative risk scores, however, do not provide any sense of the absolute magnitude of the risk. Thus, the relative ranking of a problem does not provide sufficient information for deciding whether the benefits of actions to reduce risk are worth the costs.

5.1. THE COMPOSITE RISK MODEL

Estimates of the outcomes of a risk and their probabilities may be obtained through the use of a *composite risk model*, one that integrates a model for the risk source and its releases to the environment, a model for exposure processes, and a model for consequence processes. Once the composite risk model is developed, measures of risk may be produced through four steps:

1. Specifying uncertainties in model inputs
2. Propagating input uncertainties to the uncertainties they imply over risk consequences
3. Adding and combining other sources of uncertainty
4. Displaying and interpreting uncertainties in consequences.

The complexities of coupling the models for release assessment, exposure assessment, and consequence assessment depend on the number of risk agents, subpopulations, exposure pathways, and adverse effects that must be considered. The simplest case is that of a homogeneous population facing the uncertain prospect of being uniformly exposed to a fixed level of a single risk agent that produces one adverse effect. In this case, the release model provides a probability of risk-agent release, the exposure model a probability of exposure for each individual and a resultant affected population size, and the consequence model a probability of exposure producing an effect for each exposed individual. An estimate of the total number of cases, given release, may then be obtained as the product of the exposure and effects probabilities and the population size.

In a case where there are different levels or routes of exposure that produce the same effect but at different response rates and/or different probabilities, then the estimated effects of each exposure may be summed. If the exposed population contains subgroups that differ greatly in their characteristics, then each subgroup may need to be analyzed separately. If the risk agent produces multiple effects, then each combination may have to be considered separately for each subpopulation. If there are multiple risk agents that cause different effects (as with hazardous chemical wastes), the effects of each agent on each subpopulation may need to be estimated separately. To avoid an overly complex analysis, opportunities for simplification are taken. For example, if the effects of similar chemicals in a mixture are similar or if one effect is of greatest concern because of its nature or because of the level of exposure to the risk agent causing it, it may be appropriate to aggregate the effects of the various risk agents or narrow the focus to the one agent or effect that is of greatest concern.

Although the methods for integration may seem fairly obvious once the basic logic for analysis is established, the specific details of data flow, translation, and formatting differ greatly depending on the models and requirements for the analysis. In simplest terms, model coupling requires that inputs and outputs match. For example, the risk source characteristics specified by the release model must be exactly those variables necessary for input to the exposure model. Similarly, the conditions of exposure specified by the exposure model must be those necessary to drive the consequence model. If the individual models are designed specifically for the risk assessment, then compatibility can be designed in, and model coupling will consist of little more than appropriately connecting input and output variables. If, on the other hand, the assessment uses pre-existing models that were developed for other purposes (as is often the case), model coupling can be a difficult task. Typical sources of difficulty include the use of different projection bases, coordinate systems, origins, and grid sizes.

In general, model coupling requires achieving compatibility in three areas: *temporal resolution, spatial resolution, and data consistency* (Bolton *et al.*, 1983; Braat and van Lierop, 1987b). Consistency in temporal resolution includes consistency of time horizons, temporal dynamics, and turnover times. *Time horizons* must be long enough to encompass the most slowly evolving system component. For example, in the case of acid rain, emission control measures might be implemented within a few years; however, damage to forests may continue for decades, owing to irreversible changes in forest soils. Inconsistency in *temporal dynamics* can occur if temporal averaging or limited time horizons distort the time behavior of some of the system components. For example, accounting for catastrophic failures may require representing changes that occur over minutes or seconds, while chronic health effects may occur over decades. *Turnover time* is determined by the characteristic lifetimes of the system elements. In the case of physical assets, turnover time influences the natural duration over which the asset might pose or be subject to risk. In the case of organisms, turnover time determines the maximum time that the organism might be accumulating exposures. For example, human lives extend to an average of 70 years, while tropical rain forests have turnover times of hundreds of years.

Consistency in spatial resolution includes both spatial scale and spatial dynamics. *Spatial scale* defines the area (or volume) over which data are required and estimates are generated. *Spacial dynamics* refers to the way in which things that are distributed across the spatial scale change over time. If variations over time are to be modeled (e.g., geographic patterns of releases under changing standards) care must be taken to achieve compatibility in spatial and temporal resolution. For example, if spatial variability is approximated by dividing a region into cells, as in the sulfur oxides risk assessment described in Chapter 1, then cell sizes and time steps must achieve compatibility across the various model components.

Data consistency involves aspects of source, type, level of aggregation, unit conversion, and quantity. Consistency of source of information is obviously desirable; all data that are used as input to more than one model should be taken from the same source whenever possible. To avoid logical inconsistencies, care must be exercised in mixing different types of data, such as point estimates and probability distributions or data derived based on judgmental versus classical probabilities. If conversions are needed to produce compatibility in the spatial or temporal aggregation of data, then the averaging methods used must conserve mass and energy. Care must also be taken in unit conversion; the units used in one model's outputs must be consistent with the subsequent model's input requirements. Ideally, the methods and level of detail selected to account for each link in the risk chain (Fig. 2, Chapter 1) ought to achieve compatibility in their costs and accuracies. For example, it would be inefficient to use an expensive model of the risk source that produces highly accurate, time-varying estimates of release characteristics to which the exposure model is insensitive.

Small models and large models each have their strengths and weaknesses. A model having only a small number of variables and relationships may be easier to understand, but it may not be sufficiently rich for meaningful comparison with the system it is designed to emulate. A large model may account for many more variables and may display effects that are obscured by a small model; however, it may have so many degrees of freedom that it becomes difficult or impossible to provide the necessary input data. Simple models often can serve as display and communication devices, while detailed models generally require extensive examination and explanation to be understood.

5.2. METHODS FOR ESTIMATING AND ANALYZING UNCERTAINTY

While risk assessors generally agree that probability is the preferred means for quantifying uncertainty, there is much less agreement on methods for obtaining probabilities and on what sources of uncertainty ought to be quantified. In general, the nature of the uncertainty determines the best approach for quantifying it. In most risk assessments, one of two situations exists:

1. The processes associated with the risk are sufficiently well understood that functional relationships among important variables can be presumed, but the values of some of the variables are not known.

2. The physics, chemistry, biology, or other science and engineering aspects of the risk are so poorly understood that the functional relationships among important variables cannot be presumed to be known.

Morgan (1982), among others, has summarized available means for dealing with the above cases. In the first situation, the risk assessor can use the various risk assessment methods described in this book to build and integrate release, exposure, and consequence models. If model variables are not particularly uncertain, an appropriate analytical strategy is to perform a *single-value analysis*. In such analyses, best estimates are provided as inputs for each variable, and the composite model is used to produce a best estimate of risk outcomes. Sensitivity studies may then be conducted to explore the significance of the limited uncertainty. On the other hand, if one or more of the model variables have significant uncertainty, the uncertainty about each of those variables is characterized by a probability distribution, or at least by the first few moments (e.g., mean, variance, etc.) of such a distribution. The problem of dealing with uncertainty then becomes one of how to characterize and propagate the uncertainty in the variables through these models.

Handling the second situation, in which one or more aspects of the problem are not well understood, is more difficult. Here uncertainty typically is addressed in one of three ways (Morgan, 1982):

- By performing the analysis using the model form judged on the basis of current information to be most likely or the best of the available options. Uncertainty in the value of the model's coefficients is then used as a crude way of capturing uncertainty in the model form.

- By performing an order-of-magnitude bounding analysis that is designed to determine the extent to which changes in the model form affect the assessment results so as to establish bounds on the range of possible answers.

- By performing separate analyses using a variety of competing model forms, assigning probabilities to these alternative forms, and then combining the results probabilistically. (This essentially converts a Type 2 condition to Type 1.)

5.2.1. Classical versus Bayesian Methods for Quantifying Uncertainties

As discussed briefly in Chapter 2, risk assessment methods for quantifying and propagating uncertainty through models differ significantly according to whether an objective or a subjective perspective is adopted for the analysis. The choice of perspective is critical because it not only determines the meaning assigned to probability but affects both the interpretation and quantitative values of the computed risk measures.

The *objective perspective* sees risk as a measurable property of the physical world. A risk assessment with a strong objective perspective will adopt methods based on the *classical theory* of probability and statistics. According to classical theory, probabilities are numbers associated with events. The events are interpreted as possible outcomes of repeatable experiments. For example, the event might be that a mechanical valve fails to operate correctly the third time it is called upon to function. The probability of an event occurring in a given experiment is the frequency with which it would occur in a large number of repeated experiments. More precisely, it is the value to which the long-run frequency would converge as the number of experiments increases toward infinity.

Probability numbers satisfy certain axioms. For example, the axioms state that probabilities lie between 0 and 1 and that if two events are disjoint, the probability that either will occur is the sum of the probability that the first will occur plus the probability that the second will occur. Thus, for example, the probability that a valve will fail by the third try is the probability that it fails on the first try, plus the probability that it fails on the second try, plus the probability that it fails on the third try. Although the theory requires that probabilities be assigned only to events that are outcomes to experiments, the experiments may be conceptual rather than actual experiments, that is, it is only necessary that the events could conceivably be repeated under generally similar conditions. Thus, for example, failure of a valve may destroy it, making it impossible to repeat the experiment to see if it would again fail on the third try. Nevertheless, it is possible to conceive of an identical valve that may or may not fail on the third try in a similar experiment.

The theorem in the classical theory that relates the probability of an event to its frequency in a large number of repetitions is called the *law of large numbers*. This result provides an important theoretical basis for using the observed relative frequency of an event as an empirical estimate of the event's probability. Thus, selecting the objective perspective means that the analyst will adopt a definition of probability related to the frequency with which events occur. The analyst who relies on classical theory will also tend to rely on empirical data and empirically validated models and will draw conclusions based on statistical inference. The appropriate outputs of a risk assessment adopting an objective perspective include both computed risk measures expressed in terms of estimated probabilities (i.e., frequencies with which adverse consequences occur) and measures of the uncertainties in these estimates.

The *subjective perspective* regards risk as a product of perceptions. A risk assessment with a strongly subjective perspective will adopt the view of probability often associated with the 18th century mathematician Reverend Thomas Bayes (Bayes, 1958, reprint). The *Bayesian* or *judgmental view* holds that probability is a number expressing a state of knowledge or degree of belief that depends on the information, experience, and theories of the individual who assigns it. Thus, with the subjective view, probability is a function not only of the event, but of the state of information. Different people may assign different probabilities and the probability assigned by any one person may change over time as new information is acquired.

Bayes's theory is more general than classical probability in that probabilities may be assigned to any meaningful hypothesis or proposition as well as to events. For example, an individual subscribing to the Bayesian theory of probability could assign a probability to the event "life exists on Mars." An individual who believes in only the classical theory would have difficulty with this in principle, since it is difficult to conceive of the planet Mars evolving over and over again, in some instances developing life and not in others.

Although they are subjective, judgmental probabilities are not arbitrary. Subjective probabilities must satisfy the same basic axioms as classical probabilities. Also, if a scientist says she believes the probability is 25 percent that there is life on Mars, it means that she is as confident in the statement as she is in randomly drawing a red ball from an urn containing three white balls and one red ball. The fact that judgmental probability assignments may be calibrated using frequency as a standard of reference means that judgmental probabilities may be readily interpreted and understood by others.

Bayesian risk assessment methods tend to make explicit use of expert judgment and theoretical models based on conjecture. Bayesian risk assessors generally do not provide error bands or probability estimates to measure uncertainty in reported probabilities because assigning a "degree of belief" to a "degree of belief" has little meaning. The quality of the outputs produced by a Bayesian analysis can, however, be reflected by a variety of computed measures, such as the sensitivity of those values to the range of judgments provided by different experts and measures that reflect the extent to which judgmental probabilities might change in the face of new evidence.

An oversimplification that has hampered the acceptance of even the most formal and systematic of the Bayesian methods is the belief that "objective" quantities are preferable to "subjective" quantities. Although Bayesian probabilities are "subjective" in the sense that they describe a state of knowledge rather than any property of the "real" world, they are "objective" (that is, independent of the observer) in the important sense that two "idealized" individuals faced with the same total background of knowledge would assign the same probabilities. Furthermore, an analysis free of subjective elements is impossible to obtain. Important subjective judgments required of classical methods include the form of the statistical model to be used and the definition of the population for which the sample data are considered representative. Classical methods may only appear less subjective because the subjective choices are made less deliberately. Instead of emphasizing the subjective nature of a judgment, classical methods often make choices that minimize computational complexity.

A major problem in developing probability distributions using either the classical or Bayesian perspective is representing partial dependence or correlation among uncertain quantities. Accounting for correlation among continuous probability distributions with the classical perspective can be mathematically difficult, except for certain standard named distributions, such as the normal and binormal, for which much multivariate theory exists. If the Bayesian perspective is taken and probability distributions are obtained from experts, separate, conditional distributions for a dependent uncertainty must be generated, each conditioned on specified distinct values for the quantity on which the uncertainty depends.

Both the classical and Bayesian views of risk assessment have merit, and the debate over which perspective is most appropriate for regulatory decision making has no easy answer. Bayesians regard the models and assumptions inherent in the classical approach (e.g., linear models, normal probability distributions, independence among variables, etc.) as arbitrary and not reflecting the best available information for the analysis. They therefore attempt to incorporate all available data, including judgmental data based on experience, to make maximum use of knowledge and expert judgment. Classicalists object that such an approach leaves too much to the idiosyncratic judgments of the analyst and produces analyses that cannot be fully confirmed or validated by others.

Although classicalists may be unwilling to quantify judgmental uncertainty with probabilities, they may be willing to express their confidence in computed frequency distributions or point estimates simply as a range of possibilities. Thus, for example, Spencer et al. (1985) recommend that point estimates be summarized by three intervals. The largest of these is a "total uncertainty" interval ranging from the lower statistical confidence limit obtained when judgmental parameters are set at the values that minimize the conditional lower confidence limit, to the upper statistical limit calculated at values of the judgmental parameters that maximize the conditional upper confidence limit. The other two recommended intervals are a measure of the uncertainty attributed to data-based estimates alone and uncertainty attributable to judgmental estimates alone.

Regardless of the approach taken, if a risk assessment contains both classical and Bayesian measures of uncertainty, the analysis should maintain a clear distinction between the two. As Pate (1983) notes, this will aid the interpretation and review of the risk assessment since the significance or weight that will be attributed to each source of information (e.g., statistical samples vs. different experts) is likely to vary from reviewer to reviewer.

Although the classical and Bayesian perspectives represent polar points of view, the needs and constraints of applications often require a perspective that lies somewhere between the objective and subjective extremes. Assessments of risk often must be derived indirectly using causal models designed to represent real-world systems. The validity of these models is determined both by empirical data and their subjective credibility to experts. Despite the blurring of the distinction that occurs in practical applications, the classical versus Bayesian dichotomy provides a useful framework to distinguish methods for quantifying and propagating uncertainty through risk models.

5.2.2. Methods Based on a Classical Perspective

As already discussed, some methods attempt to develop probability distributions that describe risk directly, without formally modeling release, exposure, or consequence processes. Such methods may be applicable when there is a large data base about the outcomes of concern and when the objective is to estimate the risk as it exists at a specific point in time, that is, the risk assuming that no changes occur. In this case, standard statistical analysis (e.g., as applied, in epidemiologic studies or failure analysis) may be used to estimate probability distributions. As a simple example, if over a number of years an average of 0.5 percent of a worker population has annually developed a particular form of cancer and if no changes are made to the work environment, then the estimate of the inferred risk is that 0.5 percent per year will continue to develop this cancer.

Statistical methods can be used to quantify uncertainty about the variables represented in the models developed to represent the risk source, exposure processes, and effects processes. As stated previously, the basic approach with such methods is to interpret empirical data as providing a sample from which "true" or "population" probability distributions can be estimated. These distributions are usually assumed to be specific, "named" probability distributions, such as those listed in Tables 6 and 7, which are specified by one or more parameters (for example, a mean and variance). These "population" probability distributions are developed by estimating their parameters.

Since data are generally limited, the parameters estimated using statistical methods are themselves uncertain. It is for this reason that the analyst quantifies this uncertainty by reporting for each parameter a point estimate and a standard error or, equivalently, a confidence interval. The classical theory of probability cannot serve as a basis for quantifying uncertainty in the true values of parameters because the theory applies only to situations that can be described by the outcomes of conceptual experiments. Therefore, as Raiffa (1968) notes, the careful analyst who adopts the classical perspective delicately avoids assigning probabilities to unknown parameters. Thus, as explained in Chapter 2, a 95 percent classical confidence interval does not mean that the odds are 95 to 5 that the parameter lies within the specified interval. Instead, it means that there is a procedure that associates with any set of data an interval of parameter values, and this procedure has the property that if it were applied over and over again to independent sets of data, 95 percent of the computed intervals would contain the true underlying parameter value. By specifying the classical confidence interval the analyst has stated the particular interval that happens to be associated with the set of data that were actually observed.

The key limitation for the application of classical methods is the existence of adequate data. When such data are available, the methods permit quantifying both the uncertainty associated with randomness reflected in the data base (e.g., the hourly variability of ambient air pollution concentrations) and the uncertainty associated with the limited sample size of the data base (the fact that samples provide only a limited indication of what might be learned if many more samples were taken). They do not, however, reflect uncertainty over possible changes that may have occurred since the data were collected, and they cannot readily be updated to reflect changing information. Furthermore, the methods are predicated on the assumptions inherent in the underlying statistical models.

5.2.3. Methods Based on the Bayesian Perspective

The premise of Bayesian methods is that any quantity whose value is unknown may be considered a random variable about which analysts or experts can express their uncertainty in the form of a probability distribution. Thus, the Bayesian view allows probability distributions to be assigned to parameters whose values are unknown. Confidence intervals may be constructed from such distributions and represent the fraction of the distribution lying between any two specified limits. Thus, with the Bayesian interpretation, confidence intervals may properly be interpreted as the probability that a quantity lies within the given interval. Probabilities represent an individual's belief about the world, not a specific property of the world. Bayesians believe that subjective probability distributions provide a more useful, logical, and quantitative basis for future decisions than do objective probability distributions derived through classical statistical methods (Lindley, 1970).

Methods that adopt a subjective perspective for risk estimation rely heavily on probabilities elicited from experts. Bayesians believe that individuals with the greatest knowledge and familiarity with the situation under study generally hold relevant information for risk assessment, information that is not entirely captured by a classical statistical model fit to empirical data. Hence, experts provide the logical source for subjective opinions and judgments regarding scientific and technical matters.

From a practical standpoint, the first step in applying Bayesian methods to quantify uncertainty is to assemble panels of experts. Each panel is composed of one or more individuals with expertise in the area relevant to the uncertainty to be assessed by the panel. To obtain a representative sampling of expert opinion, it is often necessary to include multiple panelists per area. Selecting a suitable cross section of unbiased credible panelists requires care. The majority of experts may have similar backgrounds that yield narrow perspectives. The including of extremists on a small panel may tend to overemphasize the credence given to such views within the professional community. Experts who disagree may have already adopted polarized positions on the topic. Even if such individuals could successfully resist incentives to bias their estimates and could provide estimates based solely on their underlying knowledge, there is the danger that the results would be held suspect by stakeholders.

Although it might be possible to directly assess a single probability distribution from a panel of experts, group assessments are generally avoided. Face-to-face interactions between panel members can create destructive pressures, such as domination by particular individuals for extraneous reasons of status or personality (e.g., persuasiveness or willingness on the part of others to give in). Thus, the probability distributions representing the opinions of a panel are best obtained by assessing probabilities from each panel member independently and then aggregating.

5.2.3.1. Probability Encoding Methods. Literature on the subject recommends that subjective probabilities be developed through a process wherein a trained interviewer elicits probability judgments from a subject through a systematic series of distinct steps. A variety of encoding procedures are available for eliciting subjective probability estimates (e.g., see,Staël von Holstein and Matheson, 1979; Van Steen, 1987; Merkhofer, 1987b). The basic types of encoding procedures are: *probability methods*, which require the subject to respond by specifying points on a probability scale that correspond to fixed values of the uncertain variable; *value methods*, which require the subject to respond by specifying points on the value scale while the probabilities remain fixed; and *probability/value methods*, which ask questions that must be answered on both scales simultaneously. (The subject essentially describes points on a probability distribution.)

Each of these encoding methods may be presented in either a direct or indirect response mode. In the *direct response method*, the subject is asked questions that require numbers as answers, for example, "What is the probability that the number of health effects is less than 20?" Probabilities may be expressed directly or in terms of odds (e.g., 1:99 rather than a probability of 0.01). In the *indirect response method*, the subject is asked to choose between two or more imaginary bets. For example, the subject might be asked, "Would you rather bet that the number of health effects would be less than 10, or bet that the number of health effects would be 10 or greater?"

Fixed-value methods are generally regarded as preferable to fixed-probability methods because they tend to produce more diffuse probability distributions and are therefore less likely to reflect overconfidence on the part of the experts

(Morgan *et al.*, 1980). A widely used probability-encoding procedure is an indirect, fixed-value method using a reference gamble. The reference gamble is typically a series of intervals defined over the range of uncertainty or a *probability wheel*. With the *interval method*, the range of uncertainty is divided into intervals (e.g., 0 to 10 deaths, 10 to 30 deaths, etc.). The intervals are adjusted until they are viewed as equally likely (i.e., it is equally likely that the value of the uncertain variable will lie within each interval). The probability wheel is a disk composed of two complementary orange and blue sectors that can be varied in angle to occupy any fraction of the disk's area. The disk may be spun in relation to a fixed pointer and will come to rest with the pointer falling in one sector or the other. The analyst adjusts the fraction of area occupied by each color until the expert is indifferent between a bet based on the uncertain variable (e.g., that the number of deaths is greater than 20) and a bet based on the wheel (e.g., that the pointer will come to rest in the orange section).

Spetzler and Staël von Holstein (1975) were the first to describe a detailed encoding process designed to help the analyst identify and reduce the effect of cognitive and motivational biases often held by subjects. This process, which makes use of a probability wheel as well as other encoding devices, consists of five stages: motivating, structuring, conditioning, encoding, and verifying. As part of the process, the analyst describes to the subject how biases can arise and the implication of those biases for estimating probabilities. Once subjects have some understanding of the biases introduced by common thought processes, typically they are anxious to take steps to avoid those biases so as to improve the internal consistency of their judgments. In addition to educating subjects, the analyst also actively tries to reduce biases, for example, by probing to identify hidden assumptions on which the assessment might be implicitly conditioned. Uncovering underlying assumptions may indicate that the encoding would benefit from disaggregation, that is, considering the probability of these underlying conditions explicitly in separate assessments and then combining the results according to the laws of probability to obtain the estimates for the desired probabilities.

The probability encoding process also attempts to use known cognitive biases to counteract one another. For example, *anchoring* and *availability* are two biases that have been identified. Anchoring refers to the tendency of individuals to produce estimates by starting with an initial value (e.g., the value regarded as most likely) and then adjusting to yield a final answer. Subjects often use this approach, for instance, when asked to provide upper 95 percent confidence limits for uncertain quantities. A bias occurs because the adjustment is typically insufficient (Tversky and Kahneman, 1974). Availability bias refers to the fact that if it is easy to recall instances of an event's occurrence (e.g., because the event is vivid or recent), then that event tends to be assigned a higher probability (Tversky and Kahneman, 1973). If the analyst believes that the subject has estimated an upper 95 percent confidence value by adjusting from a middle value, the subject could be asked to describe scenarios that would explain the high outcome. The process of visualizing extreme scenarios makes the high value seem more likely and may encourage the subject to increase the specified 95 percent confidence value (Koriat *et al.*, 198

5.2.3.2. Methods for Aggregating Expert Opinions. Methods for aggregating probability distributions obtained from members of an expert panel can be divided into two classes: *behavioral aggregation*, which involves contact and interaction among the panel members, and *mechanical aggregation*, in which the analyst uses a mathematical rule to combine the probability distributions obtained from different experts (Merkhofer, 1987b).

Behavioral methods offer the important advantage of promoting the sharing of information. Sharing knowledge reduces differences in knowledge (as opposed to differences in the way knowledge is processed) that may be responsible for differences in the assessed probability distributions. If there are several subjects whose judgments must be aggregated, the analyst typically uses a formal protocol, such as a variation of the Delphi method or the nominal group technique, to manage the information-transfer process. With the *Delphi method*, initial assessments derived independently from each panel member are circulated anonymously to the other members of the panel, along with rationales and reasons for each opinion (Dalkey, 1968; Linstone and Turoff, 1975; Runchal *et al.*, 1984). Subsequently, each member's probability distribution is reassessed. The interchange of assessments and written explanations may be repeated several times and usually produces some convergence of opinion. With the *nominal group method*, the subjects are assembled in a group where they present their initial judgments and then discuss them in a structured format designed to prevent any one expert from dominating the proceedings (Delbecq *et al.*, 1975).

Averaging is the most common mechanical aggregation method for combining probability distributions collected from different experts. Although simple averaging is used most often, differential weighting (in which the opinions of some experts are given greater weight than others') may be more appropriate in some situations. Differential weights may be chosen to reflect a decision maker's opinion of the relative expertise of the experts, or they may be based on the experts' self-ratings. One refinement is the use of Bayesian methods in which the probabilities assessed by the experts are regarded as sample data for the analyst. These new data are then used by the analyst to update his or her prior assessments (Winkler, 1968; Morris, 1974). Such methods, however, are often difficult to apply unless it is assumed that the experts' opinions are probabilistically independent of one another.

5.2.4. Methods for Propagating Uncertainty through Risk Models

The overall risk model, consisting of submodels for the risk source and its releases, exposure processes, and consequence processes, provides a means for simulating the risk process and propagating uncertainties to obtain measures of the uncertainty about consequences. Figure 26 illustrates the process.

If a Bayesian approach is taken, most probability distributions would be encoded directly from experts, although some distributions might be generated from frequency data. In this way, uncertainties due to variabilities of nature and to lack of knowledge can be combined to obtain quantitative measures of the overall uncertainty about consequences. Alternatively, an approach more consistent with classical statistics might propagate frequency distributions generated from empirical data and then superimpose judgmental bounds to reflect additional uncertainties related to lack of knowledge (e.g., Spencer *et al.*, 1985).

Numerous methods are available for converting quantitative measures of uncertainties about the values of a model's input variables into corresponding measures of the uncertainties that they induce in output variables (NRC, 1983; Marzt *et al.*, 1983; Fiksel *et al.*, 1984; Iman and Helton, 1988). No one method is always best. The choice depends on the nature of the problem and the resources available to the analyst. Important options include the method of moments, Monte Carlo methods, response surface and related methods, and probability tree methods.

5.2.4.1. Method of Moments.

The method of moments refers to various techniques that propagate and analyze uncertainty using the mean, variance, and sometimes higher-order moments of probability distributions. The functional relationship between the inputs and outputs of a risk model is normally too complex

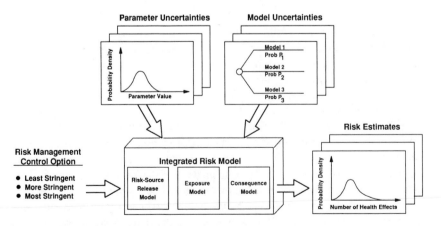

FIGURE 26.   Using an integrated risk model to obtain risk estimates

to enable an output probability distribution (or its moments) to be calculated directly from the input probability distributions (or moments). Therefore, the approach relies on approximating the risk model using a simpler function based on a *Taylor series expansion* (Cheney, 1966). The Taylor series expansion expresses deviations in a model's output value (from a specified nominal value) in terms of deviations of input values (from their nominal values) and the derivatives of the relationship between inputs and outputs (rates of change in output as a function of rates of change of inputs).

For example, with a first-order or Gaussian approximation, the actual function is approximated by a linear relationship involving first-order deviations and derivatives (the linear approximation can be visualized as a hyperplane tangent to the actual function at the nominal value). Higher-order Taylor series approximations contain powers of deviations (e.g., deviations squared) and higher-order derivatives. The Taylor series expansion essentially replaces the general functional relationship between model outputs and model inputs with a simpler form (e.g., linear, quadratic, or cubic equation) that can be solved analytically. For such simple relationships, equations are available that express the mean, variance, and other moments of the output in terms of the moments of the inputs.

Using the method of moments requires a technique for calculating the derivatives of the model. These are usually easy to derive from a computer implementation. For example, the model can be run with each uncertain input variable perturbed slightly from its nominal value. The ratio of the change in output to the change in input gives an approximation of the derivative with respect to that variable. Higher-order derivatives can similarly be approximated. For instance, second-order derivatives can be approximated by evaluating the change in output for small changes in each pair of inputs. Alternatively, computer programs are available for performing symbolic differentiation of large models (Oblow, 1983).

Once the moments of the output distribution have been calculated, a probability distribution can be selected to fit the estimated moments. In addition, methods are available for specifying confidence intervals directly in terms of specified moments (Mallows, 1956).

5.2.4.2. Monte Carlo Methods. Monte Carlo simulation provides an efficient approach for integrating and propagating probability distributions through a risk model. The method involves computing the output of the risk model for many sets of combinations of inputs. The combinations of the input values are obtained by random sampling from the distributions assigned to the input variables. Dependencies among the input variables can be accounted for by specifying the covariances between pairs of such variables. The resulting distribution of outputs is then interpreted as an approximation of the desired probability distribution.

Various versions of Monte Carlo simulation have been implemented in computer codes. In the basic approach, input values are chosen at random according to their specified distributions. The set of random values, one for each input, defines the input scenario for one simulation or "run" of the model, which yields a corresponding output value. The various output values obtained from a Monte Carlo simulation constitute a random sample for the probability distribution over the output (i.e., the output probability distribution induced by the probability distributions over the inputs). The precision of the output distribution may then be estimated from the sample of output values using standard statistical techniques. The number of runs is selected based on the cost of each run and the desired precision for the output distribution.

Several variations of the basic Monte Carlo approach are available. With *importance sampling*, values of particular importance (for example, the extreme tails of probability distributions, which correspond to scenarios that might cause a catastrophe) are sampled more often and given reduced weight to obtain improved resolution for important parts of the distributions (Clark, 1961). In *stratified sampling*, the distributions for input parameters are divided into intervals, and input values are obtained by sampling separately from within each interval instead of from the distribution as a whole. The most popular version of stratified sampling is called *Latin hypercube sampling* (McKay *et al.*, 1979). With this method, each input distribution is divided up into equiprobable intervals. Sample values are thereby constrained to cover the distribution uniformly, one from each equal probability interval. This can increase the stability of the output probability distribution if the uncertainty is dominated by only a few sources. If, on the other hand, there are many uncertain inputs contributing and the model is highly nonlinear, Latin hypercube sampling may not be much better than simple Monte Carlo.

5.2.4.3. Response-Surface and Related Methods. Since the estimation of outcome distributions often requires a large number of simulations, Monte Carlo and related forms of analysis can be costly if the risk model is complicated, and therefore time-consuming to run as a computer program. The number of computer simulations necessary to obtain reliable estimates of the distributions of the outcome variables depends most significantly on the number of uncertain input variables, their degree of probabilistic dependence or correlation, and the level of accuracy desired.

Because of the effect of model running time on the cost of analyzing a risk model, it is often important to design the model structure to minimize the computation time for multiple simulations. For example, complicated risk models are often structured to be as block-recursive as possible. A recursive model is one in which there are no simultaneous relationships that must be solved; that is, the output of any given equation in the model depends only on values from equations that have already been solved or on truly exogenous variables. More generally, it is helpful to implement the model so that each successive equation k depends only on equations 1 through $k - 1$ and on exogenous information. In a complex model, the analyst can organize subsets or blocks within the model. Even if equations within each block must be solved simultaneously, the model is block-recursive and, therefore, simpler to solve.

Response-surface methods are also sometimes used to reduce the computation time for model simulations (Downing *et al.*, 1985). The idea here is to replace the complicated risk model with a simplified approximation called a *response surface*. Typically, the approximation is a linear combination of certain simple functions whose coefficients are determined by least-squares fitting. Because the response surface is much simpler to evaluate than the original model, it is less expensive to implement.

5.2.4.4. Probability Trees. If the Bayesian perspective is taken, probability trees, rather than simulation methods, are often used for analysis because they permit the dynamic nature of events and probabilistic dependencies to be more easily addressed. Probability trees are generalizations of *event trees*. Whereas event trees typically are composed of events with two possible outcomes (the event does or does not occur), probability trees may represent uncertainties with three or more possible outcomes whose probabilities of occurrence are quantified by a discrete probability distribution. If the uncertainties are continuous, the probability tree approach may still be used if the continuous distributions are approximated by discrete ones. Typically, discrete approximations used in probability trees have between 3 and 5levels.

Figures 27 and 28 illustrate probability trees. The example is a Bayesian analysis conducted to explore the value of conducting animal tests of chloromethane, a possibly carcinogenic chemical used by industry in the manufacture of other chemicals. Figure 27 shows a probability tree indicating the accuracy of the proposed test. The numbers under the branches give the prior probabilities assumed for the unknown toxicity of the chemical (not toxic, moderately toxic, and extremely toxic) and the conditional probabilities of the possible test outcomes (no response, minimal response, and strong response).

Figure 28 shows the probability tree used to estimate risk assuming a minimal response is obtained from testing (similar trees apply for no response or strong response, the other possible test outcomes). Each node in the tree represents an uncertainty for the risk model (toxicity of the chemical, average exposure levels, and population exposed). The updated (posterior) probabilities of toxicity conditional on test outcome (probabilities on the branches emanating from the first node) were obtained using Bayes's rule—the effect of the test is to update (modify) the

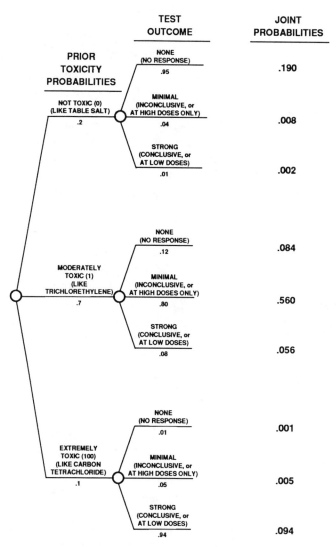

FIGURE 27.   An example probability tree for representing the accuracy of tests of the toxicity of chloromethane.

toxicity probabilities. The probabilities of the other uncertainties are independent of the test.

The risk model is utilized to obtain consequence estimates for each path through the probability tree by running the model for a set of inputs corresponding

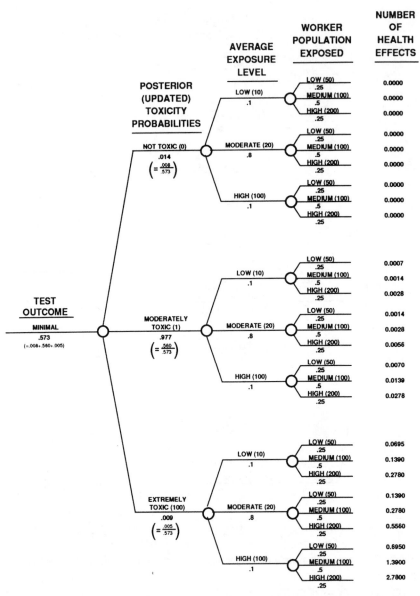

FIGURE 28.   An example probability tree for determining the effect of test outcome on the risks of chloromethane.

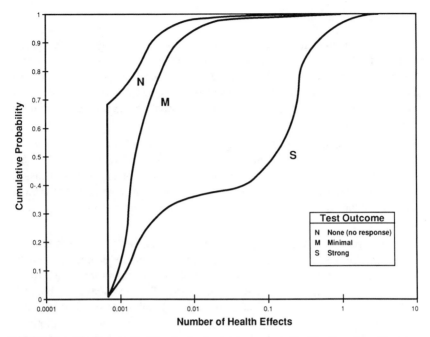

FIGURE 29.   Cumulative probability distribution for the number of health effects depending on test outcome.

to the values specified by the branches along the path. Tabulation and cumulation of the probabilities of the various end-point consequences in the tree permit the development of probability distributions describing risk. Figure 29 shows the number of health effects and probabilities obtained from the testing analysis plotted as cumulative distributions. As illustrated, the estimated risk changes significantly depending on the test outcome.

A key issue for probability trees is controlling the size of the trees. If there are more than a few uncertain variables, the number of terminal nodes that result from considering all possible permutations may cause severe computational problems, even if each uncertainty is approximated by only three discrete values. For example, if there are n uncertain variables, each discretized to m levels, a symmetric tree will have m^n end nodes. For this reason, it is important to use sensitivity analysis to identify those hopefully few uncertain variables that contribute to the bulk of the uncertainties, and to ignore the uncertainty in the rest.

5.2.5. Model Uncertainty

The major concern about models is their validity. Unfortunately, the validity (or invalidity) of a model is impossible to prove. The closest that one can come is those instances in which historical data are available for all of the inputs and outputs of the model. Then the model can be used to simulate past history—the degree to which its outputs match those that actually occurred provides a good test of the validity of the model.

In practice, the degree of validity attributed to a model rests as much on the acceptance of the model's assumptions by experts as on any quantitative test. Experts, however, frequently disagree about the form for the model. Thus, the model is itself often uncertain. Uncertainty about the form or structure of the model is generally harder to think about than uncertainty about the value of a model parameter.

One approach, mentioned previously, is to identify alternative models and assign probabilities to each. This approach has been used, for example, in a major risk assessment of nuclear power plants (NRC, 1990); the probabilities for the alternative model forms were elicited from experts. When assigning probabilities to alternative model forms, care must be taken in defining the set of possibilities. The "correct" model may not yet have been identified, so it may be tempting to assign a probability to "none of the above." Also, every model is, in a sense, wrong; by definition, a model is only a simplified version of the real world.

In some instances a metamodel (i.e., a more comprehensive model) may be defined that encompasses the alternative models as special cases. For example, debate over the form of a dose-response function may include whether a threshold exists and whether response is linearly or exponentially related to dose. A simple metamodel would include a threshold parameter and an exponential parameter that, when set to zero, reproduce nonthreshold and linear behavior. Provided that the metamodel encompasses the possible relationships, uncertainty about the model form can be converted into uncertainty about parameter values.

A basic characteristic of all models is the use of approximations that ease data and computational requirements. Examples include limited disaggregation, such as the finite grid size for modeling spatially or temporally varying values, the use of discrete probability distributions to represent continuous distributions in a probability tree, and the finite number of runs used in a Monte Carlo simulation. Uncertainties introduced by such approximations can be investigated by changing the level of detail, such as decreasing the grid size or time steps, increasing the number of levels in the discrete approximation, or increasing the number of runs in the Monte Carlo analysis. Unfortunately, such sensitivity studies can be expensive, since they often require fundamental reprogramming of the model or a substantial increase in computational complexity.

5.3. OUTPUTS OF RISK ASSESSMENT

Risk assessment has four principal outputs: (1) quantified measures of possible risk consequences and their uncertainties, especially probability distributions and their standard summary statistics (e.g., expected values of risk); (2) special summary statistics or risk indices; (3) information on the relative importance of different sources of uncertainty in the quantitative risk measures; and (4) qualitative information on the magnitude and relative importance of uncertainties not captured by the quantitative risk measures. Each of these outputs is discussed below.

5.3.1. Probability Distributions for Characterizing Risk

As noted previously, probability distributions and their standard summary statistics represent the most complete way of describing uncertainty in the potential health consequences and other consequences of concern. There are three common ways of presenting a probability distribution for an uncertain quantity: as a *probability density function* (PDF), as a *cumulative probability distribution* (CDF), or by displaying selected fractiles of the distribution, as in a *box plot*.

Figure 30 shows the PDF, the basic form for displaying probability distributions that is most familiar to many people. With the PDF, the height of the curve at any given point is proportional to the relative likelihood of the uncertain quantity having that value. Most of the standard statistics used to summarize a probability distribution can be conveniently related to the PDF. For example, the mode is the most likely value, the value where the PDF is a maximum. The median of a probability distribution is the equal probability value—the odds are 50:50 that the

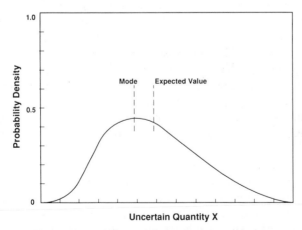

FIGURE 30.   Probability distribution displayed as a probability density function (PDF).

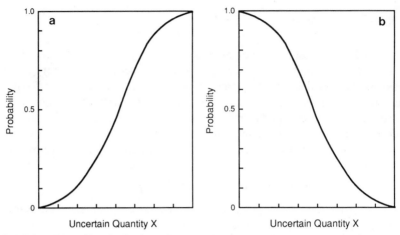

FIGURE 31.   Probability distributions displayed as (a) cumulative probability distribution and (b) complementary cumulative probability distributions (CCDF).

actual outcome value will fall above or below the median. The median is that point along the horizontal axis at which a vertical line would bisect the area under the PDF. The expected value (or mean or average) is the sum (integral) of all values weighted by their probabilities. If the shape of the PDF were cut from a piece of plywood, the expected value would be the pivot point at which the plywood would just balance.

The PDF together with its summary statistics conveniently communicate the basic features of a probability distribution. For example, a symmetric (unimodal) PDF will have the median, mean, and mode occurring at the same value, whereas a skewed PDF will have the mean removed from the mode toward the skewed side of the PDF. The amount of uncertainty expressed by a PDF is often summarized by the standard deviation. The standard deviation is computed by subtracting the mean from each possible value, squaring the result, and taking the sum (integrating) while weighting each possibility by the probability of the specified value. For a bell-shaped PDF, the mean plus or minus a standard deviation contains roughly two-thirds of the area under the PDF. The amount of skewness may be measured as the difference between the mean and the mode values divided by the standard deviation.

Figure 31a illustrates a CDF. The height of a CDF curve denotes the probability that the actual value of the uncertain quantity will be less than or equal to any value along the horizontal axis. The PDF and CDF can be derived from one another; the PDF is the derivative of the CDF, and the CDF is the integral of the PDF. Thus, the height of the PDF at any point is proportional to the slope of the CDF at that point. The CDF displays the distribution's

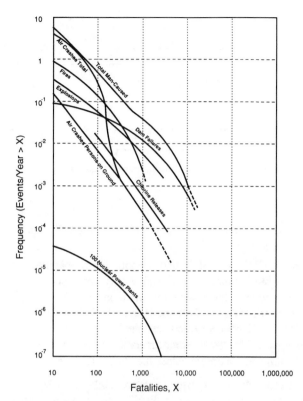

FIGURE 32. Some examples CCDFs produced as outputs of risk assessments [adapted from U.S. Nuclear Regulatory Commission (NRC, 1975)].

fractiles, which represent additional summary statistics. The "pth" fractile (e.g., 95th fractile) is defined as the value such that the probability is p that the actual value of the uncertain variable is less than that value. Thus, the 95th fractile is the point along the horizontal axis where the height of the CDF curve reaches 0.95 cumulative probability.

A variation of the CDF is the complementary cumulative probability distribution function (CCDF), shown in Fig.31b. The CCDF is simply the complement of the CDF. With the CCDF, the height of the curve gives the probability that the actual value will be greater than or equal to any value on the horizontal axis. Figure 32 shows examples of CCDFs produced as outputs of risk assessments. Depending on whether the classical or Bayesian perspective is taken, the CCDF is often called the *F–N* (*frequency–number*) *curve* or the *risk profile*, respectively. CDF and CCDF plots are often constructed on logarithmic plots because probability and

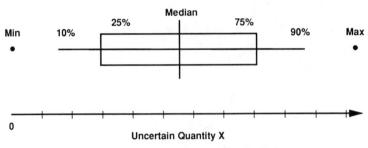

FIGURE 33.   A box plot of a probability distribution.

outcome value (e.g., number of possible fatalities) typically range over several orders of magnitude.

Whereas the CDF and PDF display the complete probability distribution, *box plots* are simpler representations that display only confidence bands constructed from specified fractiles of the distribution. With one version, shown in Fig.33, the display shows a horizontal line from the 10th to the 90th fractiles, a box from the 25th to the 75th fractiles, and a vertical line at the median. If the range of the uncertain quantity is limited to some interval, points are used to indicate the absolute minimum and maximum values that define the interval.

If the uncertain quantity is discrete, its probability distribution is often called a *probability mass function.* A discrete distribution or a distribution that contains discrete as well as continuous elements can still be represented using a CDF or PDF. An example of a situation in which a mixed distribution is useful is displaying the estimated health impact when the dose-response function contains a threshold. In such instances, there may be a finite probability that the dose may yield no adverse health effects. Discrete or mixed distributions are represented in the CDF by vertical steps, where the steps occur at the outcome values with finite probability. With the PDF, discrete probabilities are represented by vertical lines or arrows (which represent delta functions), with heights proportional to the probability mass (not density) at those points.

Although the PDF, CDF, and box plot contain similar information, each has its own advantages and disadvantages. Since the density function is the derivative of the cumulative function, it is a much more sensitive indicator of variations in probability density. This can be an advantage, if the goal is to convey small variations. It can be a disadvantage, however, if small variations represent errors introduced from the calculation process, such as sampling noise from Monte Carlo analysis or discretizing errors introduced by the finite number of paths through a probability tree. The box plot provides a simpler representation that emphasizes confidence intervals and the median, at the expense of leaving out more subtle characteristics related to the shape of the distribution.

To display uncertainty over several dependent variables, *joint probability distributions* may be plotted. Since displaying the joint probability distribution for even two dependent variables requires a three-dimensional plot, the standard approach is to select representative values for all but one uncertain quantity, and display the conditional probability distribution for the remaining quantity. As in the single-dimensional case, the distributions may be shown as a PDF, CDF, or as a box plot.

As noted previously, many risk assessments combine aspects of both the Bayesian and classical perspectives. The Bayesian proponent, for example, can introduce the classical concept of frequency into his framework by imagining a thought experiment in which the situation or action producing the risk occurs a great many times. At the end of this experiment, each possible level of consequences will have occurred many times according to some frequency distribution.

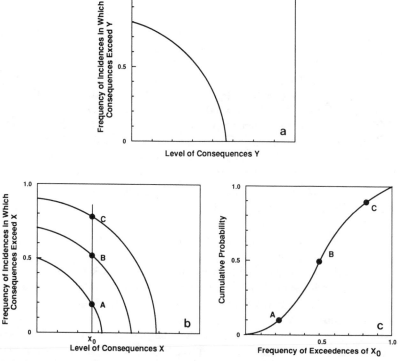

FIGURE 34.   Using families of risk curves to represent both statistical uncertainty and uncertainty due to a lack of knowledge.

Figure 34a illustrates how the results of such an experiment might be displayed as a CCDF, or risk curve, showing the frequency of consequences having magnitudes greater than any specified level. Since the experiment has not yet been conducted, the Bayesian can express his state of uncertainty about the frequency by specifying a probability distribution for alternative risk curves. Figure 34b shows a family of three such risk curves. In practice, alternative curves for the frequency of consequences of various magnitudes are produced using different assumptions for the risk model (e.g., input probability distributions provided by experts who believe in pessimistic, nominal, and optimistic scenarios).

Figure 34c shows how such a family of risk curves can be reduced to a form that makes explicit the state of knowledge or degree of belief behind each frequency curve. The conversion is based on the concept of a "cut curve." If a vertical line is drawn at any consequence level, then the intersection of this line with the family of curves leads to a cumulative probability distribution for the probability of the actual frequency of occurrences of consequences with levels less than X. Such cut curves can also be drawn to decompose a family of risk curves into its various sources of risk.

5.3.2. Risk Indices

Although probability distributions over risk consequences provide a comprehensive way of conveying the results of a risk assessment, there may be too many different types of consequences to permit the uncertainty in each to be described in this manner. Thus, it is generally convenient to reduce complexity by aggregating similar consequences into aggregate outcome measures. The aggregate measures are referred to as indices of risk. Typically, *risk indices* are single numbers (e.g., point estimates) selected to characterize some important aspect of the risk. The indices that are used, however, tend to vary depending on the type of risk.

As an example, the following are risk indices used in worker accident risk assessment. The average rate of death is defined as the average number of fatalities expected per year from accidents attributable to the risk source (Lees, 1980). The total *fatal accident rate* (FAR) is defined as the number of deaths in every 10^8 hours of exposure to risk (roughly 1,000 employee lifetimes). The FAR is typically a combined accident rate that includes various sources of risk or accident types. Otherwise, it is proportional to the average individual risk. The *individual hazard index* (IHI) is the FAR for a particular risk source or type of accident calculated for an exposure time equal to the proportion of time that an individual is actually exposed to the risk concern (Helmers and Schuller, 1982). Finally, the *equivalent social cost index* is a modification of the average rate of death that takes into account society's special aversion to accidents that produce large numbers of deaths (Okrent, 1981).

More general risk indices (used more widely than just the special area of accident risk assessment) include several common measures of individual and societal risk, in particular:

- *Individual risk*, which is the probability of a specified individual dying prematurely as a result of exposure to the risk agents. The time period of exposure must be specified. Lifetime individual risk is calculated assuming that the exposures continue over the entire lifetime of the individual (usually assumed to be 70 years).

- *Individual risk contours* show the geographical distribution of individual risk, that is, the individual risk to a (real or hypothetical) person at specified locations. Individual risk contours are usually displayed on maps as lines of constant individual risk.

- *Maximum individual risk* is the individual risk to the person experiencing the highest risk in the exposed population. If the risk source is a hazardous facility, this might be an operator working at the facility or the person living closest to the facility.

- *Average individual risk* is the individual risk averaged over the population. Some assessments take the average over the total population (even if some members are not subject to exposure) while others average over a specified subset of the total population (such as only those people whose individual risk is above a specified level). The average may also be calculated for various durations of exposure (e.g., per year, per day, or per hour of exposure).

- Various measures of *societal risk*, such as a probability distribution over the total number of fatalities in the population over a specified period of time, the expected number of fatalities as a function of location or population subgroup, and the number of individuals whose individual risk exceeds a specified level (e.g., 10^{-6} probability of death). The key distinction of most societal risk indices is the strong dependence on the number of individuals who experience the risk.

The logic used in combining and processing probability distributions and other measures depends on the situation. For example, a method commonly used for assessing risks associated with the release of hazardous substances is to calculate probability distributions for the health effects suffered by hypothetical or representative individuals located within particular geographic regions surrounding the risk source and then to combine these distributions with population density data to calculate a probability distribution for the total number of the adverse health effects. The same data may also be used to compute the annual probability that each

TABLE 22. Equations for Calculating Some Standard Risk Indices

Individual risk at location (x, y)	$IR(x, y) = \sum_{i, j} R_i\, E_{ji}(x, y)\, F_j$
Maximum individual risk	$IR^{\max} = IR(x_m, y_m)$, where (x_m, y_m) is the location where IR is the greatest
Average individual risk	$IR^{AV} = \dfrac{\sum_{x, y} IR(x, y)\, N(x, y)}{\sum_{x, y} N(x, y)} = \dfrac{F}{N}$
Total number of fatalities	$F = \sum_{xy} IR(x, y)\, N(x, y) = IR^{AV} \times N$
Fatal accident rate	$FAR = IR^{AV} \times 1.14 \times 10^4$
Equivalent social cost	$ESC = \sum_{i} C_i\, N_i^{p}$

KEY:

R_i = Probability of release scenario i

$E_{ji}(x, y)$ = Probability of exposure scenario j occurring to an individual in a geographic cell at location (x, y) given release scenerio i

F_j = Probability that exposure scenario j will result in a fatality

$N(x, y)$ = Number of people in the geographic cell at location (x, y)

N = Total number of people in the population

C_i = Probability of consequence scenario i

p = Risk aversion power factor[a]

N_i = Number of fatalities per year under consequence scenario i

[a]Values between 1.2 and 2 have been suggested (Okrent, 1981; Netherlands Government, 1985).

exposed individual may suffer a particular adverse health effect. The average over all individuals provides a measure of individual risk, whereas the average over various groups of individuals classified by location, occupation, health, and other characteristics provides a measure of the risk faced by different population groups. Table 22 provides the general equations often used for computing such risk indices.

In carcinogenic risk assessment, a common summary statistic is an upper-bound estimate for the probability that an exposed individual will contract cancer. This estimate is computed by multiplying two factors—a *lifetime average daily dose* (LADD) and a *unit cancer risk* (UCR). The LADD is a measure of the dose of the carcinogen received by an individual exposed for a substantial portion of his or her lifetime. The UCR is an estimate of the excess or added probability of cancer per unit of dose, that is, it is a measure of the carcinogenic potency of the chemical. The estimate of excess probability of cancer produced by multiplying the LADD and the UCR is an upper-bound estimate because conservatism is introduced through various assumptions used to compute the LADD and UCR. For example, the LADD may be computed for an individual who lives in a location having particularly high concentrations of the carcinogen. Oftentimes, the LADD is calculated by multiplying an estimated maximum daily dose (maximum dose the individual is likely to receive on any day during the period of his exposure) by the fraction of the total lifetime that the individual is exposed (exposed days divided by days per lifetime). Conservatism may be introduced into the UCR by using a conservative dose-response model or one designed to produce an upper-bound estimate, such as the linearized multistage model.

In noncarcinogenic chemical risk assessment, a frequently computed summary statistic is the *hazard index* (HI). The HI is the computed maximum daily dose (MDD) received by an individual, divided by a computed *acceptable daily intake* (ADI), that is,

$$HI = \frac{MDD}{ADI}$$

The ADI is usually derived from the chemical's NOEL or, if the effects observed at the lowest doses are not adverse, the *no-observed-adverse-effect level* (NOAEL). For conservatism and to account for uncertainty, a safety factor is often applied. Typically, the safety factor is 10 when extrapolating from studies involving prolonged exposure to humans, and 100 when extrapolating from results of long-term studies in experimental animals. Even larger safety factors may be used if the quality of data is questionable or if for other reasons uncertainties are particularly large (e.g., EPA, 1985c,d). Because the choice of safety factors often reflects conservatism, the level of risk for nearly everyone in the exposed population is likely to be small if the HI is less than one. However, the level of risk may also be small even if the HI is substantially greater than one.

Conservative risk indices must be used with care since they obviously introduce value judgments into risk assessment. More generally, however, the need for caution extends to all risk indices, since any method for aggregation involves value judgments. For example, aggregating automobile accident deaths into total fatalities involves making the value judgment that deaths are in some sense equal, regardless of whether death occurred instantaneously or was delayed, or whether the victim was an adult or a child.

Despite their incorporation of value judgments, risk indices are often useful means for describing and quantifying risk. Aggregating similar consequences can help decision makers by providing a coherent, explicit, and consistent measure of the magnitude of the risk outcome. Formal integration also helps decision makers avoid the costs and errors that come from intuitive combination. When complemented by similar indices that summarize the (nonrisk) costs and benefits of alternative actions for dealing with technological risks, a risk index provides one of the critical inputs for risk management.

5.3.3. Analyzing the Sources of Uncertainty

One of the main reasons for conducting a quantitative risk assessment is to be able to answer questions about the relative contribution of various sources of uncertainty in risk consequences. Such information makes it possible to compare different sources of uncertainty and can guide future research designed to reduce uncertainty.

Given a risk model, analyzing and attributing sources of uncertainty can be approached in several ways. The simplest approach is *point sensitivity analysis*, in which the derivative or rate of change of each outcome variable is computed with respect to a unit change in each input variable evaluated at nominal input values. Since this method ignores the relative range of uncertainty in input quantities, more elaborate means are generally used. For example, *parametric sensitivity analysis* involves plotting or establishing a range of output values as each input being analyzed is varied from its extreme low to high values while holding all others at nominal (or other) values. Another approach involves partitioning the uncertainty in the output according to a Gaussian approximation: the variance in an outcome distribution is divided among the inputs in proportion to the point derivative with respect to that input multiplied by its variance. Where the linear approximation is appropriate, this method may be useful for initial screening to identify the major contributors to uncertainty.

Computing *rank correlations* between outputs and inputs is also used for analyzing relative contributions to uncertainty. In this method, the output and input values are ranked and the values are replaced by their ranks before correlations are computed in the usual statistical way. An advantage of correlating ranks rather than the values of the quantities is that it makes the results independent of the measurement units chosen to quantify the variables. Another advantage is that it does not require all other inputs to be held at their nominal value, but averages the effect on each output as other quantities vary probabilistically over their entire range.

The most comprehensive means for analyzing sources of uncertainty using the risk model is *stochastic sensitivity analysis*, in which changes in the probability distributions or their summary statistics (such as expected values and variances) are explored as various input values are fixed or varied across their range. A distinction for sensitivity analysis that may be relevant for more complicated risk models is whether the analysis is *open-loop* or *closed-loop*. According to control theory, a measure of sensitivity or uncertainty importance is open-loop if it measures the sensitivity of output to changes in input assuming that decisions represented in the model do not change. If, on the other hand, decisions are adjusted to reoptimize the outcome as a function of changes in some uncertainties, then the measure is called closed-loop. Closed-loop sensitivity is a more relevant measure if decisions represented in the model are actually expected to vary as a function of some of the uncertainties in the model. An important closed-loop sensitivity measure is the expected value of perfect information (Howard, 1968). The method requires a loss function, that is, a means for valuing risk, and therefore lies in the domain of risk evaluation rather than risk assessment. Although not strictly a risk assessment method, it offers a way of comparing the importance of different sources of uncertainty in terms of a common metric of value.

5.3.4. Qualitative Uncertainty Analysis

If quantitative analysis of uncertainty is constrained by lack of time or resources to collect adequate data, seek expert judgment, or perform rigorous analyses, qualitative uncertainty analysis may still be helpful. A systematic identification and discussion of possible causes of uncertainties can be of considerable value. Rough qualitative estimates of uncertainties can provide the basis for a first approximation of the relative risk of alternative decisions and may permit an identification and rank ordering of key factors.

If, on the other hand, a detailed quantitative analysis of uncertainty has been conducted, qualitative discussion of uncertainty is still needed to clarify sources of uncertainty not adequately captured by the quantitative analysis. These sources are numerous, and not all will be accounted for by quantitative risk estimates. For example, since no satisfactory method yet exists for quantifying "unknown unknowns," no risk assessments can successfully quantify completeness uncertainties. Omitted sources of uncertainty may produce random or systematic errors and biases. Thus, to accurately convey the strength of evidence underlying a risk assessment, quantitative results must be coupled with a qualitative discussion of uncertainties that are not represented quantitatively in the results.

Despite the importance of communicating the uncertainties and limitations of analytic results, only a few conclusions exist concerning the most effective formats for accomplishing this objective. For each step of the assessment, major assumptions must be presented and the nature and magnitude of potential errors characterized. The discussion should include such topics as limitations of the data, limitations of survey design and measurement techniques, limitations of submodels, and the extent to which submodels have been validated. Any conservatisms introduced into the analysis should be clearly identified and their effects on the results should be indicated. If upper-bound risk estimates are provided, then best estimates and lower bounds should be given as well. The discussion should be sufficiently clear to allow nontechnical decision makers to form an accurate

TABLE 23. Sample Format for Qualitative Uncertainty Analysis

Component	Task	Subtask	Method	Major assumptions	Area of impact[b]	Significance[c]	Remarks
				Element of risk assessment			
Release assessment	Modeling containment failures	Delineation of accident scenarios	Event trees	[Brief statements about the major assumptions involved, methods used for identifying initiating events, accident sequences, etc.]	P	X	[Statement of conservatism, source of data, basis for selecting X, etc.]
Exposure assessment	Modeling atmospheric transport and transformation of emissions	Accounting for routine emissions	Gaussian plume model	[Brief statements about major assumptions involved and method of computation.]	C	X	[Statement of conservatism, basis for selecting X, degree and results of model calibration, etc.]

[a] Adapted from U.S. Nuclear Regulatory Commision (NRC, 1983).

[b] P = Probability or frequency; C = consequence.

[c] X can be major (M), intermediate (I), or minor (m).

understanding of the strengths and weaknesses of the analysis. At a minimum, sufficient detail must be provided to allow for peer review.

A sample of a possible format for presenting qualitative uncertainty analysis is presented in Table 23. The format and content of this example are analogous to those suggested by the Nuclear Regulatory Commission for qualitative uncertainty analysis in probabilistic risk assessment (NRC, 1983). The second and third columns in the table specify various tasks and subtasks conducted as part of the risk assessment. The next two columns list methods used and state the major assumptions and limitations associated with models, data input, and results. The "Area of impact" column indicates whether the uncertainties and limitations associated with the subtask assumptions affect primarily the estimate of probabilities or the consequences of risk outcomes. The "Significance" column labels the uncertainties associated with each subtask as having a major, intermediate, or minor impact on the total uncertainties associated with the task under consideration. This assignment of significance is based on a subjective evaluation of the uncertainty contributed by each major assumption or subtask feature to the overall uncertainty of the subtask and task. Finally, the "Remarks" column provides supplementary information, such as sources of conservatism in the assumptions, or issues related to modeling or model input adequacy, limitations, and completeness. While formats other than that of Table 23 may be equally useful, any sound qualitative discussion should include these basic types of information.

CHAPTER 6

AN EVALUATION OF THE STATE OF THE ART

Evaluating the state of the art of risk assessment is difficult. Similar to a craftsman with many specialized tools, the risk assessor has a huge variety of risk assessment methods from which to choose. If the available risk assessment methods are inadequate, the quality of risk assessments based on those methods will be limited. The use of high-quality, capable methods, however, does not necessarily ensure high-quality risk assessments. Similar to the craftsman, the risk assessor must first choose from among the available tools the one that is best for the necessary task. Furthermore, the quality of the end result depends not only on the choice of the appropriate tool, but also on the skill with which it is applied.

This chapter provides an overall appraisal of risk assessment as a scientific procedure and as an aid to decision making. The discussion is organized according to six criteria often used to evaluate formal analysis (Majone and Quade, 1980; Merkhofer, 1987a). These criteria are (1) logical soundness, (2) completeness, (3) accuracy, (4) acceptability, (5) practicality, and (6) effectiveness. The first three of these criteria, logical soundness, completeness, and accuracy, are internal criteria. They relate to the quality of the analysis and can be evaluated with reference to the scientific disciplines on which risk assessment methods are based. The last three criteria, acceptability, practicality, and effectiveness, are external criteria. They address pragmatic considerations that go beyond scientific disciplines and depend on how the method is used in the given situation.

Figure 35 summarizes these evaluation criteria and indicates some of the most important considerations under each criterion. Each of the three internal criteria poses a question about the quality of the assessment and its results. Logical soundness asks whether the risk assessment can be justified by theory and whether an application violates any fundamental theoretical assumptions. Completeness asks whether risk assessment can theoretically account for all relevant aspects of the risk and whether in practice an application produces important omissions. Accuracy asks whether the risk assessment is sufficiently precise, free from possible biases, and sensitive to assumptions that have not or cannot be tested.

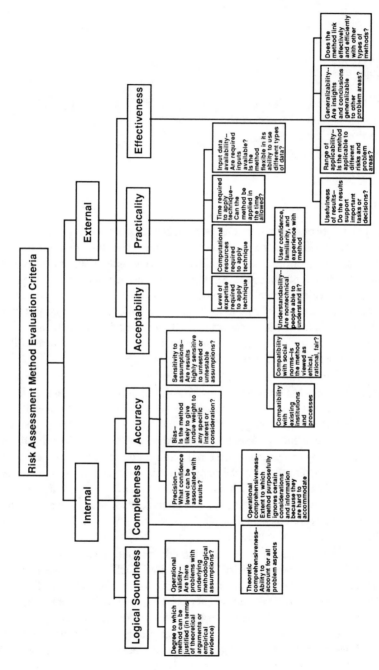

Figure 35. Criteria for evaluating risk assessment methods.

The three external criteria provide standards for judging the application of the method in a given context or situation. Acceptability requires a judgment about whether a risk assessment is understood and believed. It depends on the capabilities, perceptions, and attitudes of potential users. Practicality asks whether risk assessment can be employed in a real-world environment characterized by limited problem-solving resources and information. Effectiveness asks whether risk assessment can accomplish its intended ends; namely, producing information that improves the risk management process.

6.1. THE LOGICAL SOUNDNESS OF RISK ASSESSMENT

Logical soundness relates to whether risk assessment can be justified by theory and whether applications are likely to violate fundamental theoretical assumptions. The basic principles of risk assessment derive from well-developed mathematical disciplines such as probability theory and statistical analysis. Problems with logical soundness rarely arise from theoretical flaws in the laws of probability or statistics. Rather, logical problems in risk assessment arise because the assumptions necessary to apply these laws do not hold in specific applications. For example, the following practices raise questions for logical soundness:

- Incorrectly stating the premises or underlying assumptions for the assessment; for example, making inaccurate assumptions about whether a risk agent poses a risk to public health.
- Using data from the past to make inferences about the future without regard to whether significant changes have occurred since the data were collected.
- Using a surrogate for a phenomenon of interest, such as tests on laboratory animals to imply effects on humans, while ignoring the significant differences that exist between the surrogate and the phenomenon of interest.
- Using monitoring or probability encoding methods known to introduce random error or systematic bias and failing to account for such effects.
- Using methods of analysis based on simplifying independence assumptions that do not hold.
- Using simplified models of complex processes that reflect a biased representation of uncertain reality; for example, ignoring higher-order terms in a series expansion.
- Aggregating quantities in ways that obscure crucial dependencies, such as dependencies that tend to result in exposures to risk agents that act synergistically.

Risk assessors generally recognize the problems raised by these practices. Nonetheless, risk assessors sometimes engage in these practices because of the lack of data necessary for a logically rigorous analysis or because of limitations in available time and resources. Occasionally, logic may be violated deliberately for the purpose of manipulating the assessment to obtain results that support a preconceived point of view. Sponsors and reviewers of risk assessments can avoid such problems by insisting that crucial assumptions be clearly identified and subjected to external review and sensitivity analysis. Assumptions that dramatically alter estimated levels of risk should be validated, either through the analysis of empirical data or through persuasive theoretical arguments.

6.2. THE COMPLETENESS OF RISK ASSESSMENT

The test of completeness has two aspects: whether risk assessment can account theoretically for all relevant considerations of a risk problem and whether the use of risk assessment in practice is likely to lead to important omissions. The principal source of incompleteness in risk assessment is problem complexity coupled with inadequate scientific and technical data. If data are extensive (e.g., automobile accident data), the frequency and health consequences of risks can be analyzed through straightforward statistical analysis of the data. When data are lacking, models must be constructed. Complex situations often require complex models, complex methods for generating the inputs for the models, and complex methods for analyzing the models. Complexity increases the likelihood that important considerations may be omitted, either because they are overlooked or because the available methods for addressing them are too costly or too difficult to be applied correctly.

Often omitted in risk assessments are the human factors, including the possibility of human error (Fischhoff, 1977; Freudenburg, 1988). For example, many release and exposure assessments unquestioningly assume that people follow established procedures without deviation, that people do not deliberately or irrationally expose themselves, and that people can perform adequately under stress. Prior to the accident at the nuclear power plant facility at Three Mile Island, the possibility of operator error under emergency conditions was largely ignored in many risk assessments of accidents at nuclear power plants (U.S. President's Commission on the Accident at Three Mile Island, 1979).

Human responses to risk-protecting measures are similarly difficult to anticipate and appropriately factor into a risk assessment. For example, it is difficult to predict the public's responses to laws and regulations, such as mandatory seat belt or helmet laws. Moreover, people's responses often work at cross-purposes to actions and policies aimed at improving health or environmental quality. The example of increased effort by fishermen to catch fish above a minimum weight limit was given in Chapter 4. Another example is people's responses to the partial protection from floods offered by dams and levees. Increased residential development of flood plains often follows the construction of a dam. When a rare flood does exceed the dam's capacity, such as the 1993 flooding along the Mississippi, the damage is considerably greater than if the flood plain had been left unprotected (Slovic *et al.*, 1979).

Another common omission is unanticipated changes in the environment. Risk assessments are often predicated on assumed constancies in the external environment. These assumptions may, however, prove erroneous. For example, Fischhoff (1977) observed that the assessment of the risks associated with the construction of the Alaskan pipeline failed to foresee the consequences of the retreat of the Columbia Glacier. As the glacier retreats, it discharges large icebergs in the direction of shipping lanes for tankers loaded with North Slope oil. As another example, risk analyses of nuclear power plant designs normally assume the availability of backup power—an assumption that must be questioned in view of the Northeastern power blackout of 1965.

Whether important omissions will be made in a risk assessment is partly a function of the diligence and foresight of the risk assessor and partly a function of the capabilities and appropriateness of the risk assessment methods being used. The choice of simpler methods that omit difficult problem aspects is partly a result of the tendency of analysts to concentrate on aspects of the assessment that are easy to quantify and to omit or deemphasize aspects that are more difficult. If the analyst ignores difficult considerations, the resulting gaps in the risk model may result in risk estimates that are wrong.

Peer review provides the best means of identifying and avoiding serious omissions in risk assessment. In the natural sciences, researchers publish work in journals that require that papers be first refereed and accepted by anonymous reviewers. The approach provides a practical means for checking completeness. Peer review is beginning to be used more frequently in risk assessments; however, there are important barriers to be overcome. A detailed review of a complex risk assessment requires many different types of experts to cover all key aspects of the assessment. Furthermore, the complexity of the risk model and the time-urgent nature of many risk assessments means that the voluntary, unpaid approach effective in the general sciences will not usually work for risk assessment. Thus, peer review must be scheduled, and funding to support reviewers should be budgeted into the risk assessment process.

6.3. THE ACCURACY OF RISK ASSESSMENT

Accuracy relates to whether risk assessment produces results that correctly describe and convey risks. Much of the debate surrounding risk assessment concerns its accuracy. An accurate risk assessment must provide estimates of the risk consequences and uncertainties that are commensurate with available data, knowledge, and understanding. Lack of information does not necessarily mean that risk assessment results will be inaccurate. If a risk assessment correctly accounts for sources of uncertainty and explicitly reports their effect (e.g., by using probability distributions to describe risks), the results may indicate substantial uncertainty over risk consequences—which may be a perfectly accurate description of risk. On the other hand, if the assessment fails to recognize and properly account for significant sources of uncertainty, the risk estimates may appear more precise than is warranted. False precision represents a common inaccuracy.

Although lack of knowledge does not necessarily imply that risk estimates will be inaccurate, inaccuracies are much more likely when information and understanding are severely limited. Lack of information necessitates greater reliance on assumptions that have not or cannot be tested, and biases and errors can result if risk estimates are sensitive to such assumptions. Biases and errors also result from the inherent inadequacies of the generally more complex risk assessment methods that have been developed to overcome problems of lack of information. The most common mechanisms by which bias and errors occur include: deficiencies in data collection procedures (e.g., biases introduced through inaccuracies and omissions in reporting accident data), inaccurate data processing, the use of inappropriate assumptions for extrapolation, fitting models to sparse data, data aggregation, the use of surrogate data, relying on underqualified experts or experts who do not represent a full range of scientific opinion, discretizing continuous decision variables, utilizing models based on poor data or inadequate theory, and utilizing incomplete models (e.g., models that omit important accident scenarios in an event tree).

The magnitude of the inaccuracies introduced due to uncertainties and the inadequacies of procedures for dealing with uncertainty differ depending on the risk assessment methods employed. As indicated by the discussions in the previous chapters, the potential for inaccuracy is considerable. Figure 36 summarizes one view regarding some of the sources of uncertainty and error in methods commonly used in cancer risk assessments. Derived in part from an analysis by Cothern (1988), who attempted to define and roughly quantify the uncertainties that are an integral part of toxicological experimental design, the figure not only demonstrates the potential for underestimating uncertainties, it also suggests some of the ways that summary measures of risk, such as expected numbers of health effects, might be overestimated or underestimated.

There are several important means for countering inaccuracies in risk assessment. First, an iterative approach to risk assessment should be adopted; — initial versions of the models and assessments should be developed and tested and then modified based on the results of testing the initial models. The most important

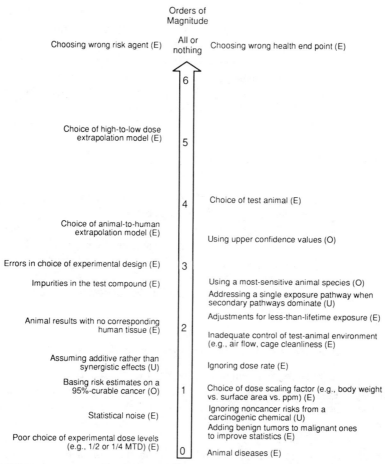

FIGURE 36.   Magnitude of typical uncertainties and errors introduced into cancer risk assessment through various sources. O = typically results in an overestimation of risk; U = typically results in an underestimation of risk; E = could result in either over- or underestimation of risk. [Based on Cothern (1988); Flamm and Lorentzen (1988).]

means for testing and guiding the evolution of the risk model is sensitivity analysis. With sensitivity analysis, those models and assumptions that are most crucial can be identified, allowing more careful checks and model refinement and elaboration to be directed at the most crucial areas. Comparing model predictions with the intuition of experts and decision makers is also useful. If models and experts disagree, then either the model is wrong or the analysis should provide a convincing argument that the experts are wrong.

To enable outside reviewers to identify and correct inaccuracies, the models, assumptions, and methods of calculation used in risk assessment must be clearly documented. Ideally, documentation should be sufficient to allow others to verify all calculations and, if necessary, replicate the results. Unfortunately, the complexity of the assessment may make detailed communication of all aspects of the assessment impossible. The most important details and assumptions, however, usually can and should be described in a short, clearly written summary.

6.4. THE ACCEPTABILITY OF RISK ASSESSMENT

Acceptability relates to whether risk assessment is understandable and compatible with the attitudes and perceptions of potential users, especially decision makers and the public. Potential users may find risk assessment unacceptable for a variety of reasons, including (1) limitations and characteristics of the data, methods, or models used in the assessment, (2) limitations and characteristics of risk assessment experts and other sources of risk information, and (3) limitations and characteristics of the intended recipients of the information. Each of these categories is discussed below.

6.4.1. Limitations Related to Risk Assessment Data, Models, and Methods

The data, models, and methods limitations that can reduce the acceptability of risk assessment are primarily those raised in the immediately preceding subsections—questions regarding logical soundness, completeness, and accuracy. The previous discussion of these issues, however, concerned the ability of risk assessment to satisfy scientific standards of acceptability. Since acceptability must be established beyond the scientific community and must include acceptance by decision makers and, often, the public, additional considerations are relevant.

The most significant problem in this area is that substantial uncertainty, when reflected in risk estimates, can reduce the perceived value of the results. Although there are well-developed theories and procedures for making decisions when consequences are uncertain (e.g., decision analysis), they are not topics about which most members of the public, or many risk managers, are familiar. Hence, the message that risk consequences are uncertain does not seem very useful to most people, even if that uncertainty can be accurately quantified.

Research has shown that, wherever possible, people attempt to reduce the anxiety generated by uncertainty through a variety of strategies (Slovic, *et al.*, 1977). Aversion to uncertainty often translates into a denial that uncertainty exists or into a marked preference for statements of fact over statements of probability. People often are unwilling to accept risk assessment because they prefer being told exactly what will happen, not what might happen (Alfidi, 1971; Fischhoff, 1983, 1985; Weinstein, 1979).

When uncertainty is great, failure of the risk assessor to convey that uncertainty produces a false sense of accuracy. But, when uncertainties are fully documented, they can be so large as to lead many to conclude that the risk assessment results are nearly useless. Examples include:

- A study by a committee of the National Academy of Sciences estimated that the expected number of bladder cancers resulting from the consumption of saccharin over a lifetime of exposure ranged between 0.22 and 1,144,000 cases (NAS–NRC, 1978).

- A study by the Department of Energy estimated that fatalities associated with emissions from coal-fired power plants ranged between 1 and 305 per year (DOE, 1981).

- A study by the Nuclear Regulatory Commission estimated that the risk of a core-melt at a nuclear power plant ranged between 1 chance in 10,000 and 1 chance in 1,000,000 (NRC, 1987b).

In the adversarial climate that surrounds most health, safety, and environmental issues, critics of risk assessment often cite such large uncertainties as grounds for rejecting risk assessment; however, risk assessment can provide valuable information and insights even when risk estimates are highly uncertain.

6.4.2. Limitations Related to Risk Assessment Experts and Others Who Provide Risk Information

Risk assessment may be perceived as unacceptable due to limitations or characteristics of risk assessment experts and others who provide risk information. These include (1) the failure of risk assessment experts and others to maintain the trust and confidence of potential users of risk assessment, (2) experts' limited understanding of public concerns and perceptions of risk, and (3) the failure of experts and others to disclose the limitations of risk assessment and resulting uncertainties.

6.4.2.1. Lack of Credibility. For 4 major reasons, risk assessors and other sources of risk information may fail to maintain the trust and confidence of potential users of risk assessment. Perhaps first among these is the fact that risk assessments can produce dramatically different results when different assumptions, data, or methods are used. Lathrop and Linnerooth (1981), for example, cite competing risk assessments of a proposal to locate a liquified natural gas (LNG) terminal at Oxnard, California. One study was funded by the city of Oxnard, the other by a company representing LNG interests. The risk estimates produced by the company-sponsored study were less than 1/300 of the estimates produced by the city of Oxnard. Widely differing results from competing risk assessments can undermine public trust and credibility. Moreover, risk assessment experts may engage in highly visible debates and disagreements about the reliability, validity, and meaning of assessment results. While debate may be constructive for the development of scientific knowledge, it is often destructive to the development of public confidence and acceptance.

Second, the technical complexity of a sophisticated risk assessment often hampers its acceptance. Risk assessors frequently use technical language and scientific jargon in communicating the results of risk assessment to decision makers and the public. Such language is not only difficult to comprehend but can also create a perception that the risk assessor is being unresponsive and evasive. For example, the statement "Drinking water contaminated with 5 parts per billion of a particular toxic substance poses a lifetime risk no greater than 10^{-6} with 95 percent probability" may be technically defensible, but it may leave individuals suspicious and confused about the meaning and relevance to their particular situation. If users do not understand the results of risk assessment, distrust and lack of acceptance are likely to result.

Third, decision makers and others may feel that risk assessment is unacceptable because it places too much power in the hands of a technical elite. Risk assessment provides technical experts with a prominent role in the decision-making process. If the risk assessment is appropriately conducted, that role is limited to providing a description of risk; however, when policy considerations are allowed to enter into the assessment process without being explicitly acknowledged, technical specialists usurp the responsibility of elected officials.

Fourth, the primary sources of most risk assessment information—government agencies and industry—often lack trust and credibility (e.g., see, Covello *et al.*, 1987). Trust and credibility are intimately linked and can be undermined by numerous factors. In the public sector, these factors include public perceptions that agency risk assessment activities are overly influenced by special interest groups, that agency assessments are inappropriately biased in favor of a particular technology, that agency risk assessors are not technically competent, or that agency experts have lied or made serious errors in the past. The enormous risk assessment responsibilities of many regulatory agencies often conflict with demands by citizens or interest groups that the agency take immediate action on a particular product, activity, or hazardous substance. Explanations by agency officials that the production of the needed risk assessment information is time-consuming, or that the risk assessment activities of the agency are constrained by resource, technical, statutory, or other limitations, are seldom perceived to be satisfactory. Jurisdictional conflicts about which agency and which level of government has the ultimate responsibility and authority leads, in many cases, to the production of multiple risk assessments, each of which might provide a different estimate of risk. The result of such confusion is often an erosion of the agency's credibility and a lack of public acceptance of the agency's risk assessment results.

6.4.2.2. Limited Understanding of Public Concerns and the Multidimensional Character of Risk. Potential users of risk assessment may find risk assessment unacceptable because the measures of risk produced in a risk assessment do not adequately reflect the concerns of the public. Risk assessment experts have often operated on the assumption that they and their audience share a common framework for judging and interpreting risk information. However, studies conducted by behavioral and social science researchers suggest that this is often not the case (Johnson and Tversky, 1984; Lindell and Earle, 1982; Covello, 1983, 1984; Renn, 1981; Slovic *et al.*, 1980a; Vlek and Stallen, 1981). One of the most important findings to emerge from this literature is that the public takes into consideration a complex array of qualitative and quantitative factors in defining and evaluating risks (Slovic *et al.*, 1980b; Vlek and Stallen, 1981; Litai *et al.*, 1983; Renn, 1981). In addition to consequence severity and probability of occurrence, which are the primary focus of most risk assessments, these factors include:

1. *Catastrophic potential.* People are more concerned about fatalities and injuries that are grouped in time and space (e.g., airplane crashes) than about fatalities and injuries that are scattered or random in time and space (e.g., automobile accidents).

2. *Familiarity.* People are more concerned about risks that are unfamiliar (e.g., ozone depletion due to emissions of fluorocarbons) than about risks that are familiar (e.g., household accidents).

3. *Understanding*—People are more concerned about activities characterized by poorly understood exposure mechanisms or processes (e.g., exposure to radiation) than about activities characterized by apparently well-understood exposure mechanisms or processes (e.g., pedestrian accidents or slipping on ice).

4. *Scientific uncertainty.* People are more concerned about risks that are scientifically unknown or uncertain (e.g., recombinant DNA experimentation) than about risks that are relatively well-known to science (e.g., actuarially documented automobile accidents).

5. *Controllability.* People are more concerned about risks that they perceive not to be under their personal control (e.g., traveling as a passenger in an airplane or automobile) than about risks that they perceive to be under their personal control (e.g., driving an automobile).

6. *Voluntariness of exposure.* People are more concerned about risks that they perceive to be involuntary (e.g., exposure to unlabeled food additives or to air or water pollutants) than about risks that they perceive to be voluntary (e.g., smoking, sunbathing, or mountain climbing).

7. *Impact on children.* People are more concerned about activities that are perceived as putting children specifically at risk (e.g., school bus accidents) than about activities not generally so perceived (e.g., adult smoking).

8. *Effects on future generations.* People are more concerned about activities that pose risks to future generations (e.g., genetic effects due to exposure to radiation) than about risks that do not pose risks to future generations (e.g., skiing accidents).

9. *Victim identity.* People are more concerned about risks to identifiable victims (e.g., a yachtsman lost at sea or a trapped coal miner) than about risks to statistical victims (e.g., statistical profiles of automobile accident victims).

10. *Dread.* People are more concerned about certain dreaded risks that evoke a response of fear, terror, or anxiety (e.g., exposure to potential carcinogens from toxic waste dumps or to nuclear radiation) than to risks that are not especially dreaded (e.g., common colds and household accidents).

11. *Institutional trust.* People are more concerned about situations where the responsible risk management institution is perceived to lack trust and credibility (e.g., criticisms of the Nuclear Regulatory Commission for its perceived close ties to industry) than they are about situations where the responsible risk-management institution is perceived to be trustworthy and credible (e.g., trust in the management of recombinant DNA risks by universities and by the National Institutes of Health).

12. *Media attention.* People are more concerned about risks that receive much media attention (e.g., airline crashes) than about risks that receive little media attention (e.g., on-the-job accidents).

13. *Accident history.* People are more concerned about activities that have a history of major and sometimes minor accidents (e.g., nuclear power plant accidents such as the accident at Three Mile Island) than about activities that have a history of no major or minor accidents (e.g., recombinant DNA experimentation).

14. *Equity.* People are more concerned about activities that are characterized by a perceived inequitable distribution of risks and benefits (e.g., offshore oil exploration) than about activities characterized by a perceived equitable distribution of risks and benefits (e.g., vaccination).

15. *Clarity of benefits.* People are more concerned about hazardous activities that are perceived to have unclear benefits (e.g., nuclear power genera-

tion) than about hazardous activities that are perceived to have clear benefits (automobile driving).
16. *Reversibility.* People are more concerned about activities characterized by potentially irreversible adverse effects (e.g., acid rain) than about activities characterized by reversible adverse effects (e.g., injuries from sports or household accidents).
17. *Personal stake.* People are more concerned about activities that they believe place them (or their families) personally and directly at risk (e.g., drinking water contamination due to local dumping of hazardous waste) than about activities that do not place them (or their families) personally and directly at risk (e.g., dumping of hazardous waste at sea or in other remote sites).
18. *Attributability.* People are more concerned about risks that are perceived to be due to human actions (e.g., industry accidents) than about activities that are perceived to be natural in origin (e.g., acts of God).

Many of the factors known to affect people's perceptions of risk, such as equity, dread, trust in institutions, and personal involvement, are difficult to include in formal risk assessments, at least as they are currently undertaken. Likely consequences of these omissions are that risk assessment results may conflict dramatically with people's intuitive beliefs, with the result that the risk assessment is distrusted, rejected, or considered irrelevant.

6.4.2.3. Failure to Disclose Limitations of Risk Assessments. Critics have often attacked risk assessments produced by government agencies and industry on the grounds that they fail to acknowledge the limitations of the assessment and the resulting uncertainties. Part of the criticism derives from a concern that the public will be misled by assessments that claim greater quantitative precision than can reasonably be justified by the quality of the data or by the current degree of scientific understanding. As stated previously, it is still more the exception than the rule for assessment results to be presented with full disclosure of the uncertainties in risk outcomes, the strengths and limitations of the assessment, and the degree to which assessment results are based on controversial assumptions and judgments.

6.4.3. Limitations Related to Potential Users of Risk Assessment Information

Research shows that lay people tend to overestimate the risks of dramatic or sensational causes of death, such as accidents, homicides, cancer, and natural disasters, and underestimate the risks of undramatic causes, such as asthma, emphysema, and diabetes, which take one life at a time and are common in nonfatal forms (Lichtenstein *et al.*, 1978; Morgan *et al.*, 1985). Several factors explain this finding, including previously mentioned availability bias, wherein the risk judgments are significantly influenced by the memorability of past events and by the imaginability of future events. As a result, any factor that makes a hazard unusually memorable or imaginable, such as a recent disaster, intense media coverage, or a vivid film, can seriously distort perceptions of risk (Lichtenstein *et al.*, 1978). Researchers have pointed out that availability bias often results in lay estimates of risk that are considerably at odds with expert estimates of the same risk (Slovic *et al.*, 1979). Other psychological biases and rules of thumb produce similar discrepancies between lay and expert estimates of risk (von Winterfeldt and Edwards, 1986).

Compounding the problem is the fact that lay people usually have difficulty understanding and interpreting probabilistic information, especially when the risk is new and when probabilities are small. This difficulty has often hampered discussions based on risk assessments of low-probability events and worst-case scenarios. Because of the difficulty lay people have appreciating the improbability of extreme but imaginable consequences, the distinction between what is remotely possible and what is probable is often blurred. Studies have also shown that many people frequently have a limited capacity for distinguishing between small probabilities (e.g., the difference between a probability of one chance in a hundred thousand and one chance in a million) and for understanding the significance of such differences (Sjoberg, 1979).

6.5. THE PRACTICALITY OF RISK ASSESSMENT

Practicality relates to whether risk assessment can be employed in a real-world, problem-solving environment when available resources and information are limited. A complete risk assessment can be expensive and time-consuming. For example, animal bioassays can cost more than $2 million and can take 2 to 5 years to complete (Hollstein *et al.*, 1979). A large fault tree/event tree model for an industrial facility can cost more than $500,000 to develop and can take more than 2 years to complete. Given these costs, risk assessments of all significant health, safety, and environmental problems would require more financial resources and personnel than realistically could be made available. Under the Toxic Substances Control Act, for example, the EPA is charged with the task of screening the roughly 70,000 chemical substances now in commercial use and the more than 1,000 chemicals that enter the market each year. To handle only the latter task the EPA would have to rule on four new chemical applications each working day, clearly an impossible job (Culliton, 1979). Similar problems face other agencies. The Consumer Product Safety Commission, for example, deals with more than 2.5 million firms, more than 10,000 products, and some 30,000 consumer deaths and 20 million consumer injuries each year.

Another factor affecting the practicality of risk assessment is its multidisciplinary nature. Multidisciplinary research requires multidisciplinary teams, which are often difficult to assemble and maintain. Experts in multidisciplinary teams often have difficulty judging the expertise of those outside of their own field of specialization. This problem is highly significant for risk assessment because the risk assessment process requires experts at one stage in the analysis to use data generated by other experts at other stages in the analysis.

Issues of practicality are best addressed by recognizing the flexibility of available strategies for conducting risk assessment. To handle information limitations, risk assessment methods can be selected according to an obvious preference order for using available data. If sufficient risk data are available to compute health-consequence frequency distributions directly, then such data provide the best basis for generating risk estimates. In the absence of statistical data on risk, preference can be given to statistical data that can be used to construct and validate release, exposure, and consequence models. In the absence of statistical data on the processes of concern, preference can be given to statistical data for similar processes that can be adopted or extended for use in or as part of a disaggregated model. In the absence of statistical data, preference can be given to data obtained from recognized and accepted technical experts; data that can be analyzed through Bayesian methods and related techniques.

Time and costs can be controlled by selecting methods that meet the time and cost constraints established for the assessment. For example, simple, "back-of-the-envelope" assessments can generally be conducted in a matter of days using unvalidated assumptions. Such methods may not produce the most precise risk estimates, but they can inexpensively produce credible risk bounds. Multidisciplinary problems can be dealt with as in other efforts requiring multidisciplinary teams. Good leadership, clear lines of authority and responsibility, and adequate mechanisms for communication and review can help overcome the difficulties of harnessing the talents of many experts.

6.6. THE EFFECTIVENESS OF RISK ASSESSMENT

Effectiveness relates largely to whether risk assessment can accomplish its intended ends; namely, producing information and measures of the level of risk that are useful in the decision-making process. Table 24 provides examples of some of the key questions that might be asked when evaluating the effectiveness of various types of risk assessment methods. While the limitations of risk assessment noted in the various sections of this chapter all potentially detract from the effectiveness of risk assessment, a variety of other factors contribute positively to the effectiveness of risk assessment.

TABLE 24. Sample Questions for Evaluating Risk Assessment Methods

Method	Internal criteria			External criteria		
	Logical soundness	Completeness	Accuracy	Acceptability	Practicality	Effectiveness
Monitoring	Are historical data representative of the future risk of concern, or have changes occurred that make historical risks irrelevant?	Are the most critical features of the risk factors of concern captured by the monitored data, or do the measurements paint only a partial picture?	How accurate are the monitored data? Are there built-in biases (due to sampling times, methods, etc.)?	Does the success of the monitoring activity depend on cooperation (from the public or other organizations) that might not be obtained?	Are the costs, time, and resources required by monitoring cost-effective and consistent with resource constraints?	Are monitoring data of use to decision makers in resolving uncertainty over the factors that make decisions difficult?
Statistical	Do the underlying statistical models involve assumptions that make sense for the application (e.g., linearity, lognormal distributions, independence, etc.)?	Are there crucial problem aspects not captured by the statistical models (e.g., uncertainties for which there are no statistical data or information possessed by experts that go beyond what can be demonstrated by hard data)?	Does the statistical analysis provide adequate measures of the uncertainties in estimates?	Are the methods unacceptable due to their technical complexity or due to lack of confidence or experience on the part of those who will use the results?	Are the data required for a statistical analysis available and are there adequate computational resources to support the analysis?	Will the results be useful to decision makers, or does the statistical analysis miss the issues of greatest concern?

Modeling	Are the basic assumptions embodied in the model logical and acceptable? Has the sensitivity of results to those assumptions been tested?	Are the models complete, or have important problem aspects been omitted (e.g., omitting the chance for human error if risks from this source dominate those represented in the model)?	Do accuracy estimates consider only model parameter uncertainty when uncertainty about appropriate model form is of more importance?	Are the models likely to be acceptable to those who must use the results of their analysis? Will accepted experts defend the structure and assumptions of the model?	Is the level of understanding of cause-effect processes sufficient to permit the development of models? Is the level of computational resources and time required to develop and run the models practical?	Can analysis of the models produce results that are of direct use to decision makers, or do they fail to address the issues of greatest concern?
Bayesian	Are the methods used adequately explained and subjected to peer review to ensure their soundness?	Have the methods failed to account for important data bases? Do the experts who provide judgmental inputs represent the complete range of relevant viewpoints?	Are the methods used likely to give undue weight to certain special interests or viewpoints? Do they adequately guard against cognitive and motivational biases that produce errors and inconsistencies in judgmental data?	Will the use of methods that highlight and make explicit the uncertainty in expert judgments create serious controversy or be unacceptable for institutional or social reasons?	Are individuals with sufficient expertise available to apply the methods? Are there recognized, accepted, and impartial experts who would be willing to provide the judgmental information necessary for a Bayesian analysis?	Do the methods address the crucial factors for decision making? Do they link effectively with other components of the risk assessment process?

First, risk assessment can provide valuable information in a form that clarifies the inherent ambiguities and uncertainties of a risk situation. Risk assessment, when properly applied, collects and analyzes information from all relevant and appropriate scientific and technical sources. The results of these analyses are then presented quantitatively; a way that can provide the clearest possible expression and understanding of adverse health, safety, or environmental consequences. Furthermore:

- Risk assessment can facilitate communication between decision makers and technical experts by providing a precise language (i.e., the mathematical language of probability and statistics) for describing the nature and extent of uncertainties in health, safety, and environmental consequences.

- Risk assessment can facilitate communication between decision makers and other interested parties by providing explicit data that are amenable to review by interested parties.

- Risk assessment can help decision makers identify the role and impact of policy considerations (e.g., social, political, economic, and legal policy judgments) in the assessment of scientific information.

- Risk assessment can help decision makers separate a complex health, safety, or environmental problem into its component, and more manageable, parts.

- Risk assessment can help decision makers identify and understand the impact of interactions and joint dependencies between variables and components of the problem that might otherwise be overlooked.

- Risk assessment can help decision makers identify research needs and set research priorities that would significantly reduce important scientific uncertainties.

- Risk assessment can help decision makers by providing a framework for explicitly examining the potential adverse consequences of alternative risk management policies or actions.

Perhaps the most common argument against the usefulness and effectiveness of risk assessment is that data and scientific understanding are often insufficient. While insufficient data and scientific understanding may rule out the use of some data-intensive risk assessment methods, it does not necessarily follow that other systematic methods designed to quantify uncertainty will not be helpful to decision makers. Furthermore, the crucial need for information about the likelihood and magnitude of possible adverse consequences and about the effectiveness of risk reduction strategies reinforces the importance of formal risk assessment. Without formal risk assessment, policies and actions will generally be based on feasibility considerations, competing interests, and intuitive and qualitative assessments. This approach is likely to be substantially less rigorous and substantially more limited than risk assessment. If properly applied, risk assessment can help inform decision makers about policies and actions that do not sufficiently protect the public or that reduce trivial risks at incommensurately high costs.

6.7. SOME RECOMMENDATIONS

Given the previous observations, we conclude with recommendations related to four topics: (1) standardizing risk assessment, (2) accounting for uncertainties, (3) dealing with value judgments, and (4) conservatism.

6.7.1. Attempts to Standardize Risk Assessment

In recent years, a variety of efforts have been made to develop standardized guidelines for risk assessment (e.g., EPA, 1984b, 1985a, 1989a). One product of these efforts has been a set of formal guidelines "describing the scientific basis for each of the many analytic steps involved in risk assessment, and specifying how the analysis at each step is to be approached" (EPA, 1984b). Some of the principal arguments for the development of standardized guidelines are achieving greater quality control, improving consistency among risk-management activities, increasing the predictability of the regulatory process, focusing attention and debate over the crucial judgmental aspects of risk assessment, fostering greater public understanding, and promoting increased administrative efficiency (NAS–NRC, 1983a). These are legitimate goals. However, the specification of risk assessment guidelines itself poses a risk and should be approached with caution.

Many of the difficulties associated with attempts to standardize risk assessment stem from (1) the different types of risks that need to be addressed, (2) the different objectives served by risk assessment, (3) the different types and amounts of analytic resources available for an assessment, (4) the different types and quality of available data, and (5) the different contexts in which risk assessment is applied and for which different risk assessment models and methods are appropriate. The descriptions and evaluations of risk assessment methods presented in this book illustrate the wide variety of analytic options available to the risk assessor. The capabilities of these methods depend heavily on available data and other resources. Methods that are useful in one situation may be counterproductive in another. As a result, standardized guidelines that require the use of particular methods or that establish the weight to be given to particular types of information may be appropriate in some instances, but in other cases may lead to significant evidence being disregarded, the generation of biased assessments, or assessments that fail to make use of all important and relevant information.

For example, consider the following guideline for carcinogen risk assessment:

If uncertainty exists over the form of the dose-response relationship at low-dose levels, then models that incorporate low-dose linearity are to be preferred.

In recent years, it has become clear that the potential for improving understanding of dose-response relationships is considerable. For instance, recognition of the distinction between administered dose and effective dose and an improved understanding of comparative metabolism and mechanisms of action provide opportunities for making more informed judgments about the validity of alternative models and assumptions. In the light of such increased knowledge, one model may appear to offer a better representation of reality than others. As a result, the risk assessor might conclude that some form other than low-dose linearity is more reflective of best scientific understanding or might find it advantageous to assign appropriate probabilities to alternative models as part of a probabilistic analysis. In addition, the risk assessor might conduct sensitivity analyses that indicate the effect on risk estimates of different model assumptions. Any standardized guideline that establishes *a priori* a preference for one model over another may bias the risk estimation process and thereby deny decision makers the most accurate, complete, and comprehensive expression of scientific knowledge.

Another concern associated with attempts to overly standardize risk assessment is that the very act of formalizing and institutionalizing scientific judgments may create the erroneous impression of a policy-free or value-free science (Wynne, 1984). Scientists often become committed to particular judgments and methods of inference through their education and patterns of professional affiliation (Johnson and Covello, 1987). These commitments can appear to have the strength of scientific fact when no such basis exists. Standardized guidelines can easily exacerbate the problem by promoting implicit policy or value considerations.

The middle course that best serves decision makers may be a strategy that includes the development of flexible risk assessment guidelines as well as restraints designed to prevent overstandardization. Flexible guidelines, designed to serve as benchmarks rather than as rules, are less likely to oversimplify the assessment process or stultify the development of scientific knowledge.

6.7.2. Accounting for Uncertainties

A crucial flaw in many risk assessments is the failure to describe and characterize adequately the uncertainties in the estimates of risk outcomes. At least five sources of uncertainty can be important: (1) *statistical uncertainty*, associated with the randomness of nature as represented in the variability of available data; (2) *parameter uncertainty*, due to imprecision in statistical estimates of model parameters made from limited or incomplete data; (3) *judgmental uncertainty*, relating to the inability of knowledgeable experts to specify precise values for model inputs for which statistical data are unavailable; (4) *model uncertainty*, resulting from a lack of understanding of physical processes or engineering behavior and failure of the models to capture the salient features of the risk; and (5) *completeness uncertainty*, resulting from the possible omission of important processes or events from the analysis.

As demonstrated in previous chapters, with the exception of completeness uncertainty, methods have been developed to account for and characterize the effects produced by each of these sources. Even so, few risk assessments explicitly address uncertainty. Most assessments compute only a single value for the level of adverse health or environmental consequences. Occasionally, statistical uncertainties are estimated and, less frequently, parameter uncertainties, provided that adequate data are available to justify the simpler statistical methods applicable when sample sizes are large. Rarely, judgmental uncertainties are quantified. Model uncertainty is almost never addressed, even qualitatively.

A risk assessment that reports only a single value for the level of adverse health or environmental consequences ignores the range of possibilities and provides decision makers with an inaccurate picture of the risk being faced. To make effective, efficient, and equitable decisions, decision makers need information not only about what adverse consequences can happen, including worst cases, but also about the relative likelihood of these consequences. Similarly, a risk assessment that omits important sources of uncertainty provides an incomplete picture of the risk. The preferences of decision makers toward various policies and actions may be strongly influenced not only by the probable range of risk consequences, but also by the potential for consequences that might fall outside of the probable range, including the probability and severity of extreme possibilities. It is therefore critical that comprehensive measures of uncertainty (e.g., probabilities, confidence intervals, or standard errors) be estimated and provided. Given the increased importance assigned to risk assessment in the regulatory decision-making process, risk assessors have a professional responsibility to present a clear and comprehensive statement of uncertainties that affect the scope and interpretation of their work.

The existence of uncertainties does not necessarily undermine the usefulness of risk assessment to decision makers. Somewhat paradoxically, it actually enhances the usefulness of risk assessment. When uncertainties are present, only a systematic and rigorous approach can produce an accurate understanding of risk. When conducted in this manner, risk assessment provides (1) a systematic approach for handling complex health or environmental problems characterized by high degrees of uncertainty, (2) a set of logically sound computational rules for manipulating and processing uncertainty, and (3) a quantitative tool for evaluating and estimating the policy implications of all assumptions and data uncertainties explicitly, consistently, and comprehensively.

6.7.3. Dealing with Value Judgments

Another consequence of a lack of knowledge is that numerous judgments must be made by researchers in the course of conducting a risk assessment. The scientific knowledge necessary to support such judgments is often extremely limited or poor in quality. In such situations, the application of risk assessment requires judgmental inferences. Inferences take the form of choices among several scientifically plausible interpretations, mathematical models, analytic assumptions, or qualitative judgments. Table 25 provides examples of the kinds of judgmental inferences that are often necessary in the conduct of a risk assessment.

Many of the judgmental inferences necessary for a risk assessment are, in effect, policy choices. For example, answers to the questions listed in Table 25 can determine the degree of policy caution or conservatism in calculating levels of risk. Policy considerations enter into risk assessment through a variety of routes, each associated with a choice or decision point. The first entry point for policy considerations is through the decision of what problems to investigate and what level of resources (e.g., financial and manpower resources) to allocate to the assessment.

Second, policy considerations enter through the choice of what adverse health or environmental consequences to assess. As noted earlier, most risk assessments have focused on cancer (e.g., Munro and Krewski, 1981). This disproportionate focus on cancer is due to a variety of factors, including the rate at which science has detected carcinogens in the environment and concomitant increases in public fears and concerns about cancer. One consequence of the overriding emphasis on cancer is that fewer risk assessment studies have been conducted on other recognized adverse health effects, such as cardiovascular, developmental, immunologic, mutagenic, neurotoxic, behavioral, reproductive, and respiratory effects. Even fewer risk assessment studies have focused on adverse effects on animals, plants, or ecosystems.

Third, policy considerations enter the risk assessment process through methodological choices and decisions that may have a subtle but significant impact on the results of an assessment. Examples include decisions and choices about what data to collect, about what data are relevant, about what methods to use, and about what simplifying assumptions to make in constructing workable models.

Finally, policy considerations enter through the selection of one risk assessment assumption over another at different stages in the risk assessment process. The lack of scientific consensus on many issues provides ample opportunity for choices based on policy considerations to significantly affect risk estimates. Researchers have identified more than 50 crucial points in a typical risk assessment where assumptions must be made in the face of insufficient scientific knowledge (NAS–NRC, 1983a). At each point, the policy consequences of selecting one assumption over another may be substantial.

The widely quoted risk assessment report by the National Academy of Sciences (NAS–NRC, 1983a) argues for the importance of maintaining a clear

TABLE 25.   Examples of Scientific and Policy Judgments Necessary for Risk Assessment

Component of risk chain	Method utilized	Example of judgment required
Releases	Monitoring	What method of interpolation or extrapolation should be used to deal with omissions or errors in the recording of data?
	Performance testing and accident investigation	How can isolated events be generalized to produce conclusions relevant to risk assessment?
	Statistical methods	How should surrogate data bases be adjusted to account for known differences between the variable of concern and the surrogate variable for which data are available?
	Modeling	What assumptions should be made concerning the nature and likelihood of externally initiated events, for example, attempts by terrorist groups to produce radioactive releases from a nuclear reactor?
Exposures	Monitoring	How should exposure measurements representing a small segment of the population be extrapolated to the entire population?
	Modeling	How should dispersion of air pollutants into the atmosphere due to convection, wind currents, etc., be represented?
Consequences	Animal tests	How should evidence of different metabolic pathways or vastly different metabolic rates between animals and humans be factored into a risk assessment?
	Epidemiology	How should risk estimates be adjusted to account for a comparatively short follow-up period in an epidemiologic study?
	Modeling	What dose-response models should be used to extrapolate from experimental doses to relevant doses?
Risk estimation	Statistical analysis	How should statistical estimates based on "independence assumptions" be adjusted to account for known but analytically untractable dependencies?
	Judgmental methods	How should differences in expert opinions be aggregated?
	Modeling	How should probability distributions over health consequences be estimated and displayed?

conceptual distinction between risk assessment and risk management, that is, between the scientific findings and judgments embodied in risk assessment and the economic, political, social, legal, and other policy considerations embodied in risk management. Despite the value of institutionally and analytically separating risk assessment from risk management, the current state of the art of risk assessment does not permit questions of science to be clearly separated from questions of policy. In practice, assumptions that have potential policy implications enter into risk assessment at virtually every stage of the process (Conservation Foundation, 1985). The ideal of a risk assessment that is free, or nearly free, of policy considerations is beyond the realm of possibility.

The degree of judgment embodied in risk assessment points to the need for structures and procedures that can maximize the soundness and objectivity of the analysis. For example, it points to the crucial importance of peer review and to the need for sensitivity analyses that evaluate the implications of different assumptions. It also points to the need for risk assessment teams, to be composed of specialists from many disciplines including engineering, physical, chemical, biological, statistical, health, and environmental sciences. Because the assessment process is inherently multidisciplinary in nature, the members of such teams must possess the ability to perform as part of a multidisciplinary unit. Managing such a team demands imagination and skillful leadership to ensure (1) that contributions of team members are consistent with their areas of expertise, (2) that the models are logically sound and appropriately integrated, and (3) that the analysis is rigorous and properly documented.

6.7.4. Conservatism

As discussed previously, risk assessments are often designed to be conservative. Conservatism is a value judgment deliberately introduced into risk assessment to account for uncertainty. Rather than attempt an explicit quantification of uncertainty, the risk assessor errs on the side of safety. In effect, the analyst produces a risk estimate that minimizes the probability that additional information will reveal that the risk estimate is too low. In providing an upper-bound estimate of risk, the analyst assumes that a more accurate estimate is unlikely to be higher and could well be lower. This conservative approach has three major drawbacks.

First, by introducing conservatism, scientists go beyond their role as providers of information. Conservatism is essentially a policy judgment, not a scientific judgment. For scientists to make such judgments is inappropriate, since it introduces value judgments into science. In contrast, it may be entirely appropriate for policymakers to act conservatively, since underestimating a particular risk may have far greater health, safety, environmental, economic, and social losses than overestimating the same risk.

Second, by introducing conservatism, scientists may produce results that are highly distorted. Major distortions can occur because conservatisms are often introduced at more than one stage in the assessment. Although each individual introduction may appear prudent, together they may produce a multiplicative cascading of biases due to the nature of the risk chain and the risk assessment process. For example, consider the various judgments scientists might make to assess the risk of a new drug that contains unavoidable impurities with possible adverse side effects. Scientists responsible for the different components of the assessment might (a) assume a conservative upper estimate for the amount of impurities in the drug, (b) assume patterns of consumption that produce a conservative upper-bound estimate of exposure, (c) calculate dose-response relationships based on animal studies using the most sensitive strain, sex, and species of animals, (d) administer the drug to laboratory animals using the most potent method of dose administration, (e) adopt conservative assumptions for extrapolating from high doses to low doses and from animal studies to humans, and (f) summarize the risk consequences in terms of the implications to the most sensitive individual. The resulting estimate of risk could easily be so overly cautious as to be misleading, particularly from the viewpoint of patients who would profit from the beneficial effects of the drug. For example, if each of the above steps introduced a factor-of-two conservatism (e.g., caused the use of a value for a factor that was twice its expected value), then the resulting risk estimate would be 64 times too large. Unless "best-scientific" estimates are also being generated, the cumulative effect of conservatisms generally cannot be estimated.

Finally, by introducing conservatism, scientists may distort the pattern of regulation and, thereby, prevent limited resources for health and safety (including regulatory agency attention) from being allocated to their highest valued uses. The problem is that the degree of conservatism varies from assessment to assessment. Different agencies or different parts of the same agency follow their own distinct procedures for estimating risks. Conservatism may lead to tighter regulation in some circumstances (where risk assessments are most exaggerated), but it may also lead to less protection in others (where risk assessments are least exaggerated). Thus, some low-level risks might be regulated too stringently, while more severe risks are tolerated. In short, conservatism in risk assessments may well lead to a pattern of regulatory decisions that produces less health and safety than would unbiased risk assessment (Nichols and Zeckhauser, 1986).

6.8. CONCLUDING REMARKS

In summary, the current practice of risk assessment admittedly has significant limitations and shortcomings. Despite these limitations and shortcomings, risk assessment still provides the best tool available for addressing health, safety, and environmental risks, and provides a logical and effective means for analyzing and evaluating limited information. Its strengths include its ability to:

- Show how different estimates of risk are derived
- Provide the logic by which different regulatory actions might reduce risk
- Present a range of plausible risk consequences reflecting uncertainty about underlying theory and data
- Reduce the range of uncertainty in decision making and identify which estimates are most likely to be accurate
- Help set priorities and develop standards
- Describe and quantify levels of risk that remain after application of risk-reduction technologies
- Provide an empirical foundation for balancing risks against benefits
- Identify subpopulations that are especially sensitive or vulnerable
- Identify crucial areas where the resolution of uncertainty can be most effective in reducing risk.

Through these means, risk assessment can reduce, though not entirely eliminate, the guesswork in health, safety, and environmental rulemaking. At the same time, it can aid decision makers in identifying those areas where research is most needed.

Even when consensus is lacking about estimates of the level of risk associated with a particular product, process, or event, risk assessment can still provide extremely useful insights. For example, it is widely recognized that assessments of the risks of a nuclear power plant accident might be in error by several orders of magnitude (NRC, 1985, 1987b). Nevertheless, these assessments have generated many important insights. They have shown, for example, that (a) on-site losses—extra costs of replacement power, the costs of cleaning and repairing the plant, and the loss of capital investment in the plant—are likely to be substantially higher than off-site losses for all but the most extreme release scenarios, (b) that the number of latent casualties from a severe accident is likely to be substantially higher than the number of acute fatalities, and that (c) in terms of overall importance, off-site property damage from severe accidents is likely to be even more serious than latent casualties. Also, these assessments have identified flaws and vulnerabilities in plant design and operation that had previously gone unrecognized (NRC, 1985). Thus, even when a risk assessment gives only a very crude measure of the level of risk, it can still be extremely valuable. It can allow the user to gain a detailed understanding of the complex cause-effect processes by which a technological system may produce adverse consequences and can identify beneficial changes in design or operations.

Finally, the rigorously analytical approach that is central to risk assessment also has important implications for the growth of scientific knowledge. Stating a risk problem in rigorous, quantitative terms ensures that critics will be able to identify and highlight questionable assumptions and flaws in the assessment. It ensures an open process through which scientists can challenge questionable theories, methods, or data, and propose new ones. Thus, risk assessment not only provides the best short-term approach for understanding specific risks, it leads naturally, over the longer term, to the improved science, capability, and resources needed to reduce all risks.

REFERENCES

Ågren, G. I., 1983, "Model Analysis of Some Consequences of Acid Precipitation on Forest Growth," in *Ecological Effects of Acid Deposition*, Report PM 1636, National Swedish Environment Protection Board, Stockholm pp. 233–244.

Ågren, G. I., and P. Kauppi, 1983, "Nitrogen Dynamics in European Forest Ecosystems: Considerations Regarding Anthropogenic Nitrogen Depositions," Collaborative Paper CP-83-28, International Institute for Applied Systems Analysis, Laxenburg, Austria.

(AIChE/CCPS) American Institute of Chemical Engineers/Center for Chemical Process Safety, 1985, *Guidelines for Hazard Evaluation Procedures*, prepared by Battelle Columbus Division for the Center for Chemical Process Safety, American Institute of Chemical Engineers, New York.

(AIChE/CCPS) American Institute of Chemical Engineers/Center for Chemical Process Safety, 1989, *Guidelines for Chemical Process Quantitative Risk Analysis*, Center for Chemical Process Safety, American Institute of Chemical Engineers, New York.

Åkland, G. G., T. D. Hartwell, T. Johnson, and R. W. Whitmore, 1985, "Measuring Human Exposures to Carbon Monoxide in Washington, D. C., and Denver, Colorado, during the Winter of 1982–83," *Environ. Sci. Technol.* **19**, 911–918.

Albert, R. E., and B. Altschuler, 1973, "Consideration Relating to the Formulation of Limits for Unavoidable Population Exposures to Environmental Carcinogens," in J. E. Ballon (ed.), *Radionuclide Carcinogenesis*, NTIS, Springfield, Virginia, pp. 233–253.

Alfidi, R. J., 1971, "Informed Consent: A Study of Patient Reaction," *J. Am. Med. Assoc. 216*, 1325.

Alstad, D. N., G. F. Edmunds, and L. H. Weinstein, 1982, "Effects of Air Pollutants on Insect Populations," *Annu. Rev. Entomol.* **27**, 369.

Ames, B., 1979, "Identifying Environmental Chemicals Causing Mutations and Cancer," *Science* **204**, 587–593.

Ames, B., R. Magaw, and L. Gold, 1987, "Ranking Possible Carcinogenic Hazards," *Science* **236**, 271–279.

Andersen, M. E., H. J. Clewell III, M. L. Gargas, F. A. Smith, and R. H. Reitz, 1987, "Physiologically-based Pharmacokinetics and the Risk Assessment Process for Methylene Chloride," *Toxicol. Appl. Pharmacol.* **87**, 185–205.

Andrews, L., and R. Snyder, 1986, "Toxic Effects of Solvents and Vapors," in C. D. Klaasses, M. O. Amdur, and J. Doull (eds.), *Casarett and Doull's Toxicology: The Basic Science of Poisons*, 3rd ed., Macmillan, New York.

Apostolakis, G., 1981, "Bayesian Methods in Risk Assessment," in J. Lewins and M. Becker (eds.), *Advances in Nuclear Science Technology*, vol. 13, Plenum, New York.

Apostolakis, G., and S. Kaplan, 1981, "Pitfalls in Risk Calculations," *Reliab. Eng.* **2**, 135–145.

Argue, A. W., R. Hilborn, R. M. Peterman, M. J. Staley, and C. J. Walters, 1983, "Strait of Georgia Chinook and Coho Fisheries," *Can. B. Fish. Aquat. Sci.*

Armitage, P., 1955, "Tests for Linear Trends in Proportions and Frequencies," *Biometrics* **11**, 375–386.

Armitage, P., and R. Doll, 1954, "The Age Distribution of Cancer and a Multistage Theory of Carcinogenesis," *Br. J. Cancer* **8**, 1.

Auer, C. M., 1988, "Use of Structure–Activity Relationships in Assessing the Risks of New Chemicals," in R. W. Hart and F. D. Hoerger (eds.), *Carcinogen Risk Assessment: New Directions in the Qualitative and Quantitative Aspects* (31 Banbury Report), Cold Spring Harbor Laboratory, Cold Spring Harbor, New York, pp. 33–41.

Auer, C. M., and D. H. Gould, 1987, "Carcinogenicity Assessment and the Role of Structure Activity Relationships (SAR) Analysis Under TSCA Section 5, *Environ. Carcinogen. Rev.* **C5**(1), 29.

Autrup, H., T. Seremet, J. Wakhisi, and A. Wasunna, 1987, "Aflatoxin Exposure Measured by Urinary Excretion of Aflatoxin B1–Guanine Adduct and Hepatitis B Virus Infection in Areas with Different Liver Cancer Incidence in Kenya," *Cancer Res.* **47**, 3430.

Bachmat, Y., B. Andrews, D. Holtz, and S. Sebastian, 1978, "Utilization of Numerical Groundwater Models for Water Resource Management," U. S. Environmental Protection Agency, EPA 600/8-78-012, Environmental Research Laboratory, Ada, Oklahoma.

Bailar, J. C. III, E. A. C. Crouch, R. Shaikh, and D. Spiegelman, 1988, "One-Hit Models of Carcinogenesis: Conservative or Not?," *Risk Anal.* **8**(4), 485–497.

Baker, W. E., P. A. Cox, P. S. Westine, J. J. Kulesz, and R. A. Strehlow, 1983, *Explosion Hazards and Evaluation*, Elsevier, New York.

Bartell, S., R. H. Gardner, and R. V. O'Neill, 1992, *Ecological Risk Estimation*, Lewis, Boca Raton, Florida.

Basta, D. J., and B. T. Bower, 1982, *Analyzing Natural Systems: Analysis for Regional Residuals—Environmental Quality Management*, Resources for the Future, Inc., Johns Hopkins University Press, Baltimore.

Bayes, T., 1958 (reprint), "Essay Toward Solving a Problem in the Doctrine of Chances," *Biometrika* **45**, 293–315.

BEIR, 1990, "Health Effects of Exposure to Low Levels of Ionizing Radiation," Report no. V of the Committee on the Biological Effects of Ionizing Radiation of the National Research Council, National Academy Press, Washington, D.C.

Berger, R. D., 1989, "Description and Application of Some General Models for Plant Disease Epidemics," in K. J. Leonard and W. E. Fry (eds.), *Plant Disease Epidemiology*, Vol. 2, McGraw-Hill, New York, pp. 125–149.

Berkson, J., 1944, "Application of the Logistic Function to Bio-Assay," *J. Am. Stat. Assoc.* **39**, 357–365.

Bhushan, B., 1975, "Analysis of Automobile Collisions," SAE Technical Paper Series, no. 750895, Society of Automotive Engineers, Warrendale, Pennsylvania.

Bischoff, K. B., 1987, "Physiologically Based Pharmacokinetic Modelling," in *Drinking Water and Health, Vol. 8: Pharmacokinetics and Risk Assessment*, National Academy Press, Washington, D. C.

Bolton, J. G., P. F. Morrison, and K. Solomon, 1983, "Risk-Cost Assessment Methodology for Toxic Pollutants from Fossil Fuel Power Plants," R-2993-EPRI, Rand Corporation, Santa Monica, California.

Bolton, J. G., P. F. Morrison, K. Solomon, and K. Wolf, 1985, "Alternative Models for Risk Assessment of Toxic Emissions," N-2261-EPRI, Rand Note, Rand Corporation, Santa Monica, California.

Boutwell, S. H., and B. R. Roberts, 1983, "Assessment Methodology for Remedial Actions in Surface Waters," Anderson-Nichols and Company, Palo Alto, California.

Boutwell, S. H., S. M. Brown, B. R. Roberts, and D. F. Atwood, 1986, *Modeling Remedial Actions at Uncontrolled Hazardous Waste Sites*, Pollution Technology Review no. 130, Noyes Publications, Park Ridge, New Jersey.

Boyce, S. G., 1978, "Multiple Benefits from Forests: A Solution to a Most Puzzling Problem," in J. Fries, H. E. Burkhart, and T. A. Max (eds.), *Growth Models for Long Term Forecasting of Timber*

Yields, publication FWS-1-78, School of Forestry and Wildlife Resources, Virginia Polytechnic Institute and State University, Blacksburg, Virginia.

Braat, L. C., and W. F. J. van Lierop (eds.), 1987a, *Economic–Ecological Modeling* (Studies in Regional Science and Urban Economics, vol. 16), Elsevier/North-Holland, Amsterdam and New York.

Braat, L. C., and W. F. J. van Lierop, 1987b, "Environment, Policy, and Modeling," in L. C. Braat and W. F. J. van Lierop (eds.), *Economic-Ecological Modeling* (Studies in Regional Science and Urban Economics, vol. 16), Elsevier/North-Holland, Amsterdam and New York, pp. 7–19.

Brenner, L., Jr., 1980, "Accident Investigations—a Case for New Perceptions and Methodologies," SAE Technical Paper Series, no. 800387, Society of Automotive Engineers, Warrendale, Pennsylvania.

Briggs, G. A., 1975, "Plume Rise Predictions," in *Lectures on Air Pollution and Environmental Impact Analysis*, American Meteorological Society.

Brown, S., S. Brett, M. Gough, J. Rodricks, R. Tardiff, and D. Turnbull, 1987, *Review of Interspecies Comparisons*, Environ Corporation, Washington, D. C.

Bunyan, P. J., M. Van den Heuvel, P. I. Stanley, and E. N. Wright, 1981, "An Intensive Field Trial and a Multi-Site Surveillance Exercise on the Use of Aldicarb to Investigate Methods for the Assessment of Possible Environmental Hazards Presented by New Pesticides," *Agro-Ecosystems* **7**, 239–262.

Burr-Doss, B., 1985, "On Errors-in-Variables in Binary Regression—Berkson Case," Technical Report no. 104, Division of Biostatistics, Stanford University, Stanford, California.

Calabrese, E. J., 1983, *Principles of Animal Extrapolation*, Wiley, New York.

Caldwell, S., D. Barrett, and S. S. Chang, 1981, "Ranking System for Releases of Hazardous Substances," in *Proceedings of the National Conference on Management of Uncontrolled Hazardous Waste Sites*, Hazardous Materials Control Institute, Silver Spring, Maryland, pp. 14–20.

Callaway, R. J., *et al.*, 1982, "Preliminary Analysis of the Dispersion of Sewage Sludge Discharged from Vessels to New York Bight Waters," U. S. Environmental Protection Agency, Corvallis, Oregon.

Canter, L. W., and R. C. Knox, 1985, *Ground Water Pollution Control*, Lewis Publishers, Chelsea, Michigan.

Carlborg, F. W., 1981a, "2-Acetylaminofluorene and the Weibull Model," *Food Cosmet. Toxicol.* **19**, 367–371.

Carlborg, F. W., 1981b, "Dose-Response Functions in Carcinogenesis and the Weibull Model," *Food Cosmet. Toxicol.* **19**, 255–263.

Carlborg, F. W., 1982, "The Threshold and Virtually Safe Dose," *Food Chem. Toxic.* **20**, 219.

Carnahan, J. V., and K. S. Krishnan, 1989, "A Bayesian Approach for Analyzing Results of Vehicle Collision Tests," *Decis. Sciences* **20**(4), 746–758.

Caswell, H., 1989, "Matrix Population Models," Sinauer Associates, Inc., Sunderland, Massachusetts.

Chankong, V., Y. Y. Haimes, H. Rosenkranz, and J. Pet-Edwards, 1985, "The Carcinogenicity Prediction and Battery Selection (CPBS) Method: A Bayesian Approach," *Mutation Res.* **153**, 135–166.

Chappelka, A. H., and M. E. Kraemer, 1988, "Effects of Air Pollutants on Plant-Insect Interactions," Proceedings of the 81st Annual Meeting of APCA, Dallas, Texas, June 19–24, Session 125, "Ecological Effects of Air Pollutants," paper no. 5.

Chen, J. J., R. L. Kodell, and D. W. Gaylor, 1988, "Using the Biological Two-State Model to Assess Risk from Short-Term Exposures," *Risk Anal.* **8**(2), 223–230.

Cheney, E. W., 1966, *Introduction to Approximation Theory*, McGraw-Hill, New York.

Clark, C. E., 1961, "Importance Sampling in Monte Carlo Analyses," *Oper. Res.* **9**, 603–620.

Clark, C. W., 1987, "Fisheries as Renewable Resources," in L. C. Braat and W. F. J. van Lierop (eds.), *Economic-Ecological Modeling* (Studies in Regional Science and Urban Economics, vol. 16), Elsevier/North-Holland, Amsterdam and New York, pp. 73–86.

Clark, C. W., and G. P. Kirkwood, 1979, "Bioeconomic Model of the Gulf of Carpentaria Prawn Fishery," *J. Fish. Res. Board. Canada 36*, 1304–1312.

Clean Air Act of 1963, as amended, Section 109, 42 U.S.C. 7414.

Clewell, H. J., and M. E. Andersen, 1985, "Risk Assessment Extrapolations and Physiological Modeling," in J. F. Stara and L. S. Erdreich (eds.), *Advances in Health Risk Assessment for Systemic Toxicants and Chemical Mixtures*, Princeton Scientific Publishing Co., Princeton, New Jersey, pp. 111–131.

Cochran, W. G., 1968, "Errors of Measurements in Statistics," *Technometrics* **10**, 637–661.

Cochran, W. G., 1970, "Some Effects of Errors of Measurements on Multiple Correlation," *J. Am. Stat. Assoc.* **65**, 22–34.

Cone, J. E., G. R. Reeve, and P. J. Landrigan, 1987, "Clinical and Epidemiological Studies," in R. G. Tardiff and J. V. Rodricks (eds.), *Toxic Substances and Human Risk; Principles of Data Interpretation*, Plenum, New York, Chap. 6., pp. 95–120

Conservation Foundation, 1985, *Risk Assessment and Risk Control*, The Conservation Foundation, Washington, D. C.

Conway, R. A. (ed.), 1982, *Environmental Risk Analysis for Chemicals*, Van Nostrand Reinhold, New York.

Cornfield, J., and N. Mantel, 1977, "Estimation of 'Safe Doses' in Carcinogenic Experiments," *Biometrics 33*, 1.

Cortese, A. D., and J. D. Spengler, 1976, "Ability of Fixed Monitoring Stations to Represent Personal Carbon Monoxide Exposure," *J. Air Pollut. Control Assoc.* **26**, 1144.

Cothern, C. R., 1988, "Uncertainties in Quantitative Risk Assessments—Two Examples: Trichloroethylene and Radon in Drinking Water," in C. R. Cothern, M. A. Mehlman, and W. L. Marcus (eds.), *Risk Assessment and Risk Management of Industrial and Environmental Chemicals* (Advances in Modern Environmental Toxicology, vol. 15), Princeton Scientific Publishing Co., Princeton, New Jersey, pp. 159–180.

Cothern, C. R., W. A. Coniglio, and W. L. Marcus, 1986, "Estimating Risk to Human Health," *Environ. Sci. Technol.* **20**(2), 111–116.

Courtemanch, D. L., and S. P. Davies, 1987, "A Coefficient of Community Loss To Assess Detrimental Change in Aquatic Communities," *Water Res.* **21**, 217–222.

Covello, V. T., 1983, "The Perception of Technological Risks: A Literature Review," *Technological Forecasting and Social Change* **23**, 285–297.

Covello, V. T., 1984, "Uses of Social and Behavioral Research on Risk," *Environ. Int.* **10**, 541–545.

Covello, V. T., and C. Hadlock, 1985, *Probabilistic Risk Assessment: The State-of-the-Art, with Special Application to Nuclear Power*, National Science Foundation, Washington, D. C.

Covello, V. T., D. von Winterfeldt, and P. Slovic, 1987, "Communicating Risk Information to the Public," in V. T. Covello, F. Allen, and J. C. Davies (eds.), *Risk Communication: Proceedings of the National Conference on Risk Communication*, The Conservation Foundation, Washington, D. C.

Cox, D. R., 1972, "Regression Models and Life Tables (With Discussion)," *J. Roy. Stat. Soc. 34*, 187–220.

Cox, D. O., and G. E. Moller, 1980, "Practical Aspects of the Engineering Problem Investigation," in *Proceedings of the American Society of Metals Fracture and Failure Sessions, 1980*, Western Metal and Tool Exposition and Conference, March 17–20, 1980, American Society of Metals.

Crane Co., 1981, "Flow of Fluids through Valves, Fittings and Pipe, Metric Edition—SI Units," Technical Paper no. 410M, Crane, New York, New York.

Crawford, N. H., 1982, "Hydrologic Transport Modeling," in K. L. Dickson, A. W. Maki, and J. Cairns, Jr. (eds.), *Modeling the Fate of Chemicals in the Aquatic Environment*, Ann Arbor Science Publishers, Ann Arbor, Michigan.

Crouch, E., and R. Wilson, 1979, "Interspecies Comparison of Carcinogenic Potency," *J. Toxicol. Environ. Health* **5**, 1095–1118.

Crump, K. S., 1981, "An Improved Procedure for Low-Dose Carcinogenic Risk Assessment from Animal Data," unpublished.

Crump, K., 1985, "Mechanisms Leading to Dose-Response Models," in P. Ricci (ed.), *Principles of Health Risk Assessment*, Prentice-Hall, Englewood Cliffs, New Jersey, pp. 235–277.

Crump, K. S., and R. B. Howe, 1984, "The Multistage Model with a Time-Dependent Dose Pattern: Application to Carcinogenic Risk Assessment," *Risk Anal.* **4**(3), 163–176.

Crump, K. S., H. A. Guess, and K. L. Deal, 1977, "Confidence Intervals and Test of Hypotheses Concerning Dose-Response Relationships Inferred from Animal Carcinogenicity Data, *Biometrics* **33**, 21–24.

Crump, K., D. Hoel, C. Langley, and R. Peto, 1976, "Fundamental Carcinogenic Processes and the Implications for Low Dose Risk Assessment," *Cancer Res.* **36**, 2973–2979.

Culliton, B. J., 1979, "Carter Addresses National Academy" (editorial), *Science* **204**, 480–481.

Dalkey, N., 1968, "The Delphi Method: An Experimental Study of Group Opinion," Rand Corporation, Santa Monica, California.

De Roos, A. M., O. Dickmann, and J. A. J. Metz, 1992, "Studying the Dynamics of Structured Population Models: A Versitile Technique and Its Application to Daphina," *American Naturalist* **139**, 123–146.

Delbecq, A., A. Van de Ven, and D. Gustafson, 1975, *Group Techniques for Program Planning*, Scott-Foresman, Glenview, Illinois.

(DOE) U. S. Department of Energy, "Liquified Gaseous Fuels Spill Test Facility," Assistant Secretary for Fossil Fuel Energy, Washington, D. C.

(DOE) U. S. Department of Energy, 1981, *Energy Technologies and the Environment*, DOE/EP-0026, National Technical Information Service, Springfield, Virginia.

Doll, R., and R. Peto, 1981, "The Causes of Cancer: Quantitative Estimates of Avoidable Risks of Cancer in the United States Today," *J. Natl. Cancer Inst. (U. S.)* **66**, 1192–1308.

Donigian, A. S., Jr., 1981, "Water Quality Modeling in Relation to Watershed Hydrology," in V. Singh (ed.), *Modeling Components of the Hydrologic Cycle*, Proceedings of the International Symposium on Rainfall Runoff Modeling, [held at] Mississippi State University, Water Resources Publications, Littleton, Colorado.

Downing, D. J., R. H. Gardner, and F. O. Hoffman, 1985, "Response Surface Methodologies for Uncertainty Analysis in Assessment Model," *Technometrics* **27**(2), 151–163.

Duan, N., 1981, "Microenvironment Types: A Model for Human Exposure to Air Pollution," SIMS Technical Report no. 47, Department of Statistics, Stanford University, Stanford, California.

Durkin, P. R., 1981, "An Approach to the Analysis of Toxicant Interactions in the Aquatic Environment," in *Proceedings of the Fourth Annual Symposium on Aquatic Toxicology*, American Society for Testing and Materials.

Easterling, R. G., F. W. Spencer, and K. V. Diegert, 1985, "Estimation, Uncertainty Analysis, and Sensitivity Analysis: Directions for RMIEP," Sandia National Laboratories, Albuquerque, New Mexico, January 4.

Efron, G. A., 1979, "Computers and the Theory of Statistics: Thinking the Unthinkable," *SIAM Rev.* **21**, 460–480.

Eisenberg, N. A., C. J. Lynch, and R. J. Breeding, 1975, "Vulnerability Model—A Simulation System for Assessing Damage Resulting from Marine Spills," U. S. Coast Guard, Office of Research and Development, Report no. CG-D-136-75, NTIS AD-015-245, Springfield, Virginia.

Eisenbud, M., 1984, *Environmental Radioactivity*, 3rd ed., Academic Press, New York.

Environ Corporation, 1986, "Elements of Toxicology and Chemical Risk Assessment: A Handbook for Nonscientists, Attorneys and Decision Makers," Environ, Council on Health and Environmental Science, Washington, D. C.

EPA (U. S. Environmental Protection Agency), 1976, "Interim Procedures and Guidelines for Health Risk and Economic Impact Assessments of Suspected Carcinogens," *Fed. Register* **41**, 24102.

EPA (U. S. Environmental Protection Agency), 1979, "Environmental Modeling Catalogue, Abstracts of Environmental Models."

EPA (U. S. Environmental Protection Agency), 1982, "Air Quality Criteria for Oxides of Nitrogen," Office of Research and Development, Research Triangle Park, North Carolina.

EPA (U. S. Environmental Protection Agency), 1984a, "Formaldehyde Determination of Significant Risk," *Fed. Register* **49**, no. 101, p. 21870.

EPA (U. S. Environmental Protection Agency), 1984b, "IRMC Issue Paper: Development of Guidelines for Assessment of Carcinogenic Risk," *Inside EPA* **5**, 15.

EPA (U. S. Environmental Protection Agency), 1985a, "Principles of Risk Assessment—A Nontechnical Review," Workshop on Risk Assessment, Tidewater Inn, Easton, Maryland, March 17–18, 1985, Washington, D. C.

EPA (U. S. Environmental Protection Agency), 1985b, "Status of Extrapolation Modeling Research Needed To Extrapolate from Animal Data to Human Risk, from High to Low Doses, and from Acute to Chronic Effects," Office of Research and Development, Washington, D.C.

EPA (U. S. Environmental Protection Agency), 1985c, "National Primary Drinking Water Regulations; Volatile Synthetic Organic Chemicals; Final Rule and Proposed Rule," *Fed. Register* **50**, 46830–46901.

EPA (U. S. Environmental Protection Agency), 1985d, "National Primary Drinking Water Regulations; Synthetic Organic Chemicals, Inorganic Chemicals and Microorganisms; Proposed Rule," *Fed. Regist.* **50**, 46936-47025.

EPA (U. S. Environmental Protection Agency), 1986a, "Superfund Public Health Evaluation Manual," EPA/540/1-86/061, Office of Emergency and Remedial Response, EPA, Washington, D. C.

EPA (U. S. Environmental Protection Agency), 1986b, "Guidelines for Carcinogen Risk Assessment," *Fed. Register* **51**, 34000, Washington, D. C.

EPA (U. S. Environmental Protection Agency), 1986c, "Guidelines for Mutagenicity Risk Assessment," *Fed. Register* **51**, 34006, Washington, D. C.

EPA (U. S. Environmental Protection Agency), 1986d, "Guidelines for Health Risk Assessment of Chemical Mixtures," *Fed. Register* **51**, 34014, Washington, D. C.

EPA (U. S. Environmental Protection Agency), 1986e, "Guidelines for Health Risk Assessment of Suspect Developmental Toxicants," *Fed. Register* **51**, 34028, Washington, D. C.

EPA (U. S. Environmental Protection Agency), 1986f, "Acid Deposition Research Program," Office of Acid Deposition, Environmental Monitoring and Quality Assurance, prepared by ICAIR Life Systems, Inc., contract no. 68-02-4193.

EPA (U. S. Environmental Protection Agency), 1986g, "New Chemical Review Process Manual," EPA 560/3-86-002, Office of Toxic Substances, Washington, D. C.

EPA (U. S. Environmental Protection Agency), 1987a, "Unfinished Business: A Comparative Assessment of Environmental Problems: Vol. 1, Overview Report," Office of Policy Analysis, Office of Policy, Planning and Evaluation, Washington, D. C.

EPA (U. S. Environmental Protection Agency), 1987b, "Unfinished Business: A Comparative Assessment of Environmental Problems: Appendix II, Non-Cancer Risk Work Group," Office of Policy Analysis, Office of Policy, Planning and Evaluation, Washington, D. C.

EPA (U. S. Environmental Protection Agency), 1987c, "Unfinished Business: A Comparative Assessment of Environmental Problems: Appendix III, Comparative Ecological Risk, a Report of the Ecological Risk Work Group," Office of Policy Analysis, Office of Policy, Planning and Evaluation, Washington, D. C.

EPA (U. S. Environmental Protection Agency), 1987d, "Unfinished Business: A Comparative Assessment of Environmental Problems: Appendix IV, An Assessment of Welfare Effects from Environmental Pollution, a Report of the Welfare Risk Work Group," Office of Policy Analysis, Office of Policy, Planning and Evaluation, Washington, D. C.

EPA (U. S. Environmental Protection Agency), 1988a, "Statistical Methods for Evaluating Ground Water from Hazardous Waste Facilities," Office of Solid Waste, Washington, D.C.

EPA (U. S. Environmental Protection Agency), 1988b, "Statistical Methods for Evaluating the Attainment of Superfund Cleanup Standards, Vol. I: Soils and Solid Media," Draft, Office of Policy, Planning, and Evaluation, Washington, D.C.

EPA (U. S. Environmental Protection Agency), 1988c, "Superfund Exposure Assessment Manual," EPA/540/1-88/001, Office of Emergency and Remedial Response, Washington, D.C.

EPA (U. S. Environmental Protection Agency), 1988d, "Selection Criteria for Mathematical Models Used in Exposure Assessments: Groundwater Models," EPA/600/8-88/075, Office of Health and Environmental Assessment, Washington, D.C.

EPA (U. S. Environmental Protection Agency), 1989a, "Risk Assessment Guidance for Superfund: Volume I—Human Health Evaluation Manual (Part A), Interim Final," EPA/540/1-89/002, Office of Emergency and Remedial Response, Washington DC.

EPA (U. S. Environmental Protection Agency), 1989b, "Soil Sampling Quality Assurance Guide" Environmental Monitoring Support Laboratory, Las Vegas, Nevada.

EPA (U. S. Environmental Protection Agency), 1989c, "Ecological Assessment of Hazardous Waste Sites: A Field and Laboratory Reference," EPA/600/3–89/013, W. W. Hicks, B. R. Parkhurst, and S. S. Baker, Jr. (eds.), EPA Environmental Research Laboratory, Corvallis, Oregon.

EPA (U. S. Environmental Protection Agency), 1989d, "Pesticide Assessment Guidelines: Subdivision M—Microbial Pest Control Agents and Biochemical Pest Control Agents," NTIS, Springfield, Virginia.

(EPRI) Electric Power Research Institute, 1987, "EMF: The Debate on Health Effects," *EPRI J.* **12**(7), 4–15.

Farquharson, F. B., 1950, "Aerodynamic Stability of Suspension Bridges, with Special Reference to the Tacoma Narrows Bridge," *Univ. of Wash. Eng. Exp. St. Bull.* **116**, Part I, Seattle, Washington.

Fauske, H. K., M. Epstein, M. A. Grolmes, and J. C. Leung, 1986, "Emergency Relief Vent Sizing for Fire Emergencies Involving Liquid Filled Atmospheric Storage Vessels," *Plant/Oper. Prog.* **5**(4), 205–208.

(FDA) U. S. Food and Drug Administration, 1982, *Toxicological Principles for the Safety Assessment of Direct Food Additivies and Color Additives Used in Food*, U.S. FDA, Bureau of Foods, Washington, D. C.

Fiksel, J. R., and V. T. Covello (eds.), 1986, *Biotechnology Risk Assessment*, Pergamon Press, New York.

Fiksel, J. R., and V. T. Covello (eds.), 1989, *Safety Assurance for Environmental Releases of Genetically Engineered Organisms*, Springer-Verlag, Berlin and New York.

Fiksel, J. R., and K. M. Scow, 1983, "Human Exposure and Health Risk Assessments Using Outputs of Environmental Fate Models," in R. L. Swann and A. Eschenroeder (eds.), *Fate of Chemicals in the Environment, Compartmental and Multimedia Models*, ACS Symposium Series 225, American Chemical Society, Washington, D. C.

Fiksel, J. R., L. A. Cox, and H. D. Ojha, 1984, "Dealing with Uncertainty in Risk Analysis," Arthur D. Little, Inc., Cambridge, Massachusetts.

Finkel, A. M., 1988, "Dioxin: Are We Safer Now Than Before?" *Risk Anal.* **8**(2), 161–165 (June).

Finney, D. J., 1952, *Statistical Methods in Biological Assay*, Hafner, New York.

Finney, D. J., 1971, *Probit Analysis*, 3rd ed., Cambridge University Press, Cambridge, England.

Finney, D. J., 1978, *Statistical Method in Biological Assay*, 3rd ed., Charles Griffin and Co., Ltd., London.

Fischhoff, B., 1977, "Cost-Benefit Analysis and the Art of Motorcycle Maintenance," *Policy Sciences* **8**, 177–202.

Fischhoff, B., 1983, "Informed Consent for Transient Nuclear Workers," in R. Kasperson and R. W. Kates (eds.), *Equity Issues in Radioactive Waste Disposal*, Oelgeschlager, Gunn and Hain, Cambridge, Massachusetts.

Fischhoff, B., 1985, "Managing Risk Perception," *Issues Sci. Tech.* **2**(1), 83–96&.

Flamm, W. G., and R. L. Lorentzen, 1988, "Quantitative Risk Assessment (QRA): A Special Problem in the Approval of New Products," in C. R. Cothern, M. A. Mehlman, and W. L. Marcus (eds.), *Risk Assessment and Risk Management of Industrial and Environmental Chemicals* (Advances in Modern Environmental Toxicology ,vol. 15), Princeton Scientific Publishing Co., Princeton, New Jersey, pp. 91–108

Food Safety Council, 1980, "Proposed System for Food Safety Assessment," Final Report of the Committee of the Food Safety Council, Washington, D. C.

Freedman, D. A., and H. Zeisel, 1987, "From Mouse to Man: The Quantitative Assessment of Cancer Risks," Technical Report no. 79, Department of Statistics, University of California, Berkeley, California.

Freudenburg, W. R., 1988, "Perceived Risk, Real Risk: Social Science and the Art of Probabilistic Risk Assessment," *Science* **242**, 44–49.

Friberg, L., G. F. Nordberg, and V. B. Vouk, 1986, *Handbook on the Toxicology of Metals*, Elsevier, Amsterdam and New York.

Fries, J. (ed.), 1974, *Growth Models for Tree and Stand Simulation*, Department of Forest Yield Research, Royal College of Forestry, Stockholm, Sweden.

Fussell, J. B., 1980, "System Reliability Engineering and Risk Assessment," University of Tennessee, Knoxville, Tennessee.

Fussell, J. B., 1981, "Advanced System Reliability Techniques for Practitioners," JBF Associates.

Fussell, J. B., and G. R. Burdick, 1977, *Nuclear Systems Reliability Engineering and Risk Assessment*, Society for Industrial and Applied Mathematics, Philadelphia, Pennsylvania.

Gage, S. J., 1979, "Statement Before the Subcommittee on Health and the Environment," Committee on Interstate and Foreign Commerce, U. S. House of Representatives, November 27.

GAO (U. S. General Accounting Office), 1991, "Toxic Substances: Status of EPA's Review of Chemicals Under the Chemical Testing Program," GAO/RCED-92-31FS, Fact Sheet for the Chairman, Environment, Energy, and Natural Resources Subcommittee, Committee on Government Operations, U.S. House of Representatives.

Gart, J., J. K. Chu, and R. E. Tarone, 1979, "Statistical Issues in Interpretation of Chronic Bioassay Tests for Carcinogenicity," *J. Natl. Cancer Inst.* **62**, 957–974.

Gately, W. V., and R. L. Williams, 1978a, *Go Methodology—Overview*, EPRI NP-765, Electric Power Research Institute, Palo Alto, California.

Gately, W. V., and R. L. Williams, 1978b, *Go Methodology—System Reliability Assessment and Computer Code Manual*, EPRI NP-766, Electric Power Research Institute, Palo Alto, California.

Gaylor, D. W., and R. L. Kodell, 1980, "Linear Interpolation Algorithm for Low-Dose Risk Assessment of Toxic Substances," *J. Environ. Pathol. Toxicol.* **4**, 305–312.

Gehring, P. J., P. G. Watanabe, and C. N. Park, 1979, "Risk of Angiosarcoma in Workers Exposed to Vinyl Chloride as Predicted from Studies in Rats," *Toxicol. Appl. Pharmacol.* **49**, 15–21.

Gillett, J. W., 1987, "Consensus Research Needs and Priorities in Environmental Risk Assessment: An Academic Perspective" presented at the SETAC Workshop held August 1987 in Breckenridge, Colorado.

Goldstein, A., L. Aronow, and S. M. Kalman, 1974, *Principles of Drug Action: The Basis of Pharmacology*, 2nd ed., John Wiley and Sons, New York.

Gompertz, D., 1980, "Assessment of Risk by Biological Monitoring," presented at the National Health and Safety Conference, London.

Gottfried, P., 1974, "Qualitative Risk Analysis: FTA and FMEA," *Prof. Safety*, October, 48–52.

Graney, R. L., 1987, "Consensus Research Needs and Priorities in Environmental Risk Assessment," presented at a workshop on Consensus Research Needs & Priorities in Environmental Risk Assessment sponsored by the Society of Environmental Toxicology and Chemistry, held, August 15–21, Breckenridge, Colorado.

Green, A. E., and A. J. Bourne, 1972, *Reliability Technology*, Wiley-Interscience, New York.

Grimsrud, G. P., E. J. Finnermore, and H. J. Owens, 1976, "Evaluation of Water Quality Models, a Management Guide for Planners," U. S. Environmental Protection Agency, EPA-600/5-76-004, Washington, D.C.

Guess, H. A., and K. S. Crump, 1976, "Low Dose Extrapolation of Data from Animal Carcinogenicity Experiments—Analysis of a New Statistical Technique," *Math. Biosci.* **32**, 15–36.

Gumbel, E. J., 1957, *Statistical Theory of Extreme Values and Some Practical Applications*, National Bureau of Standards Applied Mathematics Series 33, Bethesda, Maryland.

Hammer, W., 1972, *Handbook of System and Product Safety*, Prentice-Hall, Englewood Cliffs, New Jersey.

Hanna, S. R., G. A. Briggs, and R. P. Hosker, Jr., 1982, "Handbook on Atmospheric Diffusion," U. S. Department of Energy, DOE/TIC-11223, NTIS, Springfield, Virginia.

Harte, J., C. Holdren, R. Schneider, and C. Shirley, 1991, *Toxics A to Z: A Guide to Everyday Pollution Hazards*, University of California Press, Berkeley, California.

Hartley, H. O., and R. J. Sielken, Jr., 1977, "Estimation of 'Safe Doses' in Carcinogenic Experiments," *Biometrics* **33**, 1–30.

Harwell, M. A., and J. R. Kelly, 1986, "Ecosystems Research Center Workshop on Ecological Effects from Environmental Stresses—a Contribution to the EPA Comparative Risk Ecological Risk Workshop," Ecosystems Research Center, Cornell University, New York.

Haseman, J. D., and L. L. Kupper, 1979, "Analysis of Dichotomous Response Data from Certain Toxicological Experiments," *Biometrics* **35**, 281–293.

Hattis, D. B., 1986, "The Promise of Molecular Epidemiology for Quantitative Risk Assessment," *Risk Anal.* **6**, 181–194.

Hayne, D. W., 1984, "Development of Environmental Data Bases and Inventories," unpublished background paper prepared for the "Conference on Long-Term Environmental Research and Development," The Council of Environmental Quality, May 21–22.

Health and Welfare Canada, 1992a, *Carcinogen Evaluation*, Health & Welfare Canada, Ottawa.

Health and Welfare Canada, 1992b, *A Vital Link: Health and the Environment in Canada*, Health & Welfare Canada, Ottawa.

Helmers, E. N., and L. C. Schuller, 1982, "Calculated Process Risks and Hazards Management," *Plant/Oper. Prog.* **1**(3), 190.

Henley, E. J., and H. Kumamoto, 1991, *Probabilistic Risk Assessment: Reliability Engineering, Design, and Analysis*, IEEE Press, New York.

Hoel, D., D. Gaylor, and M. Anderson, 1983, "Implication of Nonlinear Kinetics on Risk Estimation in Carcinogesis, *Science* **219**, 1032–1037.

Hoel, D., R. Merrill, and F. Perera (eds.), 1985, *Risk Quantification and Regulatory Policy*, Banbury Report 19, Cold Spring Harbor Laboratory, Cold Spring Harbor, New York.

Hoffman, D. J., H. M. Ohlendorf, and T. W. Aldrich, 1988, "Selenium Teratogenesis in Natural Populations of Aquatic Birds in Central California," *Arch. Environ. Contam. Toxicol.* **17**, 519–525.

Hoffman, F. O., C. W. Miller, D. L. Shaeffer, and C. T. Garten, Jr., 1977, "Computer Codes for the Assessment of Radionuclides Released to the Environment," *Nucl. Saf.* **18** (3).

Hoffman, F. O., D. L. Shaeffer, C. W. Miller, and C. T. Garten, Jr. (eds.), 1978, *Proceedings of a Workshop on the Evaluation of Models Used for the Environmental Assessment of Radionuclide Releases*, CONF-770901, Oak Ridge National Laboratory, Oak Ridge, Tennessee.

Holdgate, M., 1991, "Conservation in a World Context," in I. F. Spellerberg, F. B. Goldsmith, and M. G. Morris (eds.), *The Scientific Management of Temperature Communities for Conservation*, Blackwell Scientific, Oxford, pp. 1–26.

Hollenback, J. J., Jr., 1977, "Failure Mode and Effect Analysis," SAE Technical Paper Series, no. 770740, Society of Automotive Engineers, Warrendale, Pennsylvania.

Hollstein, M., J. McCann, F. Angelosa, and W. Nichols, 1979, "Short Term Tests for Carcinogens and Mutagens," *Mutation Res.* **65**(3), 133–226&.

Holmes, B. S., and G. Sliter, 1974, "Scale Modeling of Vehicle Crashes—Techniques, Applicability, and Accuracy: Cost Effectiveness," SAE Technical Paper Series, no. 740586, Society of Automotive Engineers, Warrendale, Pennsylvania.

Howard, R. A., 1968, "The Foundations of Decision Analysis," *IEEE Trans. Sys. Science Cybernetics* **SSC-4**(3), 211–219.

Howard, R. A., 1971, *Dynamic Probabilistic Systems: Volume I: Markov Models*, John Wiley & Sons, New York.

Hylgard, T., and M. J. Liddle, 1981, "The Effect of Human Trampling on a Sand Dune Ecosystem Dominated by *Empetrum nigrum*," *J. Appl. Ecol.* **18**, 559–569.

(IARC) International Agency for Research on Cancer, 1982, *IARC Monographs on the Evaluation of the Carcinogenic Risk of Chemicals in Humans: Chemicals, Industrial Processes, and Industries Associated with Cancer in Humans* (IARC Monographs vols. 1–29), supplement no. 4, IARC, Lyon, France.

(IARC) International Agency for Research on Cancer, 1987, *IARC Monographs on the Evaluation of the Carcinogenic Risk of Chemicals in Humans: Overall Evaluations of Carcinogenicity* (Updating IARC Monographs vols. 1–42), supplement no. 7, IARC, Lyon, France.

(ICRP) International Commission on Radiological Protection, 1975, "Recommendations of the International Commission on Radiological Protection" (ICRP Publication 26), *Annals of the ICRP* **1**(3).

Iman, R. L., and J. C. Helton, 1988, "An Investigation of Uncertainty and Sensitivity Analysis Techniques for Computer Models," *Risk Anal.* **8** (1), 71–90.

Ingestad, T., A. Aronsson, and G. I. Ågren, 1981, "Nutrient Flux Density Model of Mineral Nutrition in Conifer Ecosystems," *Stud. For. Suec.* **160**, 61–71.

(IPC) Interdisciplinary Panel on Carcinogenicity, 1984, "Criteria for Evidence of Chemical Carcinogenicity," *Science* **225**, 682–687.

Iverson, S., and N. Arley, 1950, "On the Mechanism of Experimental Carcinogenesis," *Acta Pathol. Microbiol. Scand.* **27**, 773.

Jeffers, J. N. R., 1987, "Ecological Modeling: Shortcomings and Perspectives," in L. C. Braat and W. F. J. van Lierop (eds.), *Economic–Ecological Modeling* (Studies in Regional Science and Urban Economics, vol. 16), Elsevier/North-Holland, Amsterdam and New York, pp. 36–48.

Johnson, B. B., and V. T. Covello (eds.), 1987, *The Social and Cultural Construction of Risk; Essays on Risk Selection and Perception*, Reidel, Dordrecht, The Netherlands (Kluwer, Boston).

Johnson, E. J., and A. Tversky, 1984, "Representations of Perceptions of Risks," *J. Exper. Psych.: General* **113**(1), 55–70.

Johnson, K. B., P. S. Teng, and E. B. Radcliffe, 1987, "Coupling Feeding Effects of Potato Leafhopper, *Empoasca fabae*, Nymphs to a Model of Potato Growth, *Environ. Entomol.* **16**, 250–258&.

Johnson, R., and R. A. Paul, 1982, "The NAAQS Exposure Model (NEM) Applied to Carbon Monoxide" (draft report), U. S. Environmental Protection Agency, Office of Air Quality Planning and Standards, Strategies and Air Standards Division, Research Triangle Park, North Carolina.

Jones, D. D., 1977, "The Budworm Site Model," in G. A. Norton and C. S. Holling (eds.) *Proceedings of Conference on Pest Management*, CP-77-6, International Institute for Applied Systems Analysis, Laxenburg, Austria.

Kabata-Pendias, A., and H. Pendias, 1984, *Trace Elements in Soil and Plants*, CRC Press, Boca Raton, Florida.

Kadlec, R., 1989, "Field and Laboratory Event Investigation," Failure Analysis Associates, Inc., Palo Alto, California.

Kalbfleisch, J. D., D. R. Krewski, and J. Van Ryzin, 1983, "Dose-Response Models for Time-to-Response Toxicity Data," *Can. J. Stat.* **11**, 25–49.

Kamlet, M. S., S. Klepper, and R. G. Framk, 1985, "Mixing Micro and Macro Data: Statistical Issues and Implications for Data Collection and Reporting," Proceedings of the 20th National Meeting of the Public Health Conference on Records and Statistics.

Kendall, R. J., 1987, "Recommended Research Needs and Priorities," presented at a workshop on "Consensus Research Needs & Priorities in Environmental Risk Assessment"sponsored by the Society of Environmental Toxicology and Chemistry, August 15–21, Breckenridge, Colorado.

Kincaid, C. T., J. R. Morrey, and J. E. Rogers, 1983, "Geochemical Models for Solute Migration: The Selection of Computer Codes and Description of Solute Migration Processes, Vol. I," Electric Power Research Institute, Palo Alto, California.

King, W. F., and H. J. Mertz, 1973, *Human Impact Response*, Plenum, New York.

Knight, F. H., 1921, *Risk, Uncertainty and Profit*, University of Chicago Press, Chicago.

Knox, R. C., and L. W. Canter, 1980, "Summary of Groundwater Modeling in the United States," National Center for Groundwater Research, NCGWR 80-20, Norman, Oklahoma.

Kociba, R. J., 1984, "Summary and Critique of Rodent Carcinogenicity Studies of Chlorinated Dibenzo-p-Dioxins," in W. Lowrance (ed.), *Public Health Risks of Dioxins*, proceedings of a seminar held October 19–20, 1983, pp. 77–98.

Kodell, R. L., D. W. Gaylor, and J. J. Chen, 1987, "Lifetime Dose Rate for Intermittent Exposures to Carcinogens," *Risk Anal.* **7**, 339–346.

Koh, R. C., and L. N. Fan, 1970, "Mathematical Models for the Prediction of Temperature Distribution Resulting from the Discharge of Heated Water into Large Bodies of Water," U. S. Environmental Protection Agency Water Pollution Control Series, 16/30 DWD 10/70.

Koines, A., 1982, "Technical Review of Groundwater Models," Office of Solid Waste, U. S. Environmental Protection Agency, Washington, D.C.

Koren, H., 1991, *Handbook of Environmental Health and Safety: Principles and Practices*, vol. I, 2nd ed., Lewis, Grand Rapids, Michigan.

Koriat, A., S. Lichtenstein, and B. Fischhoff, 1980, "Reasons for Overconfidence," *J. Exper. Psych.: Human Learning, Memory* **6**, 107–118.

Krewski, D., and D. Murdoch, 1988, "Quantitative Factors in Carcinogenic Risk Assessment," in R. W. Hart and F. D. Hoerger (eds.), *Carcinogen Risk Assessment: New Directions in the Qualitative and Quantitative Aspects*, Banbury Report 31, Cold Spring Harbor Laboratory, Cold Spring Harbor, New York, pp. 257–273.

Krewski, D., and J. Van Ryzin, 1981, "Dose-Response Models for Quantal Response Toxicity Data," in M. Csorgo, D. A. Dowson, J. N. K. Rao, and M. E. Saleh (eds.), *Statistics and Related Topics*, North Holland Publishing Co., New York, pp. 201–231.

Krewski, D., C. Brown, and C. Murdoch, 1984, "Determining 'Safe' Levels of Exposure: Safety Factors or Mathematical Models?" Health Protection Branch, Health and Welfare, Canada, Ottawa, Ontario, Canada.

Krewski, D., D. Wigle, D. B. Clayson, and G. Howe, 1990, "Role of Epidemiology in Health Risk Assessment," in P. Band (ed.), *Occupational Cancer Epidemiology*, Recent Results in Cancer Research, vol. 120, Springer-Verlag, Berlin, pp. 1–24.

Krewski, D., J. Withey, L. F. Ku, and C. C. Travis, 1991, "Physiologically Based Pharmacokinetic Models: Applications in Carcinogenic Risk Assessment," in A. Rescigno and A. Thakur (eds.) *New Trends in Pharmacokinetics*, Plenum, New York, pp. 355–390.

Krimsky, S., and A. Plough, 1988, *Environmental Hazards: Communicating Risk As a Social Process*, Auburn House, Dover, Massachusetts.

Kurimoto, K., H. Nakaya, and K. Okada, 1981, "Modeling and Simulation of Frontal Crash Impact Response," *SAE Technical Paper Series*, no. 810793, Society of Automotive Engineers, Warrendale, Pennsylvania.

Lappala, E. G., 1980, "Modeling of Water and Solute Transport under Variably Saturated Conditions: State-of-the-Art," in *Modeling and Low Level Waste Management: An Interagency Workshop*, Oak Ridge National Laboratory, ORO-821, Oak Ridge, Tennessee.

Lathrop, J., and J. Linnerooth, 1981, "The Role of Risk Assessment in a Political Decision Process" (working paper), International Institute for Applied Systems Analysis, Laxenburg, Austria.

Lave, L. B., and G. S. Omenn, 1986, "Cost-Effectiveness of Short-Term Tests for Carcinogenicity," *Nature* **324** (6092), 29–34.

Lave, L. B., and A. C. Upton (eds.), 1987, *Toxic Chemicals, Health and the Environment*, Johns Hopkins University Press, Baltimore.

Lees, F. P., 1980, *Loss Prevention in the Process Industries*, (2 vols.), Butterworths, London and Boston.

Leung, J. C., 1986, "A Generalized Correlation for One-Component Homogeneous Equilibrium Flashing Choked Flow," *AIChE J* **32**, 524–527.

Levin, M. A., and H. S. Strauss (eds.), 1991, *Risk Assessment in Genetic Engineering*, McGraw-Hill, New York.

Lewtas, J., 1985, "Development of a Comparative Potency Method for Cancer Risk Assessment of Complex Mixtures Using Short-Term Bioassays," *Toxicol. Ind. Health* **1**(4).

Lichtenstein, S., P. Slovic, B. Fischhoff, M. Layman, and B. Coombs, 1978, "Judged Frequency of Lethal Events," *J. Exp. Psychol.: Human Learning and Memory* **4**, 551–578.

Lighthart, B., and A. S. Frisch, 1976, "Estimation of Viable Airborne Microbes Downwind from a Point Source," *Appl. Environ. Microbiol.* **31**, 700–704.

Lighthart, B., and A. J. Mohr, 1987, "Estimating Downwind Concentrations of Viable Airborne Microorganisms in Dynamic Atmospheric Conditions," *Appl. Environ. Microbiol.* **53**, 1580–1583.

Ligotke, M. W., D. A. Cataldo, P. Van Voris, and C. Novich, 1986, "Analysts Use Wind Tunnel to Study Particle Behavior in the Environment," *Research and Development* (Battelle Memorial Institute, Pacific Northwest Labs) **28**(6), 82–85 (June).

Lindell, M. K., and T. C. Earle, 1982, "How Close is Close Enough: Public Perceptions of the Risks of Industrial Facilities," *Risk Anal.* **3**, 245–254.

Lindley, D. V., 1970, *Introduction to Probability and Statistics from a Bayesian Viewpoint*, Cambridge University Press, New York.

Lindow, S. E., G. R. Knudsen, R. J. Seidler, M. V. Walter, V. W. Lanbou, P. S. Amy, D. Schmedding, V. Prince, and S. Hern, 1988, "Aerial Dispersal and Epiphytic Survival of *Pseudomonas syringae* during a Pretest for the Release of Genetically Engineered Strains into the Environment," *Appl. Environ. Microbiol.* **54**, 1557–1563.

Linstone, H. A., and M. Turoff (eds.), 1975, *The Delphi Method: Techniques and Applications*, Addison-Wesley, Reading, Massachusetts.

Lioy, P. J., and M. J. Y. Lioy (eds.), 1983, *Air Sampling Instruments for Evaluation of Atmospheric Contaminants*, 6th ed., American Conference of Governmental Industrial Hygienists, Cincinnati, Ohio.

Litai, D., D. Lanning, and N. C. Rasmussen, 1983, "The Public Perception of Risk," in V. T. Covello, W. Flamm, J. Rodricks, and R. Tardiff (eds.), *The Analysis of Actual Versus Perceived Risks*, Plenum, New York, pp. 213–224.

Lohman, P. H. M., J. D. Jansen, and R. A. Baan, 1983, "Comparison of Various Methodologies with Respect to Specificity and Sensitivity in Biomonitoring Occupational Exposure to Mutagens and Carcinogens," presented at the International Seminar on Methods of Monitoring Human Exposure to Carcinogenic and Mutagenic Agents, December 12–15, Espoo, Finland.

Loucks, D. P., 1987, "Water Quality—Economic Modeling," in L. C. Braat and W. F. J. van Lierop (eds.), *Economic–Ecological Modeling* (Studies in Regional Science and Urban Economics, vol. 16), Elsevier/North-Holland, Amsterdam and New York., pp. 135–148

Lowrance, W. W., 1976, *Of Acceptable Risk: Science and the Determination of Safety*, Kaufman, Los Altos, California.

Majone, G., 1982, "Prevention and Health Standards: American, Soviet, and European Models," *J. Health Politics Law 7*, 625–635.

Majone, G., and E. S. Quade, 1980, *Pitfalls of Analysis*, International Institute of Applied Systems Analysis, Wiley-Interscience, New York.

Mallows, C. L., 1956, "Generalizations of Tchebycheff's Inequalities," *J. R. Stat. Soc. B (London)* **18**, 139–168.

Marcus, G. H., 1983, "A Review of Risk Assessment Methodologies," Committee Print no. 98-929 0, U. S. Congress. House Committee on Science and Technology, Subcommittee on Science, Research and Technology, U. S. Government Printing Office, Washington, D. C.

Marshall, E., 1991, "A Is for Apple, Alar, and ... Alarmist?" *Science* **254**, 20–22.

Martin, J. R. (ed.), 1979, *Recommended Guide for the Prediction of the Dispersion of Airborne Effluents*, American Society of Mechanical Engineers Air Pollution Control Division, New York.

Martz, H. F., A. G. Beckman, K. Campbell, D. E. Whiteman, and J. M. Booker, 1983, *A Comparison of Methods for Uncertainty Analysis of Nuclear Power Plant Safety System Fault Tree Models*, NUREG/CR-3263, LA-9729-MS, Los Alamos National Laboratory, New Mexico.

McCormick, N. J., 1981, *Reliability and Risk Analysis*, Academic, New York.

McIntosh, M. S., 1991, "Statistical Techniques for Field Testing of Genetically Engineered Microorganisms," in M. A. Levin and H. S. Strauss (eds.), *Risk Assessment in Genetic Engineering*, McGraw-Hill, New York, pp. 219–239.

McKay, M. D., W. J. Conover, and R. J. Beckman, 1979, "A Comparison of Three Methods for Selecting Values of Input Variables in the Analysis of Output from a Computer Code," *Technometrics* **21**, 239–245.

McKone, T. E., and D. W. Layton, 1986, "Chemical Transport, Human Exposure, and Health Risk: A Multimedia Approach," in *Environmental Risk Management—Is Analysis Useful?* (Proceedings of an APCA International Specialty Conference), Air Pollution Control Association, Pittsburgh, Pennsylvania.

McLaughlin, S. B., 1985, "Effects of Air Pollution on Forests—A Critical Review," *J. Air Pollut. Control Assoc.* **35**(5), 512–540.

Mehrle, P., T. LaPoint, and C. Ingersoll, 1987, "Consensus Research Needs and Priorities in Environmental Risk Assessment," presented at a workshop on "Consensus Research Needs & Priorities in Environmental Risk Assessment" sponsored by the Society of Environmental Toxicology and Chemistry, August 15–21, Breckenridge, Colorado.

Merkhofer, M. W., 1982, "Risk Assessment: Quantifying Uncertainty in Health Effects," *Environ. Prof.* **3**, 249–264.

Merkhofer, M. W., 1987a, *Decision Science and Social Risk Management: A Comparative Evaluation of Cost-Benefit Analysis, Decision Analysis, and Other Formal Decision-Aiding Approaches*, D. Reidel, Dordrecht, The Netherlands (Kluwer, Boston).

Merkhofer, M. W., 1987b, "Quantifying Judgmental Uncertainty: Methodology, Experiences, and Insights," *IEEE Trans. Sys., Man, Cybernetics* **SMC-17**(5), 741–752.

Merkhofer, M. W., and R. J. Korsan, 1978, "Florida Utility Pollution Control Options and Economic Analysis—Volume 2: Cost-Benefit Analysis of Alternative Florida Sulfur Oxide Emissions Control Policies," SRI final report, project 5080, SRI International, Menlo Park, California.

Meyers, T. R., and J. D. Hendricks, 1986, "Histopathology," in G. M. Rand and S. R. Petrocelli (eds.), *Fundamentals of Aquatic Toxicology: Methods and Application*, Hemisphere Publishing Corp., Washington, D. C., pp. 283–331.

Miller, C., 1978, "Exposure Assessment Modeling: A State-of-the-Art Review," John F. Kennedy School of Government, Cambridge, Massachusetts.

Miller, P. E., 1987, "Long-Term Benthic Monitoring," *PPRP Project Update*, Maryland Power Plant Research Program, Department of Natural Resources, Annapolis, Maryland.

Miller, P. L., 1973, "Oxidant-Induced Community Change in a Mixed Conifer Forest," in J. A. Naegele (ed.), *Air Pollution Damage to Vegetation* (Advances in Chemistry Series no. 122), American Chemical Society, Washington, D. C., pp. 102–117

Miller, R. W., 1978, "The Discovery of Human Teratogens, Carcinogens and Mutagens: Lessons for the Future," in A. Hollaender and F. J. de Serres (eds.), *Chemical Mutagens—Principles and Methods for Their Detection*, vol. 5, Plenum, New York, pp. 101–126.

Mills, W. B., J. D. Dean, D. B. Porcella, S. A. Gherini, R. J. M. Hudson, W. E. Frick, G. L. Rupp, and G. L. Bowie, 1982, "Water Quality Assessment: A Screening Procedure for Toxic and Conventional Pollutants," EPA-600/6-82-004 (2 vols.), U. S. EPA Environmental Research Laboratory, Athens, Georgia.

Moeller, D. W., 1992, *Environmental Health*, Harvard University Press, Cambridge, Massachusetts.

Moghissi, A. A., R. E. Marland, F. J. Congel, and K. F. Eckerman, 1980, "Methodology for Environmental Human Exposure and Health Risk Assessment," in R. Hague (ed.), *Dynamics, Exposure and Hazard Assessment of Toxic Chemicals*, Ann Arbor Science Publishers, Ann Arbor, Michigan, pp. 471–489.

Moiser, J. E., J. R. Fowler, C. J. Barton, W. W. Tolbert, S. C. Myers, J. E. Vancil, H. A. Price, M. J. R. Vasdo, E. E. Rutx, T. X. Wendeln, and L. D. Rickertson, 1980, "Low-Level Waste Management: A Compilation of Models and Monitoring Techniques," ORNL/SMB-79/13617/2, Science Applications, Inc., Oak Ridge, Tennessee.

Moolgavkar, S. H., 1978, "The Multistage Theory of Carcinogenesis and the Age Distribution of Cancer in Man," *J. Natl. Cancer Inst.* **61**, 49–52.

Moolgavkar, S., and A. Dewanji, 1988, "Biologically Based Models for Cancer Risk Assessment: A Cautionary Note," *Risk Anal.* **8**(1), 5–8.

Moolgavkar, S. H., and A. G. Knudson, 1981, "Mutation and Cancer: A Model for Human Carcinogenesis," *J. Natl. Cancer Inst.* **66**, 1037–1052.

Moolgavkar, S. H., and D. J. Venzon, 1979, "Two-Event Models for Carcinogenesis: Incidence Curves for Childhood and Adult Tumors," *Math. Biosci.* **47**, 55–77.

Moorhouse, J., and M. J. Pritchard, 1982, "Thermal Radiation Hazards from Large Pool Fires and Fireballs—A Literature Review," *The Assessment of Major Hazards*, IChemE Symposium Series no. 71, IChemE, Rugby, UK, pp. 297–428 (ISBN 0–08–028768–9).

Morgan, M. G., 1982, "Uncertainty and Quantitative Assessment," in J. V. Rodricks and R. G. Tardiff (eds.), *Assessment and Management of Chemical Risks*, American Chemical Society, Washington, D. C., pp. 113–129.

Morgan, M. G., M. Henrion, and S. C. Morris, 1980, "Expert Judgments for Policy Analysis: Report of an Invitational Workshop Held at Brookhaven National Laboratory, 1979 July 8–11," Report BNL 51358, Brookhaven National Laboratory, Upton, New York.

Morgan, M. G., P. Slovic, I. Nair, D. Geisler, D. MacGregor, B. Fischhoff, B. Lincoln, and K. Florig, 1985, "Powerline Frequency Electric and Magnetic Fields: A Pilot Study of Risk Perceptions," *Risk Anal.* **5**(1), 139–150.

Morris, P. A., 1974, "Decision Analysis Expert Use," *Manage. Science* **20**(9), 1233–1241.

Mudan, K. S., 1984, "Thermal Radiation Hazards from Hydrocarbon Pool Fires," *Proc. Energy Combust. Sci.* **10**(1), 59–80 (ISBN 0360-1285).

Munn, R. E., 1973, *Global Environmental Monitoring System: GEMS*, Scientific Committee on Problems of the Environment, SCOPE 3, International Council of Scientific Unions, Paris, France.

Munro, I. C., and D. R. Krewski, 1981, "Risk Assessment and Regulatory Decision Making," *Food Cosmet. Toxicol.* **19**, 549–560.

Murphy, M. C., and A. E. Davies, 1988, "Wind Tunnel Modelling of Vehicle Emissions on Roadways as Line Sources," Proceedings of the 81st Annual Meeting of APCA, June 19–24, Dallas, Texas.

(NAS) National Academy of Sciences, 1975, *Health Effects of Chemical Pesticides*, vol. 1, National Academy Press, Washington, D. C.

(NAS) National Academy of Sciences, 1979a, *Protection Against Depletion of Stratospheric Ozone by Chlorofluorocarbons*, report by the Committee on Impacts of Stratospheric Change and the Committee on Alternatives for the Reduction of Chlorofluorocarbon Emissions, National Research Council, Washington, D. C.

(NAS) National Academy of Sciences, 1979b, *Stratospheric Ozone Depletion by Halocarbons: Chemistry and Transport*, report of a committee of the National Research Council, Washington, D. C&.

(NAS) National Academy of Sciences, 1980, *The Effects on Populations of Exposure to Low Levels of Ionizing Radiation: 1980*, Report of the Committee on the Biological Effects of Ionizing Radiation, National Academy Press, Washington, D. C.

(NAS-NRC) National Research Council, 1977, *Drinking Water and Health*, National Academy Press, Washington, D. C.

(NAS–NRC) National Research Council, 1978, *Saccharin: Technical Assessment of Risks and Benefits*, Committee for a Study on Saccharin and Food Safety Policy, National Academy of Sciences, Washington, D. C.

(NAS–NRC) National Research Council, 1980, *Principles of Toxicological Interactions Associated with Multiple Chemical Exposures*, National Academy Press, Washington, D. C.

(NAS–NRC) National Research Council, 1982, "Indoor Pollutants," U. S. Environmental Protection Agency, pub. no. EPA-600/6-82-001, NTIS pub. no. PB82180563, Washington, D. C.

(NAS–NRC) National Research Council, 1983a, *Risk Assessment in the Federal Government: Managing the Process*, NAS–NRC Committee on the Institutional Means for Assessment of Risks to Public Health, National Academy Press, Washington, D. C.

(NAS–NRC) National Research Council, 1983b, *Safety of Existing Dams: Evaluation and Improvement*, National Academy Press, Washington, D. C.

(NAS–NRC) National Research Council, 1984, *Toxicity Testing: Strategies to Determine Needs and Priorities*, National Academy Press, Washington, D. C.

(NAS–NRC) National Research Council, 1986a, *Drinking Water and Health*, vol. 6, National Academy Press, Washington, D. C.

(NAS–NRC) National Research Council, 1986b, *Acid Deposition—Long Term Trends*, Committee on Monitoring and Assessment of Trends in Acid Deposition, National Academy Press, Washington, D. C.

Nelson, R. W., 1982, "A Summary of Subsurface Fluid Flow and Contaminant Transport Models Useful in Waste Isolation Assessment," prepared for the Waste Isolation Safety Assessment Program, Battelle Pacific Northwest Laboratories, Richland, Washington.

Netherlands Government, 1985, *Environmental Program of the Netherlands 1986–1990*, Ministry of Housing, Physical Planning and Environment, Report no. VROM 85902/12-85, The Hague, The Netherlands.

NFPA (National Fire Protection Association), 1987, *Flammable and Combustible Liquids Code*, NFPA 30, National Fire Protection Association, Quincy, Massachusetts.

Nichols, A. L., and R. J. Zeckhauser, 1986, "The Perils of Prudence—How Conservative Risk Assessments Distort Regulation," *Regul.*, 13–34 (November/December).

Nisbet, I. C. T., 1980, "The Role of Exposure Assessment in Risk Evaluations: Research Needs," in C. R. Richmond, P. J. Walsh, and E. D. Copenhaver (eds.), *Health Risk Analysis: Proceedings of the Third Life Sciences Symposium*, National Academy Press, Washington, D. C., pp. 419–429

North, D. W., and M. W. Merkhofer, 1975, "Analysis of Alternative Emission Control Strategies," in *Air Quality Stationary Source Emission Control*, U. S. Senate Committee on Public Works, Serial 94-1, U. S. Government Printing Office, pp. 540–711.

(NRC) U. S. Nuclear Regulatory Commission, 1975, "Reactor Safety Study: An Assessment of Accident Risks in U. S. Commercial Nuclear Power Plants," NUREG-75/014 (WASH 1400), Washington, D. C.

(NRC) U. S. Nuclear Regulatory Commission, 1983, "PRA Procedures Guide: A Guide to the Performance of Probabilistic Risk Assessments for Nuclear Power Plants," prepared under the auspices of the American Nuclear Society and the Institute of Electrical and Electronics Engineers, NUREG/CR-2300, NTIS.

(NRC) U. S. Nuclear Regulatory Commission, 1984, "Probabilistic Risk Assessment (PRA): Status Report and Guidance for Regulatory Application, Appendix A," (draft report), Division of Risk Analysis, Washington, D. C.

(NRC) U. S. Nuclear Regulatory Commission, 1985, "NRC Policy on Future Reactor Designs: Decisions on Severe Accident Issues in Nuclear Power Plant Regulation," NUREG-1070, Office of Nuclear Reactor Regulation, U.S. Nuclear Regulatory Commission, Washington, D.C.

(NRC) U. S. Nuclear Regulatory Commission, 1987a, "Reactor Risk Reference Document, Appendices A–I: Draft for Comment," NUREG-1150, Vol. 2, Washington, D. C.

(NRC) U. S. Nuclear Regulatory Commission, 1987b, *Reactor Risk Reference Document*, NUREG-1150, vol. 1, Office of Nuclear Regulatory Research, U. S. Nuclear Regulatory Commission, Washington, D. C.

(NRC) U. S. Nuclear Regulatory Commission, 1990, "Severe Accident Risks: An Assessment for Five U. S. Nuclear Power Plants," U. S. Nuclear Regulatory Commission, Report NUREG/CR-5411, Washington, D. C.

Oblow, E. M., 1983, *An Automated Procedure for Sensitivity Analysis Using Computer Calculus*, ORNL/TM-8776, Oak Ridge National Laboratory, Oak Ridge, Tennessee.

Oday, J., 1974, "In-Depth Accident Data and Occupant Protection—A Statistical Point of View," SAE Technical Paper Series no. 740569, Society of Automotive Engineers, Warrendale, Pennsylvania.

(OECD) Organization for Economic Cooperation and Development, 1985, "The State of the Environment: 1985," OECD, Paris.

Okrent, D., 1981, "The Assessment and Perception of Risk," *Proc. R. Soc. (London) A* **376**, 133–149.

Okrent, D., 1986, "Alternative Risk Management Policies for State and Local Governments," in V. T. Covello, J. Menkes, and J. Mumpower (eds.), *Risk Evaluation and Management*, Plenum, New York, pp. 359–380.

Onishi, Y., D. L. Schreiber, and R. B. Codell, 1980, "Mathematical Simulation of Sediment and Radionuclide Transport in the Clinch River, Tennessee," in R. A. Baker (ed.), *Processes Involving Contaminants and Sediment*, Ann Arbor Science Publishers, Ann Arbor, Michigan.

Onishi, Y., R. J. Serne, E. M. Arnold, C. E. Cowan, and F. L. Thompson, 1981, "Critical Review: Radionuclide Transport, Sediment Transport, and Water Quality Mathematical Modeling; and Radionuclide Adsorption/Desorption Mechanisms," Battelle Pacific Northwest Laboratories, Richland, Washington.

Onishi, Y., S. B. Yabusaki, C. R. Cole, W. E. Davis, and G. Whelan, 1982, "Multimedia Contaminant Environmental Exposure Assessment (MCEA) Methodology for Coal-Fired Power Plants," vols. 1 and 2, Battelle Pacific Northwest Laboratories, Richland, Washington.

Orlob, G. T. (ed.), 1983, *Mathematical Modeling of Water Quality: Streams, Lakes and Reservoirs* (International Series on Applied Systems Analysis, vol. 12), Wiley, New York.

Oster, C. A., 1982, "Review of Ground-Water Flow and Transport Models in the Unsaturated Zone," Battelle Pacific Northwest Laboratories, PNL-4427, NUREG/CR-2917, Richland, Washington.

(OSTP) U. S. Office of Science and Technology Policy, 1984, "Chemical Carcinogens; Notice of Review of the Science and Its Associated Principles," *Fed. Register* **49**, 21594–21661.

(OSTP) U. S. Office of Science and Technology Policy, 1985, "Chemical Carcinogens; A Review of the Science and Associated Principles," *Fed. Register* **50** (50), 10372–10442.

(OTA) U. S. Office of Technology Assessment, U. S. Congress, 1981, "Assessment of Technologies for Determining Cancer Risks from the Environment," U. S. Government Printing Office, Washington, D. C.

(OTA) U. S. Office of Technology Assessment, U. S. Congress, 1986, "Transportation of Hazardous Materials," GPO Stock no. 052–003–01042, U. S. Government Printing Office, Washington, D. C.

(OTA) U. S. Office of Technology Assessment, U. S. Congress, 1989, Biological Effects of Power Frequency Electric and Magnetic Fields, U. S. Government Printing Office, Washington, D. C.

Ott, W. R., 1984, "Exposure Estimates Based on Computer Generated Activity Patterns," *J. Toxicol.: Clinical Toxicology* (Special Symposium Issue on Exposure Assessment: Problems and Prospects) **21**(1 and 2), 97–128.

Ott, W., and P. Flachsbart, 1982, "Field Surveys of Carbon Monoxide in Commercial Settings Using Personal Exposure Monitors," U. S. Environmental Protection Agency, no. EPA-600/4-84-019, PB-84-211291, Washington, D. C.

Overcamp, T. J., 1988, "Simple Diffusion Models for Short-Term Releases," Proceedings of the 81st Annual Meeting of APCA, June 19–24, Dallas, Texas, Session 49 and 49B, paper 2.

Park, C. N., and R. D. Snee, 1983, "Quantitative Risk Assessment: State-of-the-Art for Carcinogenesis," *Am. Stat.* **34**(4), 427–441.

Pate, M. E., 1983, "Acceptable Decision Processes and Acceptable Risks in Public Sector Regulations," *IEEE Trans. Sys., Man, Cybernetics* **SMC-13**(2), 113–124.

Patwardhan, A., R. Kulkarni, and D. Tocher, 1980, "A Semi-Markov Model for Characterizing Recurrence of Great Earthquakes," *Bull. Seis. S. Am.* **701**(1), 323-347.

Peranio, A., and A. Katz, 1970, "Establishing Motor Vehicle Accident Involvement—An Epidemiological Approach," SAE Technical Paper Series, no. 700440, Society of Automotive Engineers, Warrendale, Pennsylvania.

Perera, F., 1986, "New Approaches in Risk Assessment in Carcinogens," *Risk Anal.* **6**, 195–202.

Perera, F., 1987, "Molecular Copier Epidemiology: A New Tool in Cancer Prevention," *J. Natl. Cancer Inst.* **78**, 887–898.

Perera, F., 1988, "Molecular Dosimetry Data in Humans: Implications for Risk Assessment and Research," in R. W. Hart and F. D. Hoerger (eds.), *Carcinogen Risk Assessment: New Directions in the Qualitative and Quantitative Aspects*, Banbury Report 31, Cold Spring Harbor Laboratory, Cold Spring Harbor, New York, pp. 307–313.

Perera, F. P., R. M. Santella, D. Breener, T.-L Young, and I. B. W. Weinstein, 1988, "Application of Biological Markers to the Study of Lung Cancer Causation and Prevention," IARC Scientific Publication.

Perry, R. H., and D. Green (eds.), 1984, *Perry's Chemical Engineering Handbook*, 6th ed., McGraw-Hill, New York, New York.

Peto, R., 1978, "Carcinogenic Effects of Chronic Exposures to Very Low Levels of Toxic Substances," *Environ. Health Perspect.* **22**, 155–161.

Philipson, L. L., and J. D. Gasca, 1982, "Risk Assessment Methodologies and Their Uncertainties—Volume I, A Review of Risk Estimation Approaches," Technical Report no. 80–1398, J. H. Wiggins Co., Redondo Beach, California, pp. 3–4.

Pilz, V., and W. van Herck, 1976, "Chemical Engineering Investigations with Respect to the Safety of Large Chemical Plants," *Third Symposium on Large Chemical Plants*, European Federation of Chemical Engineering, Antwerp.

Pitblado, R. M., 1986, "Consequence Models for BLEVE Incidents," *Major Industrial Hazards Project*, Warren Center for Advanced Engineering, University of Sydney, NSW 2006, Australia (ISBN 0949269-37-9).

Pittock, A. B., 1974, "On the Representativeness of Mean Ozone Distributions," *Q. J. R. Meteorol. Soc.* **96**(407), 32.

Poje, G. V., 1987, "A Perspective on Research Needs in Environmental Toxicology and Chemistry," presented at The Society of Environmental Toxicology and Chemistry Workshop on Consensus Research Needs and Priorities in Environmental Risk Assessment, August 16–21, Breckenridge, Colorado.

Pounds, J. G., 1985, "The Toxic Effects of Metals," in P. L. Williams and J. L. Burson (eds.), *Industrial Toxicology*, Van Nostrand Reinhold, New York, pp. 197–210.

Prugh, R. W., 1988, "Quantitative Evaluation of 'BLEVE' Hazards," AIChE Loss Prevention Symposium, paper no. 74e, AIChE Spring National Meeting, March 6–10, New Orleans.

Purchase, I. F. H., 1982, "An Appraisal of Predictive Tests for Carcinogenicity," *Mutation Res.* **99**, 53–71.

Rai, D., and J. Van Ryzin, 1981, "A Generalized Multihit Dose-Response Model for Low Dose Extrapolation," *Biometrics* **37**, 341–352.

Raiffa, H., 1968, *Decision Analysis*, Addison-Wesley, Reading, Massachusetts.

Raiffa, H., and R. Zeckhauser, 1981, "Reporting of Uncertainties in Risk Analysis," in T. McCurdy and H. Richmond (project officers), *Conceptual Approaches to Health Risk Assessment*, U. S. Environmental Protection Agency, Washington, D.C.

Rall, J. E., G. W. Beebe, D. G. Hoel, S. Jablon, C. E. Land, O. F. Nygaard, A. C. Upton, R. S. Yalow, and V. H. Zeve, 1985, "Report of the National Institutes of Health Working Group to Develop Radioepidemiological Tables," NIH Publ. no. 85-2748, U. S. GPO, Washington, D. C.

Ramsey, J. C., and M. E. Andersen, 1984, "A Physiological Model for the Inhalation of Pharmacokinetics of Inhaled Styrene Monomer in Rats and Humans," *Toxicol. Appl. Pharmacol.* **73**, 159-175.

Ramsey, J. C., C. N. Park, M. G. Ott, and P. J. Gehring, 1979, "Carcinogenic Risk Assessment: Ethylene Dibromide," *Toxicol. Appl. Pharmacol.* **47**, 411–414.

Ramsey, J. C., and J. D. Young, 1978, "Pharmacokinetics of Inhaled Styrene in Rats and Humans," *Scand. J. Work, Environ. Health* **4**, 84–91.

Ramsey, J. C., J. D. Young, R. Karbowski, M. B. Chenoweth, L. P. McCarty, and W. H. Braun, 1980, "Pharmacokinetics of Inhaled Styrene in Human Volunteers," *Toxicol. Appl. Pharmacol.* **53**, 54–63.

Rasmussen, N. C., 1975, "Rasmussen on Reactor Safety," *IEEE Spectrum* **12**, 46–55.

Rasmussen, N. C., 1981, "The Application of Probabilistic Risk Assessment Techniques to Energy Technologies," *Ann. Rev. Energy* **6**, 123–138.

Reed, W. J., 1979, "Optimal Escapement Levels in Stochastic and Deterministic Harvesting Models," *J. Environ. Econ. and Manage.* **6**, 350–363.

Reijnen, M. J. S. M., and J. Van Wiertz, 1981, "Spontaneous Vegetation and Groundwater Withdrawal in a Rural Area of 370 km^3," in S. T. Tjallingii and A. A. de Veer (eds.), *Proceedings of the International Congress of Netherland Society Landscape Ecology*, Veldhoven, Pudoc Wageningen, The Netherlands, pp. 280–281.

Reitz, R. H., P. J. Gehring, and C. N. Park, 1978, "Carcinogenic Risk Estimation for Chloroform: An Alternative to EPA's Procedures," *Food Cosmet. Toxicol.* **16**(5), 511–514.

Renn, O., 1981, *Man, Technology, and Risk: A Study on Intuitive Risk Assessment and Attitudes Towards Nuclear Power*, Report Jul-Spez 115, Nuclear Research Center, Juelich, German Federal Republic.

Reynolds, S. H., S. J. Stowers, R. M. Patterson, R. R. Maronpot, S. A. Aaronson, and M. W. Anderson, 1988, "Activated Oncogenes in B6C3F1 Mouse Liver Tumors: Implications for Risk Assessment," *Science* **237**, 1309–1316 (September).

Ricci, P. F. (ed.), 1985, *Principles of Health Risk Assessment*, Prentice-Hall, Englewood Cliffs, New Jersey.

Richmond, H. M., 1987, "Development of Probabilistic Health Risk Assessment for National Ambient Air Quality Standards," paper presented at the "APCA International Specialty Conference on Regulatory Approaches for Control of Air Pollutants," Atlanta, Georgia.

Ritter, D., 1981, "Risk Analysis Research and Demonstration Act of 1981," 97th Congress, H. R. 3441.

Robertson, D., A. Bundy, R. Muetzelfeldt, M. Haggith, and M. Uschold, 1991, *Eco-Logic: Logic-Based Approaches to Ecological Modelling*, MIT Press, Cambridge, Massachusetts.

Robinson, J. D., M. D. Higgins, and P. K. Boyard, 1983, "Assessing Environmental Impacts on Health: A Role for Behavioral Science," *EIA Review* 4(1), 41–53.

Rodricks, J. V., and R. G. Tardiff (eds.), 1984, *Assessment and Management of Chemical Risks*, American Chemical Society, Washington, D. C.

Roth, H. D., R. E. Wyzga, and T. Hammerstrom, 1984, "The Use of Risk Assessment in Developing Health-Based Regulations," in S. M. Gertz and M. D. London (eds.), *Statistics in the Environmental Sciences*, ASTM STP 845, American Society for Testing and Materials, Philadelphia, pp. 46–65.

Runchal, A. K., M. W. Merkhofer, E. Olmsted, and J. D. Davis, 1984, "Probability Encoding of Hydrologic Parameters for Basalt," RHO-BW CR-145P, Rockwell International, Rockwell Hanford Operations, Richland, Washington.

Saltzman, B. E., 1987, "Environmental Monitoring of Toxic Chemicals," in L. B. Lave and A. C. Upton (eds.), *Toxic Chemicals, Health, and the Environment*, Johns Hopkins University Press, Baltimore, Maryland, pp. 71–94.

Schiermeier, F. A., 1979, "Sulfur Transport and Transformation in the Environment (STATE): A Major EPA Research Program," *Bull. Am. Meteorol. Soc.* 60, 1303–1312.

Schneider, H., and G. Beier, 1974, "Experiment and Accident: Comparison of Dummy Tests," SAE Technical Paper Series, no. 741177, Society of Automotive Engineers, Warrendale, Pennsylvania.

Schweitzer, G. E., 1982, "Monitoring to Support Risk Assessments at Hazardous Waste Sites," in F. Long and G. Schweitzer (eds.), *Risk Assessment at Hazardous Waste Sites*, American Chemical Society, New York.

Science Applications, Inc., 1981, "Tabulation of Waste Isolation Computer Models," Office of Nuclear Waste Isolation, Battelle Memorial Institute, ONWI-78, Columbus, Ohio.

(SETAC) Society of Environmental Toxicology and Chemistry, 1987, *Research Priorities in Environmental Risk Assessment*, Workshop Report, August 16–21, 1987, Breckenridge, Colorado, J. A. Fava, W. A. Adams, R. J. Larson, G. W. Dickson, K. L. Dickson, and W. E. Bishop (eds.), SETAC, Washington D. C.

Shooman, M., 1968, *Probabilistic Reliability of Engineering Approaches*, McGraw-Hill, New York.

Shultis, J. K., W. Buranapan, and N. D. Eckhoff, 1981, "Properties of Parameter Estimation Techniques for a Beta-Binomial Failure Model," NUREG/CR-2372, Nuclear Regulatory Commission, Washington, D.C.

Silvers, A., and C. Hakkarinen, 1987,"Materials Damage from Air Pollutants," *EPRI J.* 12(6), 58–59.

Sjoberg, L., 1979, "Strength of Belief and Risk," *Policy Sciences* 11, 39–57.

Slovic, P., B. Fischhoff, and S. Lichtenstein, 1977, "Behavioral Decision Theory," *Annu. Rev. Psychol.* 28, 1–39.

Slovic, P., S. Lichtenstein, and B. Fischhoff, 1979, "Images of Disaster: Perception and Acceptance of Risks from Nuclear Power," in G. Goodman and W. Rowe (eds.), *Energy Risk Management*, Academic, London, pp. 223–245.

Slovic, P., B. Fischhoff, and S. Lichtenstein, 1980a, "Informing People About Risk," in M. Maziz, L. Morris, and I. Barofsky (eds.), *Banbury Report 6*, The Banbury Center, Cold Spring Harbor, New York.

Slovic, P., B. Fischhoff, and S. Lichtenstein, 1980b, "Facts and Fears: Understanding Perceived Risk," in R. Schwing and W. A. Albers, Jr. (eds.) *Societal Risk Assessment: How Safe is Safe Enough?*, Plenum, New York, pp. 181–216.

Slovic, P., B. Fischhoff, and S. Lichtenstein, 1981, "Perception and Acceptability of Risk from Energy Systems," in A. Baum and J. Singer (eds.), *Advances in Environmental Psychology*, Erlbaum, Hillsdale, New Jersey.

Smith, J. H., W. R. Nabey, N. Bohonos, B. R. Holt, S. S. Lee, T. W. Chou, D. C. Bomberger, and T. Mill, 1977, *Environmental Pathways of Selected Chemicals in Freshwater Systems, Part I: Background and Experimental Procedures*, SRI International, Menlo Park, California.

Southworth, G. R., B. R. Parkhurst, S. E. Herbes, S. C. Tsai, 1982, "The Risk of Chemicals to Aquatic Environment," in R. A. Conway (ed.), *Environmental Risk Analysis for Chemicals*, Van Nostrand Reinhold, New York and Cincinnati, pp. 88–153.

Spencer, F. W., K. V. Diegert, and R. G. Easterling, 1985, "Uncertainty Assessment in Probabilistic Risk Assessment," presented at the International American Nuclear Society/European Nuclear Society Topical Meeting, February 24–March 1, San Francisco, California.

Spetzler, C. S., and C.-A. S. Staël von Holstein, 1975, "Probability Encoding in Decision Analysis," *Manage. Science* **22**(3), 340–358.

St. John, D. S., S. P. Bailer, W. H. Fellner, J. M. Minor, and R. D. Snee, 1982, "Time Series Analysis of Stratospheric Ozone," *Communications in Statistics, Theory, and Methods* **11** (12), 1293–1333.

Staël von Holstein, C.-A., and J. Matheson, 1979, "A Manual for Encoding Probability Distributions," final report, SRI project 7078, SRI International, Menlo Park, California.

Staley, M., 1987, "The Practice of Resource Modeling," in L. C. Braat and W. F. J. van Lierop (eds.), *Economic–Ecological Modeling* (Studies in Regional Science and Urban Economics, vol. 16), Elsevier/North-Holland, Amsterdam and New York, pp. 257–268.

Stara, J. F., and L. S. Erdreich, 1984, "Approaches to Risk Assessment for Multiple Chemical Exposures," (report of a workshop sponsored by the U. S. Environmental Protection Agency on September 29 and 30, 1982), Dynamic Corporation, NTIS PB84-182369.

Stark, R. M., and F. W. Cobb, 1969, "Smog Injury, Rot Disease, and Bark Beetle Damage in Ponderosa Pine," *Calif. Agri.* **23**, 13.

Starr, T. B., and J. E. Gibson, 1985, "The Mechanistic Toxicology of Formaldehyde and Its Implications for Quantitative Risk Estimation," *Annu. Rev. Pharmacol. Toxicol.* **25**, 745.

Stewart, D., M. Treshow, and F. M. Harner, 1973, "Pathological Anatomy of Coniferous Needle Necrosis," *Can. J. Bot.* **51**(5), 983.

Stopford, W., 1985, "The Toxic Effects of Pesticides," in P. L. Williams and J. L. Burton (eds.), *Industrial Toxicology*, van Nostrand Reinhold, New York, pp. 211–229.

Stordal, F., and I. Isakson, 1986, "Ozone Perturbations Due to Increases in N_2O, CH_4, and Chlorofluorocarbons: Two-Dimensional Time Dependent Calculations," in *Effects of Changes in Stratospheric Ozone and Global Climate*, Vol. I, Overview, U. S. Environmental Protection Agency, Washington, D. C.

Strauss, H. S., 1991, "Lessons from Chemical Risk Assessment," in M. A. Levin and H. S. Strauss (eds.), *Risk Assessment in Genetic Engineering*, McGraw-Hill, New York, pp. 297–318.

Strimaitis, D. G., R. S. Paine, B. A. Egan, and R. J. Yamartino, 1987, "EPA Complex Terrain Model Development: Final Report," EPA Contract no. G8-02-3421, Office of Research and Development, U. S. EPA, Research Triangle Park, North Carolina.

Strothmann, J. A., and F. A. Schiermeier, 1979, "Documentation of the Regional Air Pollution Study (RAPS) and Related Investigations in the St. Louis Air Quality Region," publ. no. EPA-600/4-0761, U. S. Environmental Protection Agency, Washington, D. C.

Theil, H., 1971, *Principles of Econometrics*, Wiley, New York.

Thomann, R. V., 1972, *Systems Analysis and Water Quality Management*, McGraw-Hill, New York.

Thorslund, T. W., C. C. Brown, and G. Charnley, 1987, "Biologically Motivated Cancer Risk Models," *Risk Anal.* **7**, 109–119.

Tobias, P. A., and D. C. Trindade, 1986, *Applied Reliability*, Van Nostrand Reinhold, New York.

Tomatis, L., C. Agthe, H. Barach, J. Huff, R. Montesano, R. Saracci, E. Walker, and J. Wilbourn, 1978, "Valuation of the Carcinogenicity of Chemicals: A Review of the Monograph Program of the International Agency for Research in Cancer (1971–1977), *Cancer Res.* **38**, 877–885.

Travis, C. C., C. F. Baes III, L. W. Barnthouse, E. L. Etnics, G. A. Holton, B. D. Murphy, G. P. Thompson, G. W. Suter III, and A. P. Watson, 1983, "Exposure Assessment Methodology and Reference Environments for Synfuel Risk Analysis," ESD publication no. 2232, Oak Ridge National Laboratory, Oak Ridge, Tennessee.

Travis, C. C., R. R. Killman, and J. L. Quillen, 1987, "Cancer Risk of Human Exposure to Tetrachloroethylene" (draft).

Truett, S. C., 1980, "Beaufort Sea Barrier Island-Lagoon Ecological Process Studies: Final Report, Simpson Lagoon, Part 7, Synthesis, Impact Analysis and a Monitoring Strategy," in Environmental Assessment Alaskan Continental Shelf, BLM/N OAA, OCSEAP, Boulder, Colorado.

Tversky, A., and D. Kahneman, 1973, "Availability: A Heuristic for Judging Frequency and Probability," Cognitive Psych. 4, 207–232.

Tversky, A., and D. Kahneman, 1974, "Judgment Under Uncertainty: Heuristics and Biases," Science 185, 1124–1131.

Upton, A. C., 1988, "Radiation Risk Assessment and Risk Management," in C. R. Cothern, M. A. Mehlman, and W. L. Marcus (eds.), Risk Assessment and Risk Management of Industrial and Environmental Chemicals, Advances in Modern Environmental Toxicology vol. 15, Princeton Scientific Publishing Co., Princeton, New Jersey, pp. 45–64.

U. S. President's Commission on the Accident at Three Mile Island, 1979, The Need for Change: The Legacy of TMI. U. S. Government Printing Office, Washington DC&.

Usher, M. B., 1972, "Developments in the Leslie Matrix Model," in J. N. R. Jeffers (ed.), Mathematical Models in Ecology, Blackwell Scientific, Oxford, pp. 29–60.

van der Shalie, W. H., 1987, "Research Needs in Environmental Risk Assessment," presented at a workshop on "Consensus Research Needs & Priorities in Environmental Risk Assessment" sponsored by the Society of Environmental Toxicology and Chemistry, August 15–21, Breckenridge, Colorado.

van der Zande, A. N., J. C. Berkhuizen, H. C. van Latesteijn, W. J. ter Keurs, and A. J. Poppelaars, 1984, "Impact of Outdoor Recreation on the Density of a Number of Breeding Bird Species in Woods Adjacent to Urban Residential Areas," Biol. Conservation 30, 1–39.

VanderPlank, J. E., 1963, Plant Diseases: Epidemics and Control, Academic, New York.

Van Steen, Jacques F. J., 1987, "Expert Opinion Use for Probability Assessment in Safety Studies: Main Topics and Elements of an Application-Oriented Research Program," Eur. J. Oper. Res. 32, 225–230.

Vesely, W. E., 1984, "Engineering Risk Analysis," in P. F. Ricci et al. (eds.), Technological Risk Assessment, Martinus Nijhoff, The Hague, The Netherlands, pp. 49–84.

Vesely, W. E., E. F. Goldberg, N. H. Roberts, and D. F. Haasl, 1981, "Fault Tree Handbook," NUREG/CR-0492, U. S. Nuclear Regulatory Commission, Washington, D.C.

Vieth, G. D., D. W. Kuehl, and F. A. Puglisi, G. E. Glass, and J. G. Eaton, 1977, "Residues of PCBs and DDT in the Western Lake Superior Ecosystem," Arch. Environ. Contam. Toxicol. 5, 487–499.

Vlek, C. A. J., and P. J. Stallen, 1981, "Judging Risks and Benefits in the Small and in the Large," Organ. Behav. Hum. Perf. 28, 235–271.

von Winterfeldt, D. and W. Edwards, 1986, Decision Analysis in Behavioral Research, Cambridge University Press, New York.

Wallace, L., 1979, "Use of Personal Monitors to Measure Commuter Exposure to Carbon Monoxide in Vehicle Passenger Compartments," paper no. 79-59.2, presented at the 72nd Annual Meeting of the Air Pollution Control Association, Cincinnati, Ohio, June 24–29.

Wallace, L. A., and W. R. Ott, 1982, "Personal Monitors: A State-of-the-Art Survey," J. Air Pollut. Control Assoc. 32, 601.

Wallace, L., E. Pellizzari, T. Hartwell, M. Rosenzweig, M. Erickson, C. Sparacino, and H. Zelon, 1984, "Personal Exposure to Volatile Organic Compounds: I. Direct Measurements in Breathing-Zone Air, Drinking Water, Food, and Exhaled Breath," Environ. Res. 35, 293–319.

Walton, B. T., 1987, "Ecotoxicological Research Needs for Terrestrial Biota," presented at the SETAC Workshop, Breckenridge, Colorado, August 16–17.

Weibull, W., 1951, "A Statistical Distribution Function of Wide Applicability," *J. Appl. Mech.* **18**, 293–297.

Weinstein, N. D., 1979, "Seeking Reassuring or Threatening Information About Environmental Cancer," *J. Behav. Med.* **2**, 125–139.

Weisburger, J. H., and G. M. Williams, 1981, "Carcinogen Testing: Current Problems and New Approaches," *Science* **214**, 401–407.

Whittemore, A., and B. Altschuler, 1976, "Lung Cancer Incidence in Cigarette Smokers: Further Analysis of Doll and Hill's Data for British Physicians," *Biometrics* **32**, 805–16.

Whittemore, A., and J. B. Keller, 1978, "Quantitative Theories of Carcinogenesis," *SIAM Rev.* **20**, 1–30.

(WHO) World Health Organization, 1981, *Radiofrequency and Microwaves*, Environ. Health Crit. 16, Geneva.

(WHO) World Health Organization, 1983, *Guidelines on Studies in Environmental Epidemiology*, Environ. Health Crit. 27, Geneva.

Whyte, A. V., and I. Burton, 1980, *Environmental Risk Assessment*, published on behalf of the Scientific Committee on Problems of the Environment (SCOPE) of the International Council of Scientific Unions (ICSU), (SCOPE 15), Wiley and Sons, Chichester and New York.

Wilbourne, J., L. Haroun, E. Hesetine, J. Kaldor, C. Partensky, and H. Vanio, 1986, "Response of Experimental Animals to Human Carcinogens: An Analysis Based Upon the IARC Monographs Programme," *Carcinogenesis* **7**, 1853.

Williams, G., M. F. Laspia, and V. C. Dunkel, 1982, "Reliability of the Hepatocyte Primary Culture/DNA Repair Test in Testing of Coded Carcinogens and Non-Carcinogens," *Mutation Res.* **97**, 359–370.

Williams, P. L., and J. L. Burson (eds.), 1985, *Industrial Toxicology; Safety and Health Applications in the Workplace*, Van Nostrand Reinhold, New York&.

Wilson, D. J., 1979, "The Release and Dispersion of Gas from Pipeline Ruptures," Alberta Environment Research Report, Edmonton.

Wilson, R., 1984, "Commentary: Risks and Their Acceptability," *Sci. Technol. Hum. Val.* **9**(2), 11–22.

Winkler, R. L., 1968, "The Consensus of Subjective Probability Distributions," *Manage. Science* **15** (2), 1105–1185.

Wischmeier, W. H., and D. D. Smith, 1965, "Predicting Rainfall—Erosion Losses from Cropland East of the Rocky Mountains," Agriculture Handbook 282, Agriculture Research Service, U. S. Department of Agriculture, Washington, DC.

Wischmeier, W. H., and D. D. Smith, 1978, "Predicting Rainfall Erosion Losses—A Guide to Conservation Planning," Agriculture Handbook No. 537, U. S. Department of Agriculture, Washington, D. C.

Withers, J., 1988, *Major Industrial Hazards*, Halsted Press, New York.

Working Group on Risk Assessment and Risk Management, 1992, *Risk Assessment/Risk Management: A Handbook for Use Within the Bureau of Chemical Hazards*, Health & Welfare Canada, Ottawa.

World Bank, 1985, *Manual of Industrial Hazard Assessment*, World Bank, Washington, D. C.

Wu, J. M., and J. M. Schroy, 1979, "Emissions from Spills, Monsanto Company, St. Louis, Missouri," presented at the Conference on Control of Specific (Toxic) Pollutants, February 13–16, Gainesville, Florida.

Wynne, B., 1984, "Commentary on 'Uncertainty, Ignorance, and Policy', by Jerome R. Ravetz," IIASA (International Institute for Applied Systems Analysis), Vienna, Austria.

Zanetos, M. A., 1984, "Epidemiologic Models: Applicability to Risk Assessment for Biotechnology Products," unpublished report from Battelle Laboratories, Columbus Division—Washington Operations, EPA Contract no. 68-01-6721.

Zentner, R. D., 1979, "Hazards in the Chemical Industry," *Chem. Eng. News* **57** (45), 25–27 and 30–34.

GLOSSARY

The definitions provided here reflect the context(s) within which they are used in this text. Some terms have broader or different meanings in other contexts.

absorption The penetration of one substance into or through another. In biology, the movement of a chemical from the point of initial contact across a biologic barrier (e.g., skin) into the bloodstream.

acceptable daily intake (ADI) The maximum dose of a hazardous substance that can be consumed daily without causing adverse health effects over a lifetime.

acid deposition A phenomenon wherein emissions of sulfur and nitrogen compounds and other substances are chemically transformed in the atmosphere and then deposited on earth in either a wet or dry form The wet forms, popularly called *acid rain*, can occur as rain, snow, or fog. The dry forms are acidic gases or particulates.

activity The number of nuclear decays per unit time in a sample of a radioactive substance.

acute effect An effect that results from a brief exposure or shortly after an acute exposure.

acute exposure A short exposure (possibly at high levels) of duration measured in minutes, hours, or days.

additive dose-response model A dose-response model in which the health effects attributable to exposure to particular levels of two or more risk agents are equal to the sum of the responses predicted for each agent alone.

additive effects The combined biological effects of two or more risk agents are *additive* when equal to the sum of the effects of the agents acting alone.

adduct A chemical bound to an important cellular macromolecule, such as DNA or protein.

adhesion Molecular attraction that holds the surfaces of two substances in contact.

ADI See *acceptable daily intake*.

adsorption The attachment of molecules of a gas, liquid, or dissolved solid to the surface of a solid.

advection The process by which a substance in the atmosphere is transported due to mass motion of the atmosphere.

aerosol Extremely small liquid or solid particles suspended in air.

agglomeration The process by which precipitation particles grow larger by collision or contact with cloud or other precipitation particles.

air quality standards Specified levels of pollutants prescribed by regulations that may not be exceeded during a specified time duration in a defined area.

algorithm A step-by-step procedure for solving a mathematical problem.

alpha particle The least penetrating type of radiation, composed of a helium nucleus and emitted from a material undergoing nuclear transformation.

ambient air Any unconfined portion of the atmosphere; open air; surrounding air.

ambient concentration The average amount of a substance in a particular environmental medium, usually air.

Ames test A relatively rapid and inexpensive screening procedure utilizing bacteria to determine if a substance causes mutations.

anemia A reduction of oxygen-carrying hemoglobin in the blood.

antagonistic effects Two risk agents display antagonism when their combined biological effects are less than the sum of the effects of the agents acting alone. Both agents may interfere with each other's action or only one may interfere with the the action of the other.

antibodies Blood proteins made in response to the appearance of certain types of foreign substances in the body that attack and render those substances (antigens) harmless.

aquifer An underground source of water caused by a geological formation (e.g., a layer of earth or porous stone) or group of formations.

area source A geographically dispersed collection of sources of pollution, such as automotive vehicles in an urban area.

asbestosis A chronic disease of the lungs caused by inhaling asbestos fibers. The disease makes breathing progressively more difficult and can be fatal.

asthma A condition characterized by spasms of the small muscles encircling the breathing passages and the release of excessive mucous that plugs them, leading to difficulties in breathing. Attacks of spasms may be triggered by exposures to various air pollutants.

atmospheric inversion A condition of the lower atmosphere wherein the normal decline of temperature with increasing altitude is reduced, which inhibits the normal rising of air currents and produces a stagnant air layer above the ground.

background level The level, often low, at which some substance, agent, or event is present or occurs at a particular location and time in the absence of the risk source under study.

basic event The occurrence of a fault or failure in a system component or of an external event that can initiate, or participate in, an accident sequence (i.e., a sequence of events leading to a system accident).

Bayesian updating A predictive approach for obtaining probabilistic assessments of uncertainty. A preliminary (prior) estimate of the probability of occurrence of an event is made based on available information, including subjective judgment. New information, obtained by monitoring or other means, is then used to infer a new estimate of the probability. The new estimate is derived through a mathematical formula called Bayes's rule.

becquerel A unit of activity of radiation. The mass of a radioactive substance that results in a decay rate of one atom per second.

benign tumor A tumor confined to the territory in which it arises, not invading surrounding tissue or metastasizing to distant organs. Benign tumors can usually be excised by local surgery.

benthic organisms Organisms that live in the mud or other bottom material of lakes, streams, and marine ecosystems.

beta particle An elementary particle (electron) emitted by radioactive decay. A beta particle is unable to penetrate a thin piece of paper.

binary A variable having only two possible values, such as on or off, one or zero.

bioaccumulation (biomagnification) A process whereby the concentration of certain substances in organisms increases as the organisms breathe contaminated air, drink contaminated water, or eat contaminated food.

bioactivation A metabolic process wherein a nontoxic chemical is converted to a toxic one inside the body. (See also *biotransformation*.)

bioassay The use of living organisms to measure the effect of a risk agent or condition—for example, a test for carcinogenicity in laboratory animals that includes near-lifelong exposure to the agent under test. Used interchangeably with *animal test*.

biodegradation A process wherein matter is decomposed by microorganisms.

biological modeling Models of the fate and effects of toxic pollutants in biological systems, including ecological and metabolic systems.

biomagnification factor The ratio of the concentration of a substance in an organism to that typical of its environment or food supply. See *bioaccumulation*.

biomarker A biochemical or physiological response measured in an organism that can be used to quantify exposures to risk agents or levels of stress experienced by the organism.

biota All the living material in a given area; often refers to plants and animals.

biotechnology Techniques such as genetic engineering that use living organisms or parts of organisms to produce new products (e.g., medicines, industrial enzymes), to improve plants or animals, or to develop microorganisms for specific uses (e.g., pesticides, removal of toxics from bodies of water).

biotransformation A series of chemical alterations within the body whereby a foreign substance is transformed to a more or less toxic substance. (See also *bioactivation*.)

cancer A group of diseases characterized by abnormal, disorderly, and potentially unlimited new tissue growth.

carbamate   A group of synthetic pesticides made up of carbon, hydrogen, nitrogen, and oxygen.

carcinogen   Any chemical or physical agent possessing the ability to induce cancer in living organisms.

case-control study   An epidemiologic study in which groups of individuals are selected because they do (cases) or do not (controls) have a condition under study. Comparisons between groups are generally made to analyze current or past characteristics that might have caused the condition. (See *cohort study*.)

caustic   Able to irritate, burn, or destroy tissue.

cells   The smallest structural part of living matter capable of functioning as an independent unit.

chloracne   A skin disease resembling severe acne.

chromosomes   Threadlike structures in animal or plant nuclei that carry genetic material.

chronic   Having a persistent, recurring, or long-term nature; distinguished from acute.

chronic effect   An effect of gradual onset and long duration.

chronic exposure   An exposure (usually of low concentration) of long duration, e.g., months or years.

chronic respiratory disease   A persistent or long-lasting intermittent disease of the respiratory tract.

cohort   A defined test population whose lifetime mortality or morbidity statistics have been determined.

cohort study   A study of research subjects classified on the basis of characteristics present prior to the appearance of the condition under study. The cohort groups are observed over time to determine the frequency and/or severity of the condition under study. (See *case-control study*.)

common-cause failure   A failure in which several systems or functions fail or degrade together due to a single cause.

confidence interval   The definition depends on whether a subjective or objective view of probability is adopted. With the subjective view, the confidence limit specifies limits of an uncertain quantity between which there is a specified probability of occurrence—expressed as in "the X percent confidence interval." With the objective view, the confidence limit expresses a range of values that may or may not contain the true value of an estimated parameter. The confidence limit is derived from a sample in such a way that repeated random samples would yield confidence intervals such that a specified proportion of these intervals would include the true value of the estimated parameter, assuming that the actual population satisfies the initial hypothesis.

confounding variables   Variables not of direct interest in a specified statistical study but whose variation may induce, conceal, or distort an association. The effects of confounding variables can often be reduced or controlled by appropriate selection and treatment of statistical data.

consequence assessment The process of developing a description of the relationship between specified exposures to a risk agent and the health and other consequences to the people or things exposed.

conservatism The tendency to inject a bias into an analysis, usually a weighting toward protection of human health.

contaminant Any physical, chemical, biological, or radioactive substance or matter that has been introduced to air, water, or soil.

continuous random variable (uncertainty) A random variable that can have an infinite number of values. For example, wind speed can have any value between zero and some upper limit.

continuous release The escape resulting in the introduction of a hazardous substance or energy into the accessible environment at a rate that is sustained for a prolonged period.

control An experimental group of animals or humans who were not exposed to a risk agent under study. The frequency of the disease in these individuals is used to estimate the background rate in the corresponding study group.

convection Atmospheric motions that are predominantly vertical, resulting in vertical transport and mixing in the atmosphere.

coolant A liquid or gas used to reduce the heat generated by power production in nuclear reactors, electric generators, various industrial and mechanical processes, or automobile engines.

cooling tower A structure built to help remove heat from water used as a coolant (e.g., in electric power generating plants).

core The uranium-containing heart of a nuclear reactor, where energy is released.

correlation A measure of the degree to which variables change together, usually taken to mean a linear relationship; a measure of the intensity of association.

cross-sectional study An epidemiological study design in which measurements of cause and effect are made at the same point in time.

cumulative probability distribution A curve or mathematical expression that quantifies uncertainty over a variable. It associates a probability with all values in the set of possible values. The probability associated with each value of the variable is that of the occurrence of a value less than or equal to the specified value.

curie A unit of radioactivity equal to 37 billion becquerels.

database Available, relevant raw information about a subject of concern, often maintained in a form readable by a computer.

de minimus risk From the legal maxim *de minimus non curat lex* or "the law does not concern itself with trifles." The risk below which the law is not concerned.

decay products All of the particles formed when a radioactive isotope decays. See *radioactive decay*.

degree of belief   The strength of one's faith that either empirical or subjective conditions may be valid.

Delphi method   A method designed to produce consensus estimates from a group of experts. An iterative approach is used in which a facilitator repeatedly obtains estimates from each member of the group interspersed with feedback of group responses and opinions. Group members typically remain anonymous and interact through the facilitator to minimize psychological biases in the estimates produced.

detoxification   Any process wherein a toxic is either changed into a harmless form or is removed from the body.

direct (primary) carcinogen   A chemical that acts directly and without biotransformation to cause cancer.

discrete random variable (uncertainty)   A random variable that can have only a discrete number of values or states. For example, the outcome of a toss of a coin is a discrete random variable, since it is either heads or tails.

dispersion   A scattering process. The spreading of a substance through the atmosphere via air currents and diffusion.

DNA   Deoxyribonucleic acid—the molecule in which the genetic information for living cells is encoded.

dosage (dosing) regimen   The amount of a risk agent and the route and time course over which it is administered to an organism.

dose   The amount of a risk agent that enters or interacts with an organism. An administered dose is the amount of substance administered to an animal or human, usually measured in mg/kg body weight; mg/m^2 body surface area; or ppm of the diet, drinking water, or ambient air. An effective dose is the amount of the substance reaching the target organ.

dose-response relationship   Functional relationship between the dosage level of substance received and lethality, morbidity, or level of health effect produced.

dosimetry   The measurement or estimation of doses.

ecosystem   The interacting system of a biological community and its nonliving surroundings.

effluent   Treated or untreated waste material discharged into the environment. Generally refers to wastes discharged to surface waters.

electromagnetic spectrum   A continuous sequence of a form of energy generated by objects with electric charge, such as electrons, and transmitted as a wave, including X rays, light waves, heat, and radiowaves.

electrons   The very light, negatively charged particles that may be envisioned as encircling the nuclei of atoms.

emission   Pollution discharged into the atmosphere from smokestacks, other vents, and surface areas of commercial or industrial facilities; from residential chimneys; and from motor vehicle, locomotive, or aircraft exhausts.

empirical Originating in or based on observation or experience.

endangered species Animals, birds, fish, or other living organisms threatened with extinction by man-made or natural changes in their environment. Conditions under which a species is declared endangered are specified in the Endangered Species Act.

environmental effect Effect on the living and nonliving components of the environment.

environmental fate The disposition of a substance in various environmental media such as air, water, or soil.

environmental pathway See *exposure pathway.*

enzyme A chemical produced (or synthesized) by living cells that initiates or accelerates a chemical reaction but is not itself altered by the reaction.

epidemic A widespread outbreak of disease, or a large number of cases of a disease in a single community or relatively small area.

epidemiology The study of diseases as they affect populations, including the distribution of disease, or other health-related states and events in human population; the factors (e.g., age, sex, occupation, economic status) that influence this distribution; and the application of this study to assess and control health risk.

Escherichia coli (E. coli) The common microorganism that inhabits the intestinal tracts of humans and other animals. A high concentration in water is often used as an indicator of pollution.

estuaries Regions of interaction between rivers and nearshore ocean waters, where tidal action and river flow create a mixing of fresh and salt water. These areas may include bays, mouths of rivers, salt marshes, and lagoons.

etiology The science of the origin, causes, and development of diseases.

evapotranspiration The loss of water from soil both by evaporation and by transpiration from the plants growing in the soil.

event tree analysis A systematic method for identifying and analyzing the possible effects of events using interrelationships based on "if–then" assumptions. The method is often used to estimate the failure probability of protective subsystems or of a technological system as a whole.

exceedance Violation of environmental protection standards by exceeding allowable limits or concentration levels.

expected value A summary measure of an uncertain random variable obtained by weighting all possible outcome values by their probability of occurrence and then summing. Also called *mean value.*

exponential distribution A commonly occurring probability distribution. It is often used to represent uncertainty over the time between failures of components or systems that have a constant failure rate per unit time.

exposure   An instance or condition of one or more people or things they value being open to interaction with a risk agent (e.g., an environmental contaminant or a communicable disease).

exposure assessment   The process of developing a description of the relevant conditions and characteristics of human and other exposures to risk agents produced or released by a specified source of risk.

exposure pathways   Means by which risk agents are transmitted—e.g., the route by which a given population is exposed to a toxic substance (via drinking water, air, dermal contact, etc.).

extrapolation   Prediction of the value of a variable outside the range of observation.

failure mode and effects analysis   An application of various methods for systematically analyzing all contributing component failure modes and identifying their effects on a system.

failure rate   The average frequency of failure per unit operating time.

fallout   Radioactive debris from a nuclear detonation or other source, usually deposited from airborne particulates.

fate-and-transport models   Mathematical descriptions of the movement and transformation of substances through various media.

fault or failure   An undesired action or lack of desired action that prevents a system, subsystem, or component from performing its required function.

fault tree analysis   A systematic approach used in reliability analysis of complex systems in which the probabilities of failure of individual components and the resulting chains of cause–effect consequences are estimated. The method is frequently used to estimate the probability of a major accident.

food chain   A hierarchy of organisms, each of which uses the next, lower member in the hierarchy as a food source.

fossil fuel   Natural gas, petroleum, coal, and any form of solid, liquid, or gaseous fuel derived from such materials for the purpose of creating heat.

fumigant   A pesticide dispersed as a gas or smoke, often used to disinfect interior spaces.

gamma ray   The most penetrating wave produced by radioactive decay. Gamma rays can be blocked only by dense materials such as lead.

gastrointestinal (GI)   The lower portion of the digestive system, including the stomach and the small and large intestines.

Gaussian statistical distribution   See *normal distribution*.

gavage   Forced feeding of a test animal, usually through a tube passed into the stomach.

gene   A segment of DNA that directs the synthesis of a protein. All information about the inherited characteristics of an organism is contained in its genes.

genotoxic   Capable of causing heritable changes or damage leading to heritable changes in genetic material. A genotoxic carcinogen is one that initiates cancer through a direct effect on genetic material.

gray (Gy)   A unit used to describe the amount of energy that radiation deposits in tissue; 1 gray = 100 rad.

groundwater   The supply of fresh water under the surface of the earth, usually in aquifers, that forms a natural reservoir for supplying wells and springs.

habitat   The place where humans, animals, or plants live and their surroundings, both living and nonliving.

half life   The time it takes for a quantity to decrease by half, used to describe how long radioactive isotopes take to decay.

hazard   A (potential) source of risk that does not necessarily produce risk. A hazard produces risk only if an exposure pathway exists and if exposures create the possibility of adverse consequences.

hazard (risk) identification   The process of identifying new sources of risk.

hazardous substance   Any substance that poses a threat to human health or the environment. The magnitude of the threat is potentially large but undefined and depends on whether an exposure pathway exists.

hazardous waste   Corrosive, ignitable, explosive, or toxic by-products of society that pose a hazard to humans or the environment.

health effect   An adverse deviation in the normal function of the human body resulting from exposure to a risk agent (e.g., event, activity, or substance).

heavy metals   Metallic elements (e.g., mercury, chromium, cadmium, arsenic, and lead) with high atomic weights. They can damage living organisms and tend to accumulate in the food chain.

hemoglobin   The protein in blood cells that transports oxygen. It is responsible for the red color of blood.

high-to-low-dose extrapolation   Prediction of the frequency or magnitude of an adverse health effect caused by low doses, based on the results of experiments conducted at much higher doses.

hydrocarbon   A substance made up primarily of carbon and hydrogen atoms, usually of biological origin (e.g., vegetables, petroleum, coal tar).

immediate acute effects   Immediate death or injury.

immune system   The body's defense mechanism against foreign substances. It includes white blood cells and antibodies.

in situ   In the original location. Any test conducted in the field.

in vitro   Outside living organisms (e.g., in a test tube). Any laboratory test using living cells taken from an organism.

in vivo   Within living organisms. Any laboratory test carried out on whole animals or human volunteers.

incidence   The rate at which an event occurs. In toxicology, the number of new cases of a disease within a specified period of time, often expressed per 100,000 individuals per year.

independence (also probabilistic independence)   The relationship between two or more events when knowledge of the probability or occurrence of one does not alter the probability of another.

inhalation   A dose resulting from the movement of a substance from the breathing zone through the air passageways of the lung and into the blood.

initiator   A substance that causes the first step(s) in a multistep process of carcinogenesis.

inorganic   Not of biological origin.

interspecies extrapolation   The act of applying a set of data or an individual test result from one species, under certain conditions and subject to particular dose levels of a toxic substance and application method, to another population of a different species under perhaps different conditions, dose levels, and application method.

interspecies conversion   The conversion of doses used in animal tests conducted using one species to doses that may be equivalent (in some sense) in another species, usually humans.

ionize   To remove or add one or more electrons from an atom or a molecule.

ionizing radiation   Radiation that is capable of ionizing atoms or molecules.

ions   Atoms or molecules that have lost or gained electrons so that they are electrically charged.

isotope   A form of an element having a standard number of protons in its nucleus but a specified, unique number of neutrons and, therefore, atomic weight.

judgmental probability   A number between zero and one assigned to express the likelihood of an uncertain event and which is based on personal belief. Judgmental probabilities obey the axioms of probability and are equal to objective probabilities acceptable to the assessor for a substitute gamble.

kidneys   The pair of organs responsible for filtering the blood to remove waste products of metabolism.

latency period   The time between exposure to a risk agent and the manifestation of any adverse health effects that it causes.

LD_{50}   The dose that when administered to all animals in a test (over a specified time period) is lethal to 50 percent of the animals.

leach   To dissolve and move substances through soil with percolating water.

leachate   Liquid that has percolated through a solid and has extracted dissolved or suspended materials from it.

lesion   An abnormal change in the structure of tissue due to injury or disease.

lifetime average daily dose (LADD)   A measure of the average dose of a risk agent received by an individual who is exposed for a substantial portion of his or her lifetime.

linear   Straight-line. When the statistical relationship between two variables increases on a direct unit-for-unit basis, this relationship, when plotted on a chart, will form a straight line.

log or logarithm   A function specifying the power to which a base number must be raised to produce a specified number. The logarithm to the base b of a quantity x is the power to which b must be raised to produce x. For example, the logarithm of 100 to the base 10 is 2 ($10^2 = 100$). Common bases for logarithms are 10 and a number denoted e (which is approximately 2.71828) that arises frequently in deriving formulas. Logarithms to the base 10 and e are usually denoted log and ln, respectively. Log scales are useful for expressing relationships that extend over several orders of magnitude.

logistic curve   An S-shaped curve that, if plotting dose-response relationships, is approximately linear at low doses, increases at a progressively higher rate at higher doses, and finally saturates at very high doses where the effect in question always occurs.

logistic model   A model that assumes that a dose-response relationship follows a logistic curve.

logit distribution   A probability distribution with a shape similar to the normal distribution but with a higher fraction of values at a fixed distance away from its mean.

lognormal distribution   A commonly occurring probability distribution for nonnegative quantities. A quantity having a lognormal distribution has a logarithm that has a Gaussian or normal distribution.

malignant tumor   A tumor that has invaded neighboring tissue and/or undergone metastasis to distant body sites, at which point the tumor is called a cancer and is beyond the reach of local surgery.

margin of safety   A factor added to an estimated risk level for purposes of increasing the probability that a standard based on the resultant level will provide increased protection to the general population and individual members from harmful effects of a given substance.

maximum tolerated dose (MTD)   The maximum dose that a test animal can tolerate for the duration of the experiment without serious effects on health or survival.

mean value   See *expected value*.

media   Specific environments (e.g., air, water, soil) that are the subject of regulatory concern and that may be the source of exposures to risk agents.

median   The point on a probability density function at which a vertical line bisects the area under the probability density function.

melanoma   A type of skin cancer, often fatal, that can spread quickly to other parts of the body.

metabolism All of the biological reactions taking place within a cell or an organism. An important reaction is that which breaks down complex organic compounds to free energy.

metabolite A chemical product of metabolism.

metastasis The establishment of a secondary growth site, distinct from the primary site, the occurrence of which is characteristic of a malignant tumor.

Michaelis-Menton kinetics An approximate equation relating metabolized dose v to exposure dose S: $v = V_m S/(K_m + S)$, where V_m and K_m are constants.

microbes Microscopic organisms such as tiny plants, animals, viruses, bacteria, and fungal spores, some of which cause diseases. See *microorganisms*.

microcosm An experimental, small-scale system, more or less analogous to a much larger system in terms of constitution, configuration, or development.

microorganisms Living organisms so small they usually can be seen only through a microscope.

mitigation Measures taken to reduce adverse impacts on the environment.

mode A point on a probability density function where the probability is at a maximum, i.e., goes from increasing to decreasing.

monitoring Periodic or continuous surveillance or testing to determine the characteristics of a risk source, the pollutant levels in various media, or the health status of humans, animals, and other living things.

Monte Carlo analysis The computation of a probability distribution over consequences by means of a random sampling method analogous to the game of roulette. Combinations of events and outcomes that yield possible consequences are randomly selected according to a specified probability distribution. The resulting consequences are counted and used to estimate other probability distributions.

morbidity A departure from the state of physical or mental well-being. The rate of sickness or ratio of sick persons to well persons in a population.

mortality rate The death rate, often made explicit for a particular characteristic, e.g., age, sex, or specific cause of death. A mortality rate contains three essential elements: the number of people in a population group exposed to the risk of death; a time factor; and the number of deaths occurring in the exposed population during a certain time period.

mucous membranes The mucus-secreting lining of many passageways in the body, including the nasal sinuses, respiratory tract, and gastrointestinal tract.

multihit models Dose-response models that assume that more than one interaction at the molecular level with a toxic material is necessary before effects are manifested.

multistage models Dose-response models that assume there are a given number of biological stages that occur following exposure to a risk agent—e.g., metabolism, covalent binding, DNA repair, etc.—before manifestation of the effect in question is possible.

mutagen Any substance that can cause a change in genetic material. Mutagens have the ability to induce adverse, heritable changes in the genetic material of living organisms.

mutation A change in genetic material (DNA). If it occurs in a developing sperm or egg, the mutation may be passed on to the offspring.

National Ambient Air Quality Standards (NAAQS) Air quality standards established by the EPA that apply to outdoor air throughout the U.S.

necrosis Death of one or more cells, part of a tissue, or an organ of the body.

neoplasm An aberrant new growth of abnormal cells or tissue in which the growth is uncontrollable and progressive.

neurotoxin A chemical that produces adverse effects on the nervous system.

neutrons Electrically neutral particles that, along with protons, make up the nucleus of an atom.

no-observed-adverse-effects level (NOAEL) The highest dose at which no statistically or biologically significant adverse effects are detected in a population.

no-observed-effects level (NOEL) The highest dose at which no statistically or biologically significant health effects are detected in a population.

normal distribution Also called the *normal probability distribution*, or the *Gaussian statistical distribution*. A commonly occurring probability distribution characterized by a bell shape and having a mathematical representation expressed in terms of a mean and a variance.

nuclear wastes The radioactive debris left over in a nuclear reactor after most of the original fuel has released its useful energy. May also include other radioactive waste generated from the nuclear industry.

nucleus The heavy, central portion of atoms consisting of protons and neutrons.

objective probability A number between zero and one assigned to an uncertain event based on historical trials or occurrences estimated for similar events. Probability that can be inferred from objective facts (and assumptions about relationships).

odds The ratio of probabilities of occurrence and nonoccurrence; e.g., for a throw of a fair die, the probability of a four is 1/6, and the odds are (1/6):(5/6) or 1:5.

oncogen A substance capable of producing either cancerous or benign (noncancerous) tumors.

oncogenes Genes that carry the potential for carcinogenesis.

oncogenic A substance that causes tumors, whether benign or malignant.

one-hit models Dose-response models that assume that a response is elicited after a susceptible target has been impacted once at the molecular level by a biologically effective unit of dose.

order of magnitude An expression often used in reference to calculations of environmental quantities or risk. Order of magnitude means a factor of ten. For example, 20 (2×10)

is one order of magnitude greater than 2; 200 ($2 \times 10 \times 10$) is two orders of magnitude greater than 2; and so forth.

organic matter   Matter of biological origin. Contains a high proportion of carbon atoms.

organism   Any living thing.

organochlorines   A group of organic chemicals to which varying amounts of chlorine have been added. Organochlorine pesticides can also contain oxygen and sulfur.

organophosphates   A group of organic chemicals containing phosphorus, oxygen, and sometimes sulfur. They are often used as pesticides and interfere with nerve signal transmission.

overland flow   Flow of water over a sloped surface.

particulates   Fine liquid or solid particles such as dust, smoke, mist, fumes, or smog, found in air or emissions.

parts per million (ppm), parts per billion (ppb)   A means for expressing low concentrations of pollutants in air, water, soil, human tissue, food, or other materials, according to the fraction of mass or volume occupied by the pollutant; e.g., one part salt in a million parts water.

pathogenic   Capable of causing disease.

pathogens   Microorganisms potentially harmful to humans or animals. Examples include certain bacteria, viruses, or parasites.

pathway   See *exposure pathways*.

peer review   A quality control/assurance procedure in which manuscripts, plans, or results are reviewed for technical and scientific merit by qualified experts before publication or acceptance.

percolation   The movement of water downward and radially through the subsurface soil layers, usually continuing downward to the groundwater.

permeability   The characteristic of a solid that allows it to transmit water or air. Also, the rate at which liquids pass through soil in a specified direction.

persistence   The tendency of some substances to remain unchanged in soils, water, or living organisms for extended periods of time, and, thus, to pose a long-term hazard.

pH   A measure of the acidity or alkalinity of a liquid or solid material (pH is represented on a scale of 0 to 14 with 7 representing a neutral state, 0 representing the most acid, and 14 the most alkaline).

pharmacokinetic models   Dose-response models based on the principle that biological effects are the result of biochemical interaction between foreign substances or metabolites and parts of the body.

pharmacology   Investigation of the physical and chemical properties, mechanisms of action, absorption, distribution, biotransformation, excretion, and therapeutic and other uses of drugs by observing their effects directly in animals or humans.

photochemical oxidants   Air pollutants formed by the action of sunlight on nitrogen oxides and hydrocarbons.

photochemical reaction   A chemical process stimulated by sunlight.

plume   A visible or measurable discharge of a contaminant in air or water from a given point of origin.

point estimate   A single value that summarizes a probability distribution describing some random variable.

point source   A stationary location where pollutants are discharged. Also, any single, well-confined source of pollutant (e.g., a pipe, ditch, ship, factory smokestack).

pollutant   Any material or energy entering the environment whose nature, location, or quantity produces undesired effects.

polycyclic aromatic hydrocarbons (PAHs)   Highly reactive compounds consisting of hydrogen and carbon atoms arranged in ring-like structures.

population at risk   A specific population potentially subjected to a risk source or the risk agents that it releases. A limited population that may be unique (with respect to susceptibility to the effect or to the dose) for a specific dose-response relationship.

potency   The degree of being able to cause strong physiological or toxicological effects. See *slope factor*.

precipitation   The falling out of material from the atmosphere (e.g., rain, snow, or pollution) or the settling out of suspended material from water. Also refers to the material that precipitates.

precision   The exactness with which a quantity is stated, i.e., the number of units into which a measurement scale of that quantity may be meaningfully divided. The number of significant digits is a measure of precision.

prevalence   The number of cases of a disease in existence at a given time in a specified population, usually 100,000 persons.

probability   A numerical value between zero and one and satisfying certain axioms. The number is associated with an outcome or event and specifies the likelihood of occurrence.

probability density function (PDF)   A probability distribution describing a continuous random variable. It associates a relative likelihood to the continuum of possibilities.

probability mass function   A probability distribution describing a discrete random variable. It associates with each possible value of the variable a probability of occurrence.

promoter   A substance that encourages the latter step(s) in a multistep process of carcinogenesis.

prospective study   An epidemiological study in which groups of individuals are selected in terms of whether or not they are exposed to certain factors and then are followed over time to determine differences in the rate at which disease develops in relation to exposures to the factors.

protons   Positively charged particles that, with neutrons, make up the nucleus of an atom.

proxy measure   The use of a related quantity as a surrogate or proxy for an unknown or difficult-to-measure quantity.

puff   The concentration of atmospheric pollutant resulting from a release over a short time span, typically of a few seconds or less.

pulmonary function   The performance of the respiratory system in supplying oxygen to, and removing carbon dioxide from, the body (via circulating blood). Pulmonary function tests are used to identify and locate abnormalities in performance capability.

quantification   The assignment of a number to an entity or a method for determining a number to be assigned to an entity.

rad   A unit of radiation dose; 100 rad = 1 gray.

radiation   The emission of particles or electromagnetic waves by the nucleus of an atom.

radioactive decay   The spontaneous breakup of an isotope.

radioactive substances   Substances that emit rays or particles.

radioactivity   The spontaneous decay or disintegration of unstable atomic nuclei, accompanied by the emission of radiation.

radionuclides   Radioactive elements. This class of elements may be subdivided into (a) natural radionuclides such as radium or uranium, which are normally present in the earth, and (b) artificial radionuclides, which are produced by nuclear fission.

radon   A radioactive gas created by the natural breakdown of radium in soil or rocks.

random variable   A quantity whose value or outcome is uncertain.

recombinant DNA   New DNA formed by combining pieces of DNA from different types of cells.

reference dose (RfD)   An estimate of the highest daily dosage of a risk agent that is unlikely to produce an appreciable deleterious effect in humans. The concept is used by the EPA to express a conservative threshold value for a dose-response relationship for noncarcinogenic effects.

regression analysis   An analysis based on empirical data of the relationship between a variable and one or more other variables that takes into account the degree of correlation among the variables.

release assessment   The process of developing a description of the relevant characteristics of the risk source that establish its potential for creating harm by releasing or otherwise introducing risk agents into portions of the environment accessible to people or the things they value.

reliability   The probability that a system will perform its required functions under conditions for a specified operating time.

rem   Acronym for *roentgen equivalent man*. A unit of radiation dose that accounts for the biological effectiveness of the specific type of radiation.

renal Related to the kidney.

retrospective study An epidemiological study of a group with symptoms suspected of being caused by a given toxic agent. Questionnaires, interviews, or records are used to reconstruct the exposure situation.

risk A characteristic of a situation or action wherein a number of outcomes are possible, the particular one that will occur is uncertain, and at least one of the possibilities is undesirable.

risk agents Fundamental agents for health, safety, and environmental risks, including hazardous chemicals, biological agents (e.g., viruses and bacteria), and energies (e.g., heat and noise).

risk analysis A process involving hazard identification, risk assessment, and risk evaluation.

risk assessment A systematic process for quantifying and describing the risk associated with some substance, situation, or action.

risk assessment method A systematic procedure or mode of inquiry that may be used as part of a risk assessment.

risk estimation The process of characterizing uncertainty (e.g., quantification of probabilities) and possible risk consequences.

risk evaluation The process of interpreting risks, including determining levels of risk acceptable to individuals, groups, or society as a whole.

risk management The process of selecting and implementing steps to alter levels of risk.

RNA Ribonucleic acid. A molecule that carries the genetic message from DNA to a cell's protein-producing mechanisms. Similar to, but chemically different from, DNA.

runoff The part of precipitation, snow melt, or irrigation water that runs off the land into streams and other surface water. It can carry pollutants from the air and land into the receiving waters.

saturated zone A subsurface area in which all pores and cracks are filled with water under pressure equal to or greater than that of the atmosphere.

saturation (effect) A phenomenon causing the response in a dose-response relationship to level off at high doses (i.e., no longer to increase with increasing dose).

screening (hazards) A process of hazard identification whereby a standardized procedure is applied to classify products, processes, phenomena, or substances with respect to their potential for creating risk.

sedimentation A process whereby solids settle out of water by gravity.

sediments Soil, sand, and minerals washed from land into water, usually after rain. Sediments pile up in reservoirs, rivers, and harbors, sometimes destroying fish-nesting areas and homes of water animals and clouding the water.

sensitivity analysis   A method used to examine the behavior of a model by systematically measuring the deviation in its outputs produced as each input, parameter, or assumption is varied from its nominal or base-case value.

sievert (Sv)   A unit of radiation dose that accounts for the biological potency of the specific type of radiation; equals 100 rem.

silt   Fine particles of sand or rock that can be picked up by the air or water and deposited as sediment.

simulation   The use of a physical model (e.g., a microcosm) or an analytical model (i.e., set of equations) to approximate the action of a real system.

sink   A location where pollutants are collected by means or processes such as absorption. The opposite of *source*.

skew   The asymmetry of a probability density function. The skew is to the side of the mode under which lies the greatest area.

slope factor   The slope of a linear dose-response function. A measure of the increase in response (e.g., incidence of cancer) resulting from a unit increase in dose. Also called *potency, potency factor*, or *unit cancer risk*.

smelter   A factory that extracts a metal from its ore through heating.

smog   A complex collection of chemicals formed in the atmosphere from reactions between nitrogen oxides and hydrocarbons.

soluble   Able to dissolve in a liquid.

solvents   Substances (usually liquid) capable of dissolving or dispersing other substances.

sorption   The action of soaking up or attracting substances.

source   A location where pollutants are emitted, e.g., a chimney stack.

stack   A chimney or smokestack; a vertical pipe that discharges used air.

standard deviation   A measure of dispersion or variation. The square root of the variance. Often used because it is in the same units as the random variable itself and can be depicted on the same axis as the probability density function of which it is a characteristic.

stationary source   A fixed, nonmoving producer of pollution; mainly power plants and other facilities using industrial combustion processes.

subjective probability   See *judgmental probability*.

surface impoundment   In-ground ponds for treating, storing, or disposing of liquid hazardous waste.

surface water   All water naturally open to the atmosphere (rivers, lakes, reservoirs, streams, impoundments, seas, estuaries, etc.), and all springs, wells, or other collectors that are directly influenced by surface water.

synergism Production of an effect by two or more agents acting together that is greater in magnitude than the sum of the effects that would be produced by each agent individually.

synergistic effects The combined biological effects of two risk agents are synergistic when the combined effects are greater than the sum of the effects of each agent acting alone.

system A complex entity composed of many, often diverse, things or parts and the relationships among them or their characteristics. A system is typically conceptualized as consisting of subsystems. A system may also be a part of a larger system.

systemic effects Refers to the toxic action of a substance at sites remote from the point of initial contact, which implies that absorption and distribution have occurred.

tailings Residue of raw materials or waste separated out during the processing of mineral ores.

target organ The specific organ affected by a dose of a toxic substance. Not necessarily the organ receiving the highest concentration.

technological risk Risks created by technology.

teratogen Substance that causes birth defects (malformation or serious deviation from normal development of embryos and fetuses).

thermal pollution Discharge of heated water from industrial processes that can affect the life processes of aquatic organisms.

threshold A point of discontinuity in the relationship between two or more quantities, e.g., between a dose and a response. One condition (e.g., no response) exists below the discontinuity and a different one above it. Usually, the effect is absent below the threshold but occurs or increases rapidly above it.

threshold dose Minimum application of a given risk agent required to produce a measurable response.

time-to-response The time required to produce a specific, measurable condition.

tolerance The capacity to withstand a toxic dose without adverse effects on normal growth or function.

tolerance distribution models Dose-response models that assume that under constant environmental conditions there is a threshold dose below which each individual will not elicit a specific response. Although these thresholds are not known for specific individuals, it is assumed that they can be described for the population by a frequency distribution.

topography The physical features of a surface area, including relative elevations and the position of natural and man-made features.

toxic Harmful to living organisms.

toxic substance A substance that, when introduced into or absorbed by a living organism, destroys life or injures health.

toxicity   A measure of the degree of harm caused by a specified exposure of human, animal, or plant life to a substance.

toxicokinetics   The mechanism by which chemical or physical change causes toxic effects.

toxicology   The study of adverse effects of chemicals on living organisms.

transpiration   The process by which water vapor is lost to the atmosphere from living plants. The term is also applied to the quantity of water thus dissipated.

tumor   Any abnormal growth of tissue in which growth is uncontrolled and progressive. A neoplasm.

ultraviolet (UV) light   A form of high-energy, invisible light capable of causing tissue damage.

uncertainty   A situation where a number of possibilities exist and one does not know which of them has occurred or will occur.

unit cancer risk (UCR)   A measure of the carcinogenic potency of a chemical. An estimate of the excess or added probability that an exposed individual will develop cancer due to continuous exposure to one unit of dose. The measure assumes a linear relationship between dose and incremental probability at low dose levels. See *slope factor*.

unsaturated zone   The area above the water table where the soil pores are not fully saturated, although some water may be present.

urban runoff   Stormwater from city streets and adjacent domestic or commercial properties that may carry pollutants of various kinds into the sewer system and/or receiving water.

variance   A measure of the variability of a random variable. The mean of the squares of the deviations from the mean of the distribution.

virus   The smallest form of microorganisms capable of causing disease.

volatile   Capable of readily evaporating under normal conditions.

volatile organic compounds (VOCs)   Carbon-containing substances that readily produce fumes and tend to interact with nitrogen oxides in the atmosphere to produce photochemical smog. Includes benzene, trichloroethylene (TCE), and many common solvents.

watershed   The land area from which water drains into a stream.

Weibull distribution   A commonly occurring probability distribution that is often used to represent uncertainty in the time between failures of components or systems. It represents an extension of the exponential distribution and can accommodate a wide variety of failure rate curve shapes.

weight-of-evidence criteria   Criteria used to indicate the extent to which available data indicate that an agent is a carcinogen in humans. For example, the EPA has established the following classifications: (A) carcinogen, with sufficient evidence from epidemiological studies; (B1) probable carcinogen, with limited evidence from epidemiological studies; (B2) probable carcinogen, with sufficient evidence from animal studies; (C) possible carcinogen, with limited evidence from animal studies in the absence of human data; (D) not classifiable as to carcinogenicity, owing to inadequate evidence; (E) evidence of noncarcinogenicity, with no evidence of carcinogenicity in at least two adequate animal tests in different species, or in both adequate animal and epidemiological studies.

wet deposition The removal of atmospheric particles to the earth's surface by rain, fog, or snow.

whole-body dose A radiation dose calculated by dividing the energy of radiation deposited anywhere in the body by the total mass of the body.

X ray A type of radiation within the electromagnetic spectrum that is capable of inflicting biological damage. X rays have many applications in medicine and industry.

INDEX